Epidemics and War

Epidemics and War

The Impact of Disease on Major Conflicts in History

REBECCA M. SEAMAN, EDITOR

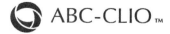

An Imprint of ABC-CLIO, LLC

Santa Barbara, California • Denver, Colorado

Library of Congress Cataloging-in-Publication Data

Names: Seaman, Rebecca M., editor.
Title: Epidemics and war : the impact of disease on major conflicts in
  history / Rebecca M. Seaman, editor.
Description: Santa Barbara, California : ABC-CLIO, LLC, [2018] | Includes
  bibliographical references and index.
Identifiers: LCCN 2017049950 (print) | LCCN 2018005269 (ebook) | ISBN
  9781440852251 (eBook) | ISBN 9781440852244 (hardcopy : alk. paper)
Subjects: LCSH: Epidemics—History. | Communicable diseases—History. |
  War—Medical aspects.
Classification: LCC RA649 (ebook) | LCC RA649 .E65 2018 (print) | DDC
  614.4/9—dc23
LC record available at https://lccn.loc.gov/2017049950

ISBN: 978-1-4408-5224-4 (print)
      978-1-4408-5225-1 (ebook)

22 21 20 19 18   1 2 3 4 5

This book is also available as an eBook.

ABC-CLIO
An Imprint of ABC-CLIO, LLC

ABC-CLIO, LLC
130 Cremona Drive, P.O. Box 1911
Santa Barbara, California 93116-1911
www.abc-clio.com

This book is printed on acid-free paper ∞

Manufactured in the United States of America

If Leon Trotsky was even half right, and war—or failure in war—is the locomotive of history, then epidemics—or a failure to stem them—might be described as the underground train of history, unseen on the surface of history, but affecting millions as it fans out quietly but lethally. *

—Howard Phillips

This volume is dedicated to my parents, Don and Ruth Kelley. Their determination to give each of their children educational opportunities paved the way for me to study my inherited love of history. Their own careers, based in the sciences, and in particular my mother's nursing career, encouraged me to explore history from an interdisciplinary approach. Finally, their own experiences during World War II created an appreciation for the complexity of war and its impact on society. Collectively, their influence helped give birth to this volume.

—Rebecca M. Seaman

---

* Howard Phillips, "The Last Plague: Spanish Influenza and the Politics of Public Health in Canada," Review, *American History Review* 119, no. 3 (2014): 883, accessed June 14, 2017, https://academic.oup.com/ahr/article/119/3/883/13510/Mark-Osborne-Humphries-The-Last-Plague-Spanish.

Contents

Preface

The purpose of this book was not to write a detailed analysis of any war or battle, as that would be far too deep and time-consuming for such a brief volume. Nor was the book intended to present a detailed medical analysis of any of the included diseases that formed the basis of epidemics studied. Instead, this volume tried to pull together elements of both specialties, providing essential information to help the reader understand the importance of place, timing, conditions, and the interaction of humans and environment in producing wars and epidemics. As a result of my own research on diseases that affected Native Americans, *Epidemics and War: The Impact of Disease on Major Conflicts in History* incorporates disease experiences from around the globe and across the ages. The volume is inherently tied to military history and benefited from my recent opportunity to attend the Military History Instructor's Course (MHIC) at Ft. Leavenworth, Kansas.

This volume was designed with individual stand-alone chapters; each chapter provides the context for a war and epidemic covered within. However, the introductions to each group of chapters (parts I–IV) provide insights that will help readers better understand the difficult concepts and complexities associated with each chapter of that particular section of the text. Consequently, readers are encouraged to read the section introduction before tackling any chapter within that section. The epilogue helps pull the various chapters together, preferably as a summary once the entire book is digested.

Certain threads emerged as the chapters came together for this work: the impact of reforms, the importance of the size of armies on health and disease, the relationship of humans to their environments, and the basic responses of human nature to war and epidemics. The constant seeking of knowledge that led to reforms in military strategies, structures, and medical care during wars and peacetime was an important thread that can be found in almost every chapter in the book. The conditions of war consistently provided the necessary elements that facilitated the spread of various epidemics. These conditions and epidemics also encouraged military and medical personnel to seek improvements to prevent such reoccurrences. Depending on the knowledge available, these attempts appeared useless in some instances, and even damaging in others. However, the gradual compilation of knowledge over the ages indeed resulted in the improvement of hygiene, nutrition, and medical care and the prevention or reduction of widespread contamination. The consequent decline in deaths due to disease, in comparison to the deaths due to combat, is a clear indication of such advancements.

Another thread that consistently emerged in the chapters was the importance of numbers during the conscription or recruitment of military forces. The rapid and dramatic mobilization of great armies and navies consistently played a significant role in the advent of epidemics, but one that could be countered with proper preparation, resources, and support. Unfortunately, despite the best intentions and the most progressive policies, history is not linear and does not always result in consistent improvements. Different societies and geographies created inconsistencies in experiences and in the sharing of knowledge gained through the experience of wars. As the chapters dealing with more recent conflicts reveal, increased medical knowledge, improved military practices, and medical reforms were often incapable of countering the suddenness and disruptiveness that continues to plague (pun intended) modern militaries and societies during times of war.

While other threads weave their way through various chapters, the remaining two that are important to note here include the interactions of humans with their environments during periods of war and basic responses of human nature. Even the most hygienic of individuals fell into the practice of tolerating conditions that perpetuated disease. Part of this was again due to the number of people brought together during warfare, and part was due to exhaustion—mental and physical. The potential for war to pollute the environment, to cross sections of land repeatedly, eradicating vegetation and disrupting the natural processes that normally assist in the prevention of disease, was part of the detrimental human interactions with their environment. Additionally, the movement of people into regions that exposed them to new disease vectors, bacteria, viruses, fungi, protozoa, and other causal factors of epidemics increased the opportunities for new contagions. Combined with these new contagions were the human responses to previously unknown and often frightening diseases.

People often react to new and deadly illnesses with irrational responses. The chapters attempted to capture some of these responses, from perceptions of divine retribution, to racist or bigoted stereotypes and scapegoats, to superstitious remedies and rituals. Even the more recent actions to provide fresh air and clean up the physical environment of ill and wounded soldiers were based on the incorrect belief that the miasmas, or odors, associated with swamps, garbage, and human waste were the cause of such diseases as the Antonine Plague, cholera, and the Black Death, among others. While the actions were beneficial, the flawed reasoning did not address the bacteria responsible for the underlying epidemics. The human interaction with the environment and human responses to disease consistently played a role in how disease was understood and addressed in each chapter of the volume.

Many people helped this volume come together, from the publishing staff at ABC-CLIO to the individual contributors and the library and archival staff that helped support each of them across the United States and even abroad in the United Kingdom. I wish to thank in particular the staff at Olympic College's Haselwood Library as well as the staff at the Sylvan Road branch of the Kitsap County Library system. Special thanks is owed to Lt. Col. Edward J. Gawlik III, a former professor of military science at Elizabeth City State University, for encouraging and supporting me in the teaching of military history for the ROTC and in receiving the valuable training from MHIC at Ft. Leavenworth. The experience of shooting muzzle-loaded weapons with the accompanying black powder at MHIC provided new insight into how the conditions of battle affected the health of combatants.

Three other individuals were invaluable in the completion of this volume. Dr. Hilary Green and Mr. Joshua Seaman provided instrumental assistance in giving needed feedback and extra pairs of eyes to catch errors. I cannot thank them enough for their professionalism and constant support. Of course, I could never have accomplished this task without the constant and loving support of my husband, Jack, who put up with long nights of research and editing. He gracefully endured my repeated requests to listen to me reread sections aloud, although he did insist that the more descriptive entries not be read near meal times.

The contributors and I hope these chapters will give all readers an appreciation for the intricacies of wartime circumstances and the associated complexities of diseases. Historical events were affected through the interplay of the two experiences. Some of the events encountered in the chapters, both the conditions of wars and related difficulties of the accompanying epidemics, are well-known today, while others are not. Many, if not all, are misunderstood to some extent in how the events, factors, and circumstances joined to create devastating and lasting impacts on the surrounding societies and history.

Rebecca M. Seaman

Part I

Contested Epidemics during Well-Known Conflicts: Introduction

Rebecca M. Seaman

> Any ancient account of a disease will be couched in the language of a prescientific era, and no matter how intelligent, authoritative, and perceptive its author may be, an account will always be a product of its author's culture, beliefs, and notions.[1]
>
> —Jennifer Manley

Studying the connections and impacts of wars and epidemics is a complex project. Doing so for diseases that have only been identified in recent medical and historical research adds layers to that complex task. The undertaking becomes almost impossible, or at least fraught with uncertainties, when studying conflicts and epidemics from the distant past that still have no confirmed identity. Despite this reality, "Humans seem to insist on seeking reasons or causes for disease: for its incidence, its origin, its course, its outcome."[2]

Historian Andrew Cunningham has recently raised the question of legitimacy, the possibility or even the desirability of retrospective diagnosis of these past, unknown epidemics. Cunningham correctly indicated that diseases are experienced biologically and socially. While the biological element may be capable of a retrospective diagnosis—if evidence is found that has not been contaminated by the passage of time and exposure to the environment—its impact on the society completely depends on the context of time. Later medical diagnoses may provide a more "correct" biological identity, but nonetheless cannot change how the society experienced the disease at the time of its outbreak.[3]

The presumption that modern analyses are superior to earlier medical interpretations often results in the tendency for medical historical research to discount earlier interpretations and diagnoses as simply means of coping with disease. The need to translate eyewitness accounts, especially those from ancient and classical languages, results in multiple interpretations, often with conflicting descriptions of symptoms and even the chronology of events. Linguistic translations are not the only issue. Debates circulate regarding the motives of authors for primary accounts. Historical dependence on primary document accounts therefore comes under close scrutiny and demands the usage of additional physical evidence to substantiate diagnoses.

Missing evidence, or at least evidence assured of no contamination, is a common problem when researching unknown epidemics from the past. The following three chapters cover three wars and epidemics of unknown origin, wherein researchers have connected graves of victims from the diseases studied. Paleomicrobiology, the study of remnants of microbial DNA in ancient but well-preserved human tissue, can be used when there is a usable sample available. However, when studying viruses, the ability to trace connections biologically across the ages is virtually impossible. Moreover, for those unidentified epidemics of more recent origin, such as the 16th-century English sweating sickness, legal implications often block access to burial evidence that may help shed light on a retrospective diagnosis. This leaves modern scholars with only the existing written accounts to identify the disease. This method of diagnosis, complete with its accompanying conundrums, is known as paleopathology.[4]

The Roman physician Galen blended the Hippocratic humoral theories[5] with the Pythagorean theory—which took the four basic elements of Greek thought and combined them with the physiologic qualities of dry, moist, cold, and hot. This approach served as an improvement over the previous primary usage of empirical analysis. Yet, the trend of physicians and historians for the next several centuries to defer to Galen's theories hindered opportunities to review historical analysis of prior epidemics while physical evidence might have remained available.[6]

The physical evidence and historical documents that remain available today, though requiring critical analysis, present a series of common themes when studying unknown epidemics, especially those corresponding to concurrent wars. For those epidemics targeted in the next three chapters, all three lack the influence of modern medical knowledge, thanks to their ancient, classical, and early modern occurrences. The eyewitness accounts typically focused on attempted cures as well as a litany of presumed symptoms rather than what is now considered disease presentation and analysis of diffusion. Consistently, superstitions and mystical understandings of the emergence of epidemics appeared in eyewitness accounts and in many later historical documents. Often, the outbreaks of such epidemics were closely associated with guilt, especially the guilt of one side involved in the ongoing war. This is evident in all three epidemics studied in this section. Finally, the identities of unknown epidemics are intricately affected by the cultural perceptions of the time. The Greek Plague of Athens and the Antonine Plague of Rome were both understood through the lens of fate and balance; even Christianity's role came into play in the Antonine Plague.

Missing evidence, conflicting interpretations, and contradictory timelines pose problems in diagnosing epidemics from the past. These factors also hamper historians in their analysis of impacts and correlations between the epidemics and the ongoing wars of the time. The Plague of Athens occurred in the early years of the war with Sparta and resulted in the deaths of large numbers of Athenian citizens, leaders, and soldiers. However, modern scholars continue to debate the connection between the plague and Athens's eventual loss to Sparta almost three decades later. Similarly, while there is confirmed evidence of the existence of the Antonine Plague, modern scholars continue to debate the impact of the plague on Rome's military and economy and the extent of the trauma within the Roman Empire. With the more recent occurrence of English sweating sickness, there is ironically even more confusion and uncertainty. The timelines of the outbreak, as well as consistent reports of where the disease occurred and who was affected, leave historians conflicted as to how the epidemic is connected to the military conflict at the end of the Hundred Years' War.

The following three chapters focus on these events and their associated epidemics. Readers will benefit from a succinct analysis of each disease's symptoms and corresponding probable identities debated as well as the discussion by historians and medical researchers who have weighed in on the debates. Additionally, the context of the epidemics in relation to the accompanying wars is provided. Considering the lack of sufficient evidence, the authors of these chapters do not attempt to definitively identify the diseases; instead, they present the leading options, supporting information, and, where appropriate, information that undermines various theories.

NOTES

1. Jennifer Manley, "Measles and Ancient Plagues: A Note on New Scientific Evidence," *Classical World* 107, no. 3 (Spring 2014): 395–396.
2. Andrew Cunningham, "Identifying Disease in the Past: Cutting the Gordian Knot," *Asclepio* 54, no. 1 (2002), 13.
3. Cunningham, "Identifying Disease in the Past," 14.
4. Cheston B. Cunha and Burke A. Cunha, "Great Plagues of the Past and Remaining Questions," in *Paleomicrobiology: Past Human Infections*, ed. Didier Raoult and Michel Drancourt (Berlin: Springer-Verlag, 2008), 1–3.
5. The humoral theory references the explanation of differences in character and health through the study of the four primary humors: phlegm, yellow bile, black bile, and blood. Health was determined by examining the balance of these humors in afflicted individuals.
6. Darlene Berger, *A Brief History of Medical Diagnosis and the Birth of the Clinical Laboratory: Part 1, Ancient Times through the 19th Century* (July 1999), 2, accessed April 8, 2017, http://www.academia.dk/Blog/wp-content/uploads/KlinLab-Hist/LabHistory1.pdf.

Chapter 1

Plague of Athens: A Fate More Terrible Than the Spartans, 430–426 BCE

Christopher Howell

Such was the grievous calamity which now afflicted the Athenians; within the walls their people were dying, and without, their country was being ravaged. In their troubles they naturally called to mind a verse which the elder men among them declared to have been current long ago: "A Dorian war will come and a plague with it."[1]

—Thucydides

In the annals of human history, there is no more famous and yet enigmatic epidemic than the Plague of Athens, which struck the Greek city-state between 430 and 426 BCE. Though it is not the first epidemic noted in ancient history, it is currently the oldest observed and best-recorded epidemic. The long-standing conflicts between Sparta, Athens, and the Persian Empire raged across the fifth century, culminating with the Second Peloponnesian War of 431–404 BCE. Within a year of the war's start, a plague descended upon Athens. The war and the epidemic are inextricably intertwined in the minds of most researchers precisely because they represent that most common pairing of human civilization catastrophes: war and disease. Yet, there remains no consensus on the cause of the plague nor of its impact on the war. In part, the vast distance of time is to blame. However, the main source of information on the war and epidemic, the unfinished *Peloponnesian Wars* by Thucydides, provides some clues and difficulties as well as conditions or variables common at the time, 2,400 years ago.

Remarkably, both the "father of medicine," Hippocrates, and one of the fathers of history, Thucydides (a survivor of the epidemic), were present. Yet, neither the clues left by the Hippocratic-trained medical community nor the main primary source, Thucydides's *Peloponnesian Wars*, has enabled modern researchers to conclusively identify the primary medical cause of the epidemic. Indeed, Thucydides's role in the analysis of the Plague of Athens presents a conundrum. Thucydides was well-informed regarding medical terminology used in Classical Greece. As a general and historian, he was also an excellent observer and recorder of his observations.

He contracted and survived the plague, adding his own experiences to his documentation of the disease. Nonetheless, limited existing knowledge of clinical diagnosis during the Peloponnesian War combined with the difficulty in translating the nuances of Classical Greek by historians and medical researchers today leave modern experts grasping for a firm diagnosis. The variables contributing to the difficulty in identifying the Plague of Athens are impacted by the bias of the sole primary resource. Though attempting to be objective, Thucydides inevitably associated his own experience with the disease as the norm for others, introducing subjectivity to his interpretation of the symptoms. His additional experience during the war, and resulting exile by Athens, likely shaped his views of the time, in line with Greek thinking regarding balance and fate. As a result of these factors, even the plague's definitive impact on the larger war between Athens and Sparta (431–404 BCE) remains elusive.[2]

Origins of the Plague amid the Great Peloponnesian War

The stage for the Athenian plague was set in the early years of the Great Peloponnesian War. This conflict was a renewal of a long-standing conflict between terrestrial Sparta and maritime Athens. In the backdrop, Persia awaited the results of the inter-Greek conflict, having already invaded the region twice in the same century, with varying levels of success and failure. When the renewed conflict with Sparta began, the Athenian tyrant Pericles ordered the Athenian population of 300,000 inside the city walls while he sent the animals to Euboea Island. Athens relied on its seaport Piraeus for importing all needed provisions. Conditions became crowded, with the accompanying lowering of hygiene and lessening of dietary health. The stage was set for not just the calamity of war but also the spread of any disease.

In the second year, as Spartan troops arrived to renew the siege, an unknown epidemic spread from Piraeus to the main city. Thucydides reported that the disease only affected Athenians.[3] The epidemic is estimated to have killed 25–33 percent of the Athenian population packed within the city-state's walls. Among those casualties was the leader of classical Athens, Pericles, along with much of his family. Two major epidemic episodes occurred in quick succession, the first in 430–428 BCE and another in 427–426 BCE.[4]

According to Thucydides, the invasion of Attica by Sparta and its allies forced the sizeable Athenian population into the confines of the polis's walls and the long wall built by the Athenians to the port in Piraeus. Most refugees had to live outdoors, and the crowded conditions resulted in the deterioration of hygiene and increased close contact, and therefore transference of any contagious disease. Limited food supplies further compromised the immune systems of the population, who were already traumatized by the increased stresses of war and dislocation. Cut off from inland resources, Athens became completely dependent on resources acquired through its port. While other Greek city-states in the region did not report the new epidemic at the time, Egypt, Ethiopia, Lemnos, and Persia reported similar outbreaks—all regions that traded with Athens. As the disease spread through each age group, the city was unable to dispose of the bodies, further adding to the problems of hygiene and contagion.[5] Although the disease apparently did not hit the Spartan alliance, it did travel with Athenian troops in a later siege of Potidaea, devastating 30 percent of the Athenians in the siege but reportedly no Potidaeans inside the walls. Finally, the plague, which lessened after its first two-year run, reemerged for a second time in 427–426 BCE. Thucydides, who came down with the plague, survived and later attempted to gather exact population losses, albeit from a distance, as he had been exiled for poor military command performance. This second outbreak killed 4,400 hoplite soldiers, 300 horsemen, and an untold but vast number of civilians.

The Plague of Athens attacked all age sets and health levels, military and civilian. No one, not doctors, priests, sailors, the elderly, nor children, healthy or ill, was safe. Thucydides noted the demoralizing nature of this and the flight of doctors from the Hippocratic school of medicine, though later sources contradict him.[6] Even Pericles, the leader of Athens during the Peloponnesian War with Sparta, and his family fell to the epidemic.

Such a catastrophic epidemic should have collapsed Athens after these two episodes. Yet, Sparta, too, was in trouble. The Spartans kept their alliance forces back from an actual attack on Athens, greatly fearing the spread of the disease to their troops and back to their homeland on the Peloponnesus. Simultaneously, Athens had considerable success at sea by raiding the Spartan homeland and its allies. Such Spartan losses and those of its allies shook the foundation of Spartan power. Sparta struggled to keep its alliances intact in the face of the enormous Athenian maritime reach. The imbalance in methods of fighting the war—the naval strategy utilized by Athens versus the landed strategy of Sparta—combined with the impact of the disease on Athens and the fear of disease by the Spartans, managed to prolong the war and counter the disastrous effects of the disease on the Athenians.

Symptoms Observed

Thucydides's record of observations that he had associated with the Plague of Athens is quite similar to Galen's, a Roman who later recorded the symptoms and treatments of those who had contracted the mysterious Antonine Plague during the late Roman Empire rule of Marcus Aurelius in the third century CE. These observations by Thucydides were formulated on the Hippocratic method of the day and further influenced by his survival as well as Athens at large. His goal was prognosis rather than diagnosis.[7] Unfortunately, the result for later historians was a documentation of all symptoms without the ability to determine whether some of the observed symptoms were the result of other illnesses or whether they were varying levels of presentations of the same disease.

According to this "scientific" father of history, symptoms rapidly appeared on the first day of the disease: a burning fever, inflamed or bleeding throat and tongue, and red eyes.[8] By the second day, victims had runny noses, hoarseness, sneezing, and a cough. By days three and four, the cough had become violent and moved into the chest, accompanied by stomachaches, vomiting, and skin rashes. The description of the rash is problematic in that the translation often changes the description significantly.[9] The interpretation concerning the color of the rash alone, by translators as well as medical researches millennia later, has led to divergent diagnoses.

By the fifth day, patients' skin was hot to the touch and extremely sensitive, and their thirst could not be quenched. Most patients died around day six, with those surviving becoming sleepless and plagued by uncontrollable diarrhea. By the second week of illness, the discoloration of genitals, fingers, and toes indicated that patients had suffered from tissue necrosis or gangrene. Thucydides reported some patients in the second week suffering from blindness and memory loss. He also asserted that those who had managed to survive to that point were impervious to later outbreaks of the same disease.[10] However, an examination of other translations and portions of his work indicates the possibility that Thucydides referenced the "folly of hope" regarding future immunity to the current plague and other diseases.[11]

The disease variables (measurable attributes) associated with the Plague of Athens correlate to a number of other diseases. An exhaustive search of past research and published hypotheses from classical times until today reveals a dizzying array of possible diseases as the cause, despite the detailed symptom and progression observations left by Thucydides.[12] These include smallpox, measles, bubonic plague, influenza typhus, glanders, ergot toxin, typhoid fever, bacterial infection, Lassa fever, scarlet fever, and alimentary toxic aleukia. All share some similar symptoms.

Several diseases could have caused the Plague of Athens. Epidemic typhus (also known as jail or war typhus), smallpox, measles, and typhoid fever all spread via simple human contact. Smallpox, eradicated in 1978, was the early leader among researchers, as it has killed perhaps 300 million people, or more, in history.[13] Epidemic typhus is another common suggestion now, with measles a strong third. Typhoid fever is also possible, based on the much-debated findings of it in three Plague of Athens burial remains via scientific genetic testing.[14] We should also recognize the nature of evolutionary change, as many epidemic infectious diseases are of the DNA variety and may experience limited genetic change through time, but some are of the RNA variety and mutate rapidly. Thus, it is possible the culprit of the Athenian plague no longer exists or exists in a form currently unrecognizable.[15]

Modern Theories and Retrospective Diagnoses

Yet, modern research continues to attempt a definitive diagnosis, for who can resist the allure of a two-and-a-half-millennium-old mystery? The recent research trends of the last few decades focus on epidemic diseases spread via simple human contact. These include epidemic typhus, smallpox, an ancient form of measles, and typhoid fever. In the last few years, Ebola and avian flu outbreaks have had researchers exploring those candidates as well.[16] Finally, the concept of multiple diseases, with one primary, has gained footing.

Both typhus and typhoid fever are caused by bacteria, and smallpox (*Orthopoxvirus* genus) and measles (Paramyxoviridae family) are viral. Epidemic typhus moves via infected body lice and cloth. The presence of lice in the general population, documented through observations of pruritus (severe itching), makes the diagnosis of typhus plausible.[17] The conditions of overcrowded Athens give further support for such a possibility. Smallpox, spread by cough droplets and by contaminated bedding or clothing, provides another likely suspect. The presence of smallpox in Classical Greece is debated, as a clear description separating smallpox from measles was not available until the Middle Ages. Certainly, the crowded conditions of Athens and the sharing of equipment, utensils, clothing, and even bedding during a period of war provided an ideal setting for spreading smallpox. Another option, typhoid fever, is spread via water and food supply via *Salmonella* bacteria. The limitation of Athens's resources to those acquired through Piraeus could account for contamination through the food supply, and certainly typhoid fever existed in the Greek population at the time. However, the descriptions and timeline of symptoms provided by Thucydides seem to preclude typhoid as the primary culprit, though it might have been present and contributed to some of the symptoms observed.[18]

Scarlet fever is another possible culprit. Presenting suddenly early on with a fever, red eyes, runny nose, and sore throat, the disease is often accompanied by a livid red throat and tongue, convulsions, and vomiting and includes a rash that starts on the head and then spreads over the body and appendages, much in line with Thucydides's record. Yet, the death rate associated with the plague far exceeds the expected death rate of a scarlet fever epidemic. Thus, all the above are reasonable fits for the historical context at Athens at the start of the Peloponnesian War in 431–430 BCE. However, these diseases fail to conclusively demonstrate evidence supporting any as the sole or even primary cause of the plague as described by Thucydides.

Marks against more recent suggestions of Ebola include the lack of proof of its existence in the Classical Greek era. Avian flu, another recent possible culprit, is usually associated with certain animal populations that were absent in Athens during the siege. Yet, marks against the four top candidates of epidemic typhus, typhoid fever, smallpox, and measles also exist. The absence of pox marks in contemporary descriptions is an issue, but smallpox is known to have existed before the time of Athens (the mummy of Rameses V, for instance). Researchers have also pointed out that not all pox cases come with pox marks. Smallpox and measles tend to attack the young or elderly and do not often reach 25 percent death rates today, but these diseases did cause higher death tolls in prevaccination times. Measles accounts for the most clinical symptoms recorded, according to infectious disease specialist Burke Cunha, followed by smallpox.[19]

Robert Littman, who has devoted a lifetime of research to the subject, has evolved his opinion over time to eliminate measles, malaria, and other diseases by using math modeling of paleopathology and epidemiology. He suggests measles would last only a few months—and not five years—in a population of 300,000.

Littman does like smallpox, typhus, arboviral diseases, and the plague, but not typhoid fever.[20] The common sources of imported grain could be a source for typhoid fever or diseases such as ergotism, but the water sources differ from sea-level Piraeus wells to the stream, river, and cistern water of upland Athens, some 26 miles inland, undermining the plausibility of contamination through water. Lice that spread typhus were noted in Greek ports such as Corinth at this time. Furthermore, the continued pestilence to 426 BCE and the conferred immunity also fit typhus and smallpox according to immunologist Erika Hammerlund, while typhoid fever survivors earned only short-term immunity (one year) according to microbiologist S. Sarasamboth.[21]

Hippocrates (460–377 BCE) is given credit for contextualizing the study of epidemics in his work *Airs, Waters, Places*, and fellow classical thinker Democritus (460–370 BCE) is given credit for the theory of invisible particles spreading diseases. Thucydides, for his part, left us a Hippocratic-inspired description of the epidemic and war in *The Peloponnesian Wars*.[22] Indeed, it was the Plague of Athens that helped set in motion the study of epidemics and their impact, especially in war or military history. Today, ironically, though the science of epidemiology begun in the Hellenic world provides our best chance at understanding morbidity and mortality frequency and determinants in a given population, we still have no consensus on the epidemic that hit Athens.[23]

The dilemma that continues regarding the identification of the Plague of Athens should not surprise modern researchers. Even Thucydides warned us this would be the case in his writings:

> As to its probable origin or the causes which might or could have produced such a disturbance of nature, every man, whether a physician or not, will give his own opinion. But I shall describe its actual course, and the symptoms by which anyone who knows them beforehand may recognize the disorder should it ever reappear. For I was myself attacked, and witnessed the sufferings of others.[24]

We cannot be sure, but ancient sources suggest Thucydides stopped his account of his work around 411 BCE, after writing much of it in exile after 424 BCE while communicating or visiting with both Athenian and Spartan sources.[25] Unfortunately, there is no surviving complete version or original of his unfinished work on the plague and war. Instead, we draw upon various fragmentary copies over many later centuries. Most date from the 10th–14th centuries CE, and a few papyrus fragments from Egypt date back to about 500 years after the Plague of Athens.[26] Researchers of ancient manuscripts suggest that most of these later copies seem to have derived from two or more earlier works.[27] What is certain is just how tenuous and fragmentary our knowledge is of the author's life, of his original and unfinished primary source on the war, and thus of our knowledge of the Plague of Athens.

Despite the incomplete and inconclusive Plague of Athens's research, hope emerged in 2006 with the genetic testing and identification of typhoid fever, or at least *Salmonella*, from three skeletons recovered from a likely burial associated with the plague. Though debate surrounds the findings, as it should in any serious academic scientific context, it represents the only actual scientific genetic evidence so far, and that alone makes it worthy of mention.[28] So, at the very least, the findings of Manolis Papagrigorakis (professor and orthodontist) and Christos Yapijakis (geneticist) represent a possible way forward with genetic data derived from contextualized archaeological remains. Similar finds have now taken place for both the 14th century CE Black Death and the 5th century CE "Plague of Justinian" with *Yersina pestilis,* or bubonic plague, research. The ancient strain of typhoid fever may have mutated or adapted or even been spread by the Spartans in a form of bioterrorism.[29] Still, as Littman and others have pointed out, the sample size is far too small to be in any way representative and could simply be an indication of a known endemic disease that presented while the main unknown culprit ravaged the population of Athens.[30]

Robert Littman has arguably put in more work on the etiology of the epidemic that hit Athens than anyone else. Using philology, clinical diagnosis, and epidemiology, Littman has shifted his explanation from smallpox alone toward typhus and arboviral diseases, and he has not ruled out the bubonic plague. Nonetheless, his work discounts the likelihood of measles and typhoid fever as possible causes of the epidemic. Interestingly, a University of Maryland conference called in 1999 to solve the dilemma also identified typhus as the likely culprit. It even went so far as to present an anonymous historic patient (Pericles) with symptoms to determine the consensus prognosis: epidemic typhus was the answer.[31]

Historical Debates of the Causes and Effects of the Plague of Athens

Ancient researchers also debated the causes and effects of the Plague of Athens. Galen, himself a great physician in Roman Empire times during the Antonine Plague (165–168 CE), also referenced Thucydides's account. Galen described that Roman epidemic and commented on the similarity of the rash form of the Antonine Plague to that described from the Plague of Athens.[32] Galen's description is suggestive, though not conclusive, of smallpox for the Antonine Plague. Pliny the Elder, Galen, and Aetius contradict Thucydides's suggestion that Hippocrates, Acron, and Empodocles remained on or returned to Athens and stayed the epidemic by using fire to cleanse the air.[33] Plutarch and Pliny, writing 500 years later, echoed other ancient researchers who believed "bad air" was the cause of plagues and that balancing humors or fluids in the body on an individual basis was a treatment. For the treatment of entire communities, the use of fire to cleanse the air was again suggested. Thucydides, however, seems ambivalent, acknowledging attempts to stop the disease while also writing that physicians were unable to cope with the plague:

> For a while physicians, in ignorance of the nature of the disease, sought to apply remedies; but it was in vain, and they themselves were among the first victims, because they oftenest came into contact with it. No human art was of any avail, and as to supplications in temples, enquiries of oracles, and the like, they were utterly useless, and at last men were overpowered by the calamity and gave them all up.[34]

While ancient and modern specialists have failed to identify the causes of the plague, we do have a reasonable record of its death toll and, through that information, assertions of its wartime impact. As indicated previously, the Plague of Athens, based on its rolling death toll of roughly 30 percent, would seem to have brought down the Athenian empire during the Peloponnesian War. For instance, the epidemic impact on Athenian designs to besiege Potidaea suggest a major military impact:

> In the same summer, Hagnon, the son of Nicias, and Cleopompus[,] the son of Cleinias, who were colleagues of Pericles in his military command, took the fleet which he had employed and sailed forthwith against the Thracian Chalcidians and against Potidaea, which still held out. On their arrival they brought engines up to the walls, and tried every means of taking the town. But they did not succeed; nor did the result by any means correspond to the magnitude of their armament; for thither too the plague came and made dreadful havoc among the Athenian troops. Even the soldiers who were previously there and had been in good health caught the infection from the forces under Hagnon. But the army of Phormio escaped; for he and his 1,600 troops had left Chalcidice. And so Hagnon returned with his fleet to Athens, having lost by the plague out of 4,000 hoplites 1,050 men in forty days. But the original armament remained and prosecuted the siege.[35]

Here we find a roughly 25 percent death rate in 40 days, and reportedly only for Athenians. Logically, this should have helped collapse the Athenian war effort and led to a Spartan victory and the war's end. But that is not what happened.

A simple examination of the timeline of the Peloponnesian War reveals the Plague of Athens epidemic occurred as only one episode in over a century of conflict between Athens, Sparta, and the Persian Empire. The plague accounted for just four more years in this age-old contest. When viewed in this context, the Plague of Athens, while a significant event, appears to have had no real bearing on the outcome of the Second Peloponnesian War of 431–404 BCE, which was the focus of Thucydides's unfinished history. After its surrender to Sparta in 404 BCE, Athens then reinstituted democracy and rebuilt its sea power along with the much hated (by Sparta) long wall system by 395 BCE. This was the same wall that had alarmed the Spartans and their allies, as it connected Athens with the port of Piraeus, and became the focal point of the Plague of Athens from a distribution perspective. Even more telling, the century-long conflicts involving Athens, Sparta, and Persia are found both *before* and *after* the Plague of Athens event of 430–426 BCE. From a military history perspective, this is hardly the timeline of an epidemic that collapsed Athens or elevated the Spartan alliance to victory.

Yet, following the Plague of Athens, the Athenian alliance became involved in Syracuse and Sicily in 427 BCE and off and on again in 422 BCE. Devastated by the plague, Athens became split between the "peace" party, or pro-Spartan party, led by Niceas and the "war" party led by Alcibiades.[36] This internal rift led to a peace treaty, never honored, between Athens and Sparta in 421 BCE, followed by a massive set of seaborne expeditionary forces into Sicily by both sides in the battle of

Syracuse 415–413 BCE led by Alcibiades. The Spartans and their allies responded by reinforcing Syracuse, and the key battle of the Peloponnesian War was set.

All of these activities occurred a decade after the Plague of Athens had supposedly brought the Athenian and Greek world to its knees. Despite the spectacular failure for Athens in the Syracuse expedition, with losses of almost 50,000 men, 250 ships, and untold amounts of bullion, the war continued. In 411 BCE, the mighty Persian Empire, long a background player in Greek city-state power, funded the Spartan navy, and Athens superiority at sea seemed doomed. Nevertheless, Athens scored a major sea victory by destroying the Spartan fleet at Arginusae in 406 BCE, thereby keeping grain shipments from Asia Minor open to Athens.[37] Once again, Sparta turned to Persia as Spartan naval commander Lysander rebuilt the Spartan alliance fleet and engaged the Athenian alliance off Aegospotami in 405 BCE. Surprisingly, the Spartans caught the Athenian fleet resupplying on the beach, and losses were finally insurmountable for the Athenians, with over 150 ships captured and 3,000 plus sailors executed. Finally, in exhaustion, Athens surrendered in 404 BCE.[38] The continuation of the war long after the heavy loss of life and morale during the Plague of Athens leads to assertions that the epidemic had no lasting impact on the war. Yet, it was the continuation of the war on the heels of the plague, and the repeated losses despite expectations of potential Athenian victory, that ultimately exhausted Athens and resulted in its decision to surrender to its age-old enemies.

Even this surrender did not last long, leaving the epidemic impact on war in further doubt for some. As Sparta proved unable to govern the unruly Greek world any better than Athens, Persia achieved economically what it could not with military might in the earlier Persian Wars of 490–476 BCE. Athens was removed from its dominant trade position in the Mediterranean in favor of the Persian seafaring allies: the Phoenicians of Byblos, Sidon, and Tyre. Yet, all three powers found themselves in economic exhaustion and military overextension. Sparta, Athens, and Persia were ripe for invasion. Soon, a new military might arose in the 300s BCE in Macedon, led by Phillip II and later his son, Alexander the Great. Both made any memory of the Plague of Athens and the economically exhausting Sparta, Athens, Persia rivalry obsolete as they brought the Greek and Persian worlds down in a way not even the Plague of Athens could.[39]

Combined Impact of the Plague and War in Athens

If there is a lesson from the Plague of Athens and the Peloponnesian War for us today, and for later wars and epidemics that followed, it is that the intertwined nature of conflict and disease are not so easily unwrapped. The association exists, but the exact etiology, impact, and historical significance are much harder to understand than a superficial examination would suggest. No doubt the Spartan command, well versed in the art of war and the role of disease, kept waiting for an Athenian collapse from the epidemic Plague of Athens. Although disease had devastated the population and morale, and divided the polis in its approach to fighting the war, it did not lead to the collapse of Athens. Not the losses at Syracuse, the rival factions in Athens, or even the repeated problems of revolts, alliance changes, and multiple Plague episodes on Athens alone brought the polis down. Persian gold seems to be the key resource that broke the back of the Athenian whale, only to see it reemerge in 395 BCE.[40] The century-long conflict of the big three powers in the eastern Mediterranean theater left each power blinded to the rise of Macedonia, a "barbarian" kingdom that nevertheless conquered and united all three power regions in a way that a century of conflict and almost a decade of disease could not.

Disease and war are usually recipes for collapse and chaos. The Plague of Athens was but a part of a more complex, historic record of power shifts. Researchers from ancient times forward have speculated on the etiology of the disease known as the Plague of Athens and its wartime impact without consensus. Researchers mostly identify epidemic typhus, smallpox, or, to a lesser extent, measles with the Plague of Athens. Other considerations include scarlet fever or the presence of multiple diseases. These epidemic diseases have repeatedly ravaged human civilization in similar conditions. Recent suggestions of additional diseases, such as Ebola, and the recent finds of Typhoid fever in three skeletal remains continue to muddy the waters.[41] Despite millennia of unanswered questions, historians continue to seek answers to this puzzle.

Perhaps if Thucydides had lived to finish his work on the war or if he had more time to see the aftereffects, or lack thereof, concerning the outcome of the Plague of Athens and the Peloponnesian War of 431–404 BCE, his analysis and linkage of the two would have proceeded differently. But perhaps not, as the association of the two in time and space was undeniable; yet, the cause and effect, if any, remains unidentifiable.

NOTES

1. Thucydides, "The Plague," trans. Benjamin Jowett (Oxford: Clarendon Press, 1900), accessed August 31, 2017, http://www.perseus.tufts.edu/hopper/text?doc=Thuc .+2.47& fromdoc=Perseus%3Atext%3A1999.04.0105.

2. James Longrigg, "The Great Plague of Athens," *History of Science* 18 (1980): 209, SAO/ NASA Astrophysics Data System, accessed August 31, 2017, http://articles.adsabs .harvard.edu/cgi-bin/nph-iarticle_query?bibcode=1980HisSc..18..209L&db _key=AST&page_ind=0&data_type=GIF&type=SCREEN_VIEW&classic=YES.

3. Various rationales may account for Thucydides's assertion that only Athenians died from the disease. His work, written after he was exiled from Athens, may reflect his own bias against the Athenian leadership of the period and utilize a Greek perception of balance and fate underlining his account. It is also quite likely that Thucydides, providing an eyewitness account, reported only the deaths of which he was aware. This would account for the omission of reports of similar outbreaks in Egypt and elsewhere in the Mediterranean region.

4. See Donald Kagan, *The Peloponnesian War* (2003), by Penguin Books, for the definitive modern history overview for the lay reader based on his four-volume tome. See Victor Hanson, *A War Like No Other: How the Spartans and Athenians Fought the Peloponnesian*

War (2005), by Random House, for the historical military context. See Morgen Hansen, "Athenian Population Losses 431–403 B.C. and the Number of Athenian Citizens in 431 B.C.," in *Three Studies in Athenian Demography* (Copenhagen, Denmark: Munkgaard Historisk-Filosopfiske Meddelelser, 1988), lvi; and Robert Littman, "The Plague of Athens: Epidemiology and Paleopathology," *Mount Sinai Journal of Medicine* 76 (2009): 456–467, for medical context and population estimates.

5. Thucydides, "Plague of Athens," in *History of the Peloponnesian War*, trans. Benjamin Jowett, ed. A Peabody (Boston: Lothrop & Co., 1883). This was originally in 13 books but modernized to 8 books. References by book number and passage number (2:47–2:52, 2:58, and 3:87) are the main passages with information on the Plague of Athens in Thucydides's unfinished work now known as "Peloponnesian Wars."

6. A number of translations of Thucydides's "Peloponnesian Wars" exist, but we rely here on two tested translations that give readers a sense of the variance and difficulty in translating ancient sources. See Thucydides, *History of the Peloponnesian War*, 47, and compare with the same passage describing symptom progression from Thucydides, *History of the Peloponnesian War to 411 BCE*, trans. Rex Warner (1954; repr., London: Penguin Books, 1972), 152–153. Historians utilizing these varying interpretations continue to debate the meaning and possibility of bias or translation error.

7. Longrigg, "The Great Plague of Athens," 210–212.

8. The disease symptom daily progress is drawn from the work of D. L. Page, "Thucydides's Description of the Great Plague at Athens," *Classical Quarterly* 3 (1953): 109–110; and Burke A. Cunha, "The Cause of the Plague of Athens: Plague, Typhoid, Typhus, Smallpox, or Measles?," *Infectious Disease Clinics North America* 18 (2004): 33–34, accessed September 16, 2017, https://doi.org/10.1016/S0891-5520(03)00100-4. Page's work on pages 109–110 contains only his English translation of the classical Greek terms used for disease symptom progression. His philology study with Greek term discussion, the short English translation summary of the symptom progression (109–110), and English-language terminology notes stretch across pages 29–43, accessed August 31, 2017, http://www.jstor.org/stable/637025.

9. See Adam Parry, "The Language of Thucydides' Description of the Plague," *Bulletin of the Institute of Classical Studies* 16 (1969): 106–107 and 118, for discussion on the Hippocratic School in the writings of Thucydides, accessed August 31, 2017, http://onlinelibrary.wiley.com/doi/10.1111/j.2041-5370.1969.tb00667.x/abstract. See Lee T. Pearcy, "Diagnosis As Narrative in Ancient Literature," *American Journal of Philology* 113, no. 4 (Winter 1992): 595, accessed August 31, 2017, http://www.jstor.org/stable/295542, for additional linguistic issues centered on medical terms, writing style, etc., in ancient literature. See Jody Ruben Pinault, "Hippocrates and the Plague," in *Hippocratic Lives and Legends* (Leiden, the Netherlands: E. J. Brill, 1992), 35–37.

10. Main clinical and epidemiological variables in Thucydides's description of the Plague of Athens epidemic follow Page, "Thucydides's Description," 109–110; Thucydides, "Plague of Athens," 2:49–51; and Cunha, "The Cause of the Plague of Athens," 33–34.

11. G. W. Bowersock, "The Personality of Thucydides," *Antioch Review* 25, no. 1, Special Greek Issue (Spring 1965): 144.

12. From classical times forward, over 50 researchers have proposed at least 31 diseases singly or in combination as the cause of the Plague of Athens. The author of this chapter referenced information following the tabulations by David T. Durack et al., "Hellenic Holocaust: A Historical Clinico-Pathologic Conference," *American Journal of*

Medicine 109 (2000), 393, Table 1; and tables from Cunha, "The Cause of the Plague of Athens," 29–43. Additionally, an exhaustive search of all published literature in multiple languages resulted in 50 researchers and 31 diseases total.

13. Michael Oldstone, *Viruses, Plagues, & History* (New York: Oxford University Press, 2010), 306.

14. The hotly debated findings of typhoid fever in three Plague of Athens burial skeletons centered on the quality of the scientific process of the samples. Unfortunately, this takes away from the larger issue of the extremely small, anecdotal size of the samples. Three cases of typhoid fever, endemic to the Athens region, would not be statistically significant among perhaps 90,000 Plague of Athens victims, assuming a 30 percent death rate among 300,000. See M. Papagrigorakis et al., "E. DNA Examination of Ancient Dental Pulp Indicates Typhoid Fever as a Probable Cause of the Plague of Athens," *International Journal of Infectious Diseases* 10 (2006): 206–214; M. Papagrigorakis and C. Yapijakis, P. Synodinos, "Ancient Typhoid Epidemic Reveals Possible Ancestral Strain of *Salmonella enterica* serovar Typhi," *Infection, Genetics and Evolution* 7 (2007), 126–127; M. Papagrigorakis et al., "The Plague of Athens: An Ancient Act of Bioterrorism?," *Biosecurity and Bioterrorism: Biodefense Strategy, Practice, and Science* 11, no. 3 (September 2013): 228–229, for initial findings. For critique and replies, see Beth Shapiro, "No Proof That Typhoid Caused the Plague of Athens (A Reply to Papagrigorakis et al.)," *International Journal of Infectious Diseases* 10 (2006): 334–340, in International Society for Infectious Diseases, letters to the editor, accessed August 31, 2017, http://ac.els-cdn .com/S1201971206000531/1-s2.0-S1201971206000531-main.pdf?_tid=481bc36e -8f24-11e7-82c9-00000aacb362&acdnat=1504277345_278565821f4a0200da459ae 9aaf906c9.

15. A. Froland, "The Great Plague of Athens 430 BCE," *Danish Medicine History Journal* 38 (2010): 63–80; Longrigg, "The Great Plague of Athens," 18:221; and J. C. F. Poole and A. Holladay, "Thucydides and the Plague of Athens," *Classical Quarterly* 29 (1979): 282–283.

16. For the Ebola candidacy, see Bernard, "Ebola in Greece?," *British Medical Journal* 313, no. 7054 (August 17, 1996): 430; and Powel Kazanjian, "Ebola in Antiquity?," *Clinical Infectious Diseases* 61, no. 6 (2015): 964–965; for references on Ebola beyond the Athens's plague, see 963–998 for a full discussion, accessed August 31, 2017, http://cid .oxfordjournals.org/content/61/6/963; and responses to letters to the editor http://cid .oxfordjournals.org/content/early/2015/08/20/cid.civ605.full. For the Avian flu candidacy, see Karen Spence, "The Epidemic That Killed Pericles: Contextual and Paleopathological Analysis of the 5th Century BCE Plague of Athens via Primary Resources and Modern DNA Sequence-Based Identification Strategies of Dental Pulp from a Mass Grave at Kerameikos: A Novel Offering of Compelling Evidence of Avian Influenza as the Causative Agent of the Plague of Athens" (master's thesis, University of Leicester, 2013), the Classical Mediterranean School of Archaeology and Ancient History.

17. Cunha, "The Cause of the Plague of Athens," 32.

18. Cunha, "The Cause of the Plague of Athens," 37.

19. Cunha, "The Cause of the Plague of Athens," 38.

20. Littman, "The Plague of Athens," 456–467; David M. Morens and Robert J. Littman, "Epidemiology of the Plague of Athens," *Transactions of the American Philological Association* 122 (1992): 293–300; Robert J. Littman and M. L. Littman, "Galen and the Antonine Plague," *American Journal of Philology* 94, no. 3 (1973): 243–245; and Robert

J. Littman and M. L. Littman, "The Athenian Plague: Smallpox," *Transactions and Proceedings of the American Philological Association* 100 (1969): 261.

21. See Hammerland et al., "Antiviral Immunity Following Smallpox Virus Infection: A Case-Control Study," *Journal of Virology* 84, no. 24 (December 2010): 12754. Published online 2010, October 6, accessed August 31, 2017, https:/ncbi.nlm.nih.gov /pmc/articles/PMC3004327. See also S. Sarasomboth et al., "Systemic and Intestinal Immunities after Natural Typhoid Infection," *Journal of Clinical Microbiology* 25, no. 6 (1987): 1088.

22. Sarah Boslough, ed., *Encyclopedia of Epidemiology* (Thousand Oaks, CA: Sage Publications, 2008), 318–319.

23. Boslough, *Encyclopedia of Epidemiology*, xxxv.

24. Thucydides, "Plague of Athens," 2:48.

25. Hanson, *A War Like No Other*, 68–82; Kagan, *The Peloponnesian War*, xxiv. Both modern authors do much to illuminate the little we know about the life of Thucydides, from his own work and from contemporary Greek and later Roman sources on his life.

26. Herbert Fox, *Thucydides Histories: Book III* (Oxford: Clarendon Press, 1901), ix.

27. Bernard P. Grenfell and Arthur S. Hunt, *The Oxyrhynchus Papyri, Part I* (London: Egypt Exploration Society, 1898), 39–44.

28. See Papagrigorakis et al., "E. DNA Examination," 10:206–214; Papagrigorakis, Yapijakis, and Synodinos, "Ancient Typhoid," 7:126–127; Spence, "The Epidemic That Killed Pericles," 26–29.

29. Papagrigorakis, Yapijakis, Synodinos, "Ancient Typhoid," 7:126–127; and Papagrigorakis et al., "The Plague of Athens," 228–229.

30. Littman, "The Plague of Athens," 76:456–467.

31. Littman, "The Plague of Athens"; Littman and Morens, "Epidemiology of the Plague of Athens," 271–272; and Littman and Littman, "The Athenian Plague: Smallpox," 100:261. See also Durack et al., "Hellenic Holocaust," 394, for results of the innovative findings.

32. Littman and Littman, "Galen and the Antonine Plague," 253.

33. Jody R. Pinault, "How Hippocrates Cured the Plague," *Journal of History of Medicine and Allied Sciences* 41, no. 1 (1986): 52–75, doi:10.1093/jhmas/41.1.52; and Pinault, *Hippocratic Lives and Legends*, 36–40.

34. Thucydides, *History of the Peloponnesian War*, 2:47–48.

35. Thucydides, *History of the Peloponnesian War*, 2:58.

36. Donald Kagan, *The Peace of Nicias and the Sicilian Expedition* (Ithaca, NY: Cornell University Press, 1981), 17–18.

37. Debra Hamel, *The Battle of Arginusae: Victory at Sea and Its Tragic Aftermath in the Final Years of the Peloponnesian War, Witness to Ancient History Series* (Baltimore, MD: Johns Hopkins University Press, 2015).

38. Kagan, *The Peloponnesian War*, 471–480.

39. Kagan, *The Peloponnesian War*, 471–480.

40. Kagan, *The Peloponnesian War*, 333, 357.

41. Kazanjian, "Ebola in Antiquity?," 964–965.

Chapter 2

The Antonine Plague: Unknown Death within the Roman Empire, 165–180 CE

Brenda Thacker

This pestilence must have raged with incredible fury; and it carried off innumerable victims. As the reign of M. Aurelius forms a turning point in so many things, and above all in literature and art, I have no doubt that this crisis was brought about by that plague . . . The ancient world never recovered from the blow inflicted upon it by the plague which visited it in the reign of M. Aurelius.[1]

—B. G. Niebuhr

The Antonine Plague, which lasted from 165 CE to at least 180 CE, is a classic example of contagious diffusion and the dilemma of researching an unidentified disease. Brought into the Roman Empire from an unknown source, the pandemic caused widespread death and fear throughout the Mediterranean. The disease, which has yet to be conclusively identified, was apparently new to the existing population. This lack of exposure meant there was no immunity, creating a virgin-soil epidemic. This left people extremely vulnerable, as was the case with so many epidemics during the life of the empire.[2] The Antonine Plague, one of many case studies, illustrates the connection between human conflict and disease. The armies of Rome, involved in a war with the Parthian Empire, were the first population group documented as contracting the infection. It was through Rome's armies that the pestilence quickly spread throughout the empire. The deaths caused by the Antonine Plague also made it difficult for Marcus Aurelius, the emperor after whom the epidemic is named, to effectively fight a war against various barbarian tribes following the plague's ravages. In this case, the connection to human conflict was twofold. Not only did a military campaign help to introduce the disease to the Roman Empire, but its aftermath also influenced the ability of the Romans to wage war.

Historians and physicians have speculated about the culprit of the Antonine Plague, but the actual contagion has yet to be identified. Although commonly referred to as a *plague*, the word is used as a general term, synonymous with *epidemic* or *pandemic*. Paleomicrobiology is used when there is a reliable sample available. Unfortunately, no such sample exists for the Antonine Plague. To date, no remains have been found that are suitable for testing. This leaves modern scholars with only the existing written accounts to identify the disease: paleopathology.[3] The pestilence behind the Antonine Plague has been difficult to pin down. This is due in large part to a scarcity of firsthand descriptions of the disease that allow for a modern diagnosis as well as the universality of some of the symptoms recorded.

Symptoms and Associations with the Antonine Plague

For diagnosing the Antonine Plague, the writings of Galen are indispensable. The epidemic has sometimes been referred to as the Plague of Galen, rather than the Antonine Plague, for this reason. Galen, a second-century physician, lived and practiced medicine in Rome during the initial outbreak there, sometime in 166 CE. He was also a witness to an outbreak in Aquileia, a city in northern Italy, around 168 CE.[4] Before looking at efforts to identify the disease, Galen's description needs to be summarized. The physician noted three key symptoms he associated with the plague. The first was a rash, sometimes black, accompanied by ulcers and followed by scabbing. The second was a fever, something that Galen most closely associated with the plague. The third was diarrhea, which was also often black in color. Other recorded symptoms included nausea, vomiting, bad breath, a cough, and internal ulcers or bleeding. Galen also made connections between the progression of certain symptoms and chances of survival.[5] However, Galen was not writing with his future audience and modern researchers in mind, and his descriptions of the disease are not always clear.

Because of the difficulty in diagnosing based on observations, early scholars often avoided the question altogether. Instead, they chose to focus on demographic, economic, or cultural impacts. Barthold Niebuhr, in the third volume of his famous *Lectures on the History of Rome*, proclaimed that, "the ancient world never recovered from the blow inflicted upon it by the [Antonine] plague."[6] H. M. D. Parker, in his *History of the Roman World*, agreed with this assessment, stating that the plague "contributed perhaps more than any other factor to the decline of the Empire."[7] J. F. Gilliam's article on the plague first reviewed the body of primary sources available to historians and then concluded with a statement on its impact. There was no attempt to determine which disease might have caused the epidemic, although Gilliam mentioned earlier scholars who had postulated theories in their works.[8]

Problems with Retrospective Diagnoses

Writing in the 19th and 20th centuries, a select few scholars argued in favor of a handful of different infectious diseases. Smallpox was the evident favorite. August Hirsch, whose *Handbook of Geographical and Historical Pathology* was published in 1883, placed the Antonine Plague in a sequence of possible smallpox outbreaks in the ancient and late antiquity worlds.[9] In *Disease and History*, Frederick

F. Cartwright supported the consensus that the "plague of the physician Galen" was possibly the earliest recorded appearance of smallpox.[10] William H. McNeill, in his history of epidemiology, agreed with this assessment.[11] Also deserving of mention is Abu Becr Mohammed ibn Zacariya ar-Razi, more commonly known as Rhazes, a 10th-century Persian physician. Rhazes was the first to document a difference between smallpox and measles. He argued quite strongly for the identification of Galen's plague as smallpox.[12] Only Arturo Castiglioni, writing in 1969, went against the trend and diagnosed it as either typhus or bubonic plague after analyzing the available primary sources.[13] Nonetheless, these scholars often failed to elaborate on why they had identified particular diseases as the source of the plague. The exception is Rhazes, who was a physician rather than a historian.

"Galen and the Antonine Plague," written by R. J. and M. L. Littman in 1973, was possibly the first paper to attempt a differential diagnosis of the Antonine Plague. The Littmans pointed out that the central problem with using Galen as a chief source centers on his purpose for writing about the disease. The emphasis was on treatment, not diagnosis, and Galen only mentioned symptoms when they tended to indicate which potential cures worked best.[14] Nonetheless, the Littmans' historical analysis of Galen's writings strongly favored smallpox for a number of reasons. When looking at the three diseases considered—smallpox, typhus, and bubonic plague—the first symptom that helped to narrow down the possibilities was the rash. In describing the Antonine Plague, Galen reported a rash that covered the entire body. This is true of smallpox and typhus but not bubonic plague. Whether the rash is flat or raised is the second difference. Although Galen was not always clear, he did note the existence of pustules. Galen also described the presence of ulcers sometimes accompanying the rash. This corresponds to a particular disease type known as "hemorrhagic smallpox." Littman connected other symptoms recorded by Galen to hemorrhagic smallpox, including the gastrointestinal symptoms that might indicate internal bleeding. Taken together, this makes an effective case for the diagnosis.[15] Littman also went on to guess a higher mortality than had been previously estimated, based on what is now known about the virulence of smallpox in different areas. Historically, smallpox outbreaks often resulted in 10 percent of the infected individuals dying. The Antonine Plague lasted for approximately 23 years, and so the estimated death total ranges from 7 million to 10 million.[16]

Although Cheston B. and Burke A. Cunha approached the question from a medical point of view, they arrived at the same conclusion in a 2008 chapter surveying the plagues of Athens, Marcus Aurelius, and Justinian. They, too, eliminated measles as a possibility based on the type of rash described by Galen. They also addressed the problem of immunity. Smallpox, like other viral diseases, leaves survivors with lasting protection. The only way to account for the plague resurfacing decades later is if it managed to find large enough populations or areas that had previously been untouched.[17] This was possible, but only a careful reading of the texts could confirm it. The authors were firmly convinced that the Antonine Plague was caused by smallpox. A similar 2010 study on the origins of the measles virus dates its appearance to the 11th and 12th centuries CE, making measles a biological improbability.[18]

Today, smallpox seems to be the most commonly accepted diagnosis for the Antonine Plague. However, confirmation of such a diagnosis requires the testing of human remains. If the identification of smallpox is correct, it can tell us a lot about the plague's place in the history of infectious diseases. Smallpox's closest viral relative is cowpox, suggesting that the process of domestication caused it to evolve and jump species. The earliest presumed descriptions of the disease come from India and are dated to the first through the fourth centuries CE, and maybe even earlier. The disease likely traveled westward through trade, which saw an uptick around the same time. The Mediterranean world at the turn of the first millennium CE experienced relatively little exposure to infectious diseases of epidemic proportions.[19] Whether or not it was smallpox, it is entirely possible that the Antonine Plague was the debut of a new disease in the West.

Historical Debates Regarding the Antonine Plague

Fortunately, historians are not required to know the cause of an epidemic to examine its impact. The works of several different authors from antiquity, Galen included, allow the piecing together of a historical timeline of the Antonine Plague and its progression through the Roman Empire. Of course, a few problems with these sources are worth noting.

First, no single resource covers the plague in its entirety. Some give information about the origins and impact of the epidemic on the empire, and others simply note its existence and general severity. Aside from one resource, there are no death counts from which to guess a mortality rate. This factor makes it difficult to determine the extent to which the Antonine Plague affected the population. Even after combining the various accounts, historians are left with relatively little definitive information.

Second, it is difficult to judge the accuracy of the information contained within the various resources. To date, no material evidence has been found that affirms the existence of the Antonine Plague's origin and identity. It is possible, even likely, that the historians and biographers who recorded something about the plague embellished or fabricated their accounts. As such, the individual accounts should be taken with a grain of salt. Regardless, it is clear that the Antonine Plague did occur, even if the actual disease remains elusive, and that the plague was a monumental event for the Mediterranean world. While the details are questionable, the written sources demonstrate that the plague was widespread and deadly. Also of great significance, the Antonine Plague was directly connected to the Roman Empire's military conflicts during the reign of Marcus Aurelius.

Military Actions and Politics as a Stage for the Antonine Plague

Marcus Aurelius and Lucius Verus, co-emperors of the Roman Empire beginning in 161 CE, were judged by Cassius Dio to be well matched. Marcus Aurelius was an intellectual who was perhaps more interested in attending lectures than running an empire. Lucius Verus, the younger of the two, had the aggressive character necessary for conducting military campaigns in person. When the tension between Rome and Parthia snapped in the same year, it was clear which ruler would lead troops to the eastern frontier. Vologases IV of Parthia initiated the conflict by invading Armenia and overthrowing its pro-Roman ruler, replacing him with a relative named Pacorus. The Parthians went on to defeat M. Sedatius Severianus, the governor of Cappadocia (eastern Anatolia), at Elegia. The entire affair lasted only three days. Next to fall was Attidius Cornelianus, the interim governor of Syria. The way was then clear for the Parthians to invade Roman territory.[20]

In 162 CE, Verus was dispatched to Antioch to establish his campaign headquarters and raise troops. He was apparently in no rush, as the emperor managed to set aside time for "hunting in Apulia, travelling about through Athens and Corinth accompanied by orchestras and singers, and dallying through all the cities of Asia."[21] Marcus Aurelius also arranged for the replacements of Severianus and Cornelianus. Severianus's successor, Statius Priscus, came to Cappadocia from Britain. Priscus may have beaten Verus to the eastern front. Once there, he was successful in recovering Armenia for Rome in 163 CE. With Rome's focus on the east, Vologases sent his own forces against Osrhoene, a Roman client kingdom in northern Mesopotamia that sat between the two great empires. However, Verus was not fazed. Roman troops immediately moved to take two cities on the Parthian side of the Euphrates, and the two armies clashed at Sura the same year.[22]

After spending a year preparing for the invasion of Parthia, Verus made his move. In 165 CE, Osrhoene was decisively liberated, sending the Parthians retreating east.[23] Osroes, the Parthian general who had been so victorious at the beginning of the war, was forced to swim across the Tigris River when the city of Nisibis fell to Roman forces; he was able to save himself by hiding out in a nearby cave.[24] General Avidius Cassius, leading a second army, devastated the Parthians at Dura Europus and took the city for Rome rather than raze it. He then moved south to the final stage of the campaign.

To reach a decisive victory, there were two final targets in Parthia. The first was the capital of Ctesiphon, on the east bank of the Tigris River. Cassius burned Vologases's palace and occupied the city. The second, on the opposite side of the river, was the ancient city of Seleucia. Initially, the Seleucians surrendered and opened their gates to the Roman army. Cassius, however, chose to break the truce and destroyed the city completely. Although one source claims this was simply a response to Seleucia betraying the peace first, the decision permanently tarnished Cassius's military career.[25] Whether this was deserved, the war with Parthia had reached its conclusion.

Unfortunately for Cassius and Verus, the destruction of Seleucia was not the only thing to haunt them upon their return to Rome. The Antonine Plague entered the historical record during Rome's conquest of the Parthians. One source places the plague's ultimate origin in Ethiopia. From there, it spread north to Egypt and then moved into the Parthian Empire. There is no estimate given for how long this process took, but it is possible the plague was already present in Nisibis when the Roman army besieged the city.[26]

The city of Seleucia was another recorded point of outbreak, although the details seem fantastical. According to the biographer of Lucius Verus, "a pestilential vapour arose in a temple of Apollo from a golden casket which a soldier had accidentally cut open, and that it spread thence over Parthia and the whole world."[27] This occurred during Rome's invasion following the city's surrender. A similar story was written much later by Ammianus Marcellinus, who wrote that the plague was unleashed during the sacking of the city by Roman soldiers searching for valuable treasure hidden in the temple. In this account, Marcellinus suggested the "secret science of the Chaldeans" originally contained the plague in Seleucia.[28] These tales seem more mythology than history, but they show that many believed the Roman army to be responsible for awakening a deadly plague. Certainly, the belief existed that the plague spread because Cassius acted wrongly in destroying Seleucia. In this sense, the Antonine Plague was Rome's punishment.

Rome's infrastructure and efficient troop movements made the disease's spread easier. Brought back by returning soldiers and dispersed along the empire's extensive trade system, the plague moved into Europe. It arrived in Rome in 166 CE, and it struck as far away as Gaul and the Rhine frontier.[29] Two other discoveries—excavations of mass graves from the Roman site of Glevum (modern-day Gloucester) and the city of Tomis in the Balkan province of Moesia Inferior—suggest that these areas also experienced heavy casualties as a result of the epidemic.[30] Orosius, writing much later in the fifth century CE, credited the Antonine Plague with emptying Italy so that "nothing remained but ruins and forests."[31] The epidemic devastated populations without regard to class. Upper classes were in as much danger as anyone else. In Smyrna, a city in modern-day Turkey now known as Izmir, the writer Aelius Aristides nearly died from the plague at this time. His servants all became ill before him, and he recorded that even animals died from the disease. Aristides managed to recover, albeit slowly.[32] There is no suggestion of why he survived when others did not, but he was lucky.

Marcus Aurelius, always the stoic, used the plague in his *Meditations* to make a comparison with a diseased mind.[33] However, he understood how desperate the situation was and did what he could to calm the population. As the plague ran its course through the capital, the death rate was so high that bodies were removed by the wagonload. With the Roman system facing an unprecedented number of deaths, the empire enacted new laws regulating burial practices. Such laws focused on the theft and sale of sepulchers, suddenly a concern in the face of so many dead.[34] Families could no longer inter bodies close to one's home or even transport victims through towns out of fear of their diseased state. The emperor honored the most illustrious of the deceased with statues. He also sponsored public funeral rights for lower-class victims of the plague.[35] The responses of other public figures were not nearly as palliative. One well-known oracle, Alexander of Abonutichus, reportedly offered a verse to anyone seeking protection from the plague, instructing them to display the verse above a door to shield anyone inside. Lucian, a rhetorician and satirist during the plague, noted that Abonutichus's verse was wholly ineffective, possibly due to overconfidence in such a measure.[36] Another public figure, his name unknown, climbed a fig tree on the Campus Martius and prophesied the end of the world. A central part of this prediction was that he would fall from the tree and transform into a stork. When the appointed time came, he fell, and a stork was pulled from underneath his robe. Despite the anxiety that the stunt had caused, the man was pardoned.[37]

Despite the legal reforms, public honors, and attempts at prophesying relief, a second and possibly more deadly plague occurred at the opening of the reign of Commodus (180–192 CE). The most illustrious victim of this renewed epidemic was Marcus Aurelius himself. Though it does not appear that the emperor succumbed to the Antonine Plague, the combined ravages of the plague and repeated frontier invasions upon his forces wore him down. After years of ill health, he finally died from lingering ailments of the stomach and chest. Yet, Aurelius spoke of the plague shortly before his death in 180 CE. His biography states that he took steps to keep Commodus, his heir, away from his sick bed in case his illness was highly contagious and fatal.[38] Cassius Dio claimed that this disease was "the greatest of any" he knew; at the height of the outbreak, Rome lost 2,000 people a day.[39] It is difficult to determine whether this was a recurrence of the Antonine Plague; if it was, Cassius Dio's account suggests the returning plague was far worse than the initial outbreak. Historians do not know if this second epidemic spread throughout the empire, but it did hit other parts of the Italian peninsula. Both men and animals died in high numbers.

At the suggestion of his physicians, Commodus fled to the town of Laurentum, 25 miles south of Rome, with the hope of isolating himself from the plague. Disease and environment were viewed as closely linked, and the countryside was believed to be free of disease. Those unable to make such a journey used scent for protection. Romans were instructed to protect themselves from illness by cleansing the air with incense and herbs. Others took the ritual one step further and kept their ears and noses constantly filled with perfume. However, as with Alexander's magical verse, these precautions reportedly had no effect.[40]

Rome's conflict with Parthia was central to the impact the Antonine Plague had on society. The timing of the Roman troops' return from the east facilitated the rapid spread of the plague. However, if warfare was the impetus for the outbreak and spread of the epidemic, the epidemic was equally influential on the empire's ability to wage war. In late 166 or early 167 CE, just as the Parthian war came to a close and the plague reached Rome, a second conflict broke out on the northern frontier. The Langobardi and Obii had crossed the Danube River into the province of Pannonia. Two commanders—Marcus Vindex leading the cavalry and Candidus leading the infantry—managed to push the invaders back out of Roman territory. Iallius Bassus, the governor of Pannonia, received a delegation of 11 representatives, one for each tribe waiting just beyond the border; they were led by the Marcomannic king, Ballomarius. A peace was arranged, and the war appeared to be over before it had even begun.[41]

The timing of the peace was fortunate with regard to the simultaneous spread of the plague. The impact of the Antonine Plague on the ability of Rome to raise necessary troops was noted by multiple sources. The empire's army, having carried the disease back from Parthia, was hit harder than the general population. From Orosius, we learn that "the Roman army and all its legions stationed far and wide in their winter quarters lost so many men that the Marcomannic war . . . could not have been waged without the fresh levy of troops," an effort that lasted three years.[42] Marcus Aurelius was praised for his handling of the Marcomannic Wars in the face of a shortage of able-bodied men following the plague.[43] One source described him as being "of all virtues and of celestial character, and was thrust before public calamities like a defender." This reference to public calamities included not only the epidemic but also a host of natural disasters.[44] Historian Arthur E. R. Boak believed that Rome's declining population resulted in a manpower shortage in the third century CE, which in turn was prompted by the plague and casualties of war. Boak refuted the idea that the empire ever rebounded from this decline, with the cycle of the depleted workforce undermining military and farming efforts over the next centuries.[45]

This process of disease and warfare precipitating a decline began in 168 CE, when Marcus Aurelius and Verus established their headquarters in Aquileia, a town in northern Italy. By this time, the Marcomanni and other tribes had begun to resume their attacks along the frontier, breaking the peace made the year before. The show of power by Rome along the frontier persuaded some recalcitrant tribes to ask for forgiveness. In the case of the Quadi, a tribe whose king had died, they claimed that the co-emperors could choose their tribal successor as a sign of their submission. Despite these small victories, Verus hesitated to continue north. The prefect Furius Victorinus had died, along with part of the troops he had commanded. This event, mentioned in the biography of Marcus Aurelius, does not give any details; the common assumption is that they were lost in battle. However, the Antonine Plague is just as likely to have been the cause.[46] If that is the case, then the epidemic affected more than just recruitment numbers, resulting in the attempted change of military strategy along Rome's increasingly fragile frontier.

Whatever the cause, Verus's attempt to stop Rome's northern advance was overruled. Not convinced of the thorough defeat of the tribes, Marcus Aurelius continued over the Alps and began preparations for a military campaign. The focus was on defending Italy and Illyricum, the province along the northeastern coast of the Adriatic. Accompanying the Roman forces was the physician Galen, who was likely there to address continued threats of the Antonine Plague to Roman plans. Galen wrote that there were many deaths at this time, and he advised the emperors to return to Rome for the winter. Alternatively, the biography of Verus states that the co-emperor was unhappy on the frontier and longed for "the pleasures of the city." Tragically, Verus never again enjoyed the urban life. While on the road, he suffered a stroke. After three days of being incapacitated, the co-emperor Verus died. Marcus was left to direct the Marcomannic War alone.[47]

The emperor continued with Verus's body to Rome, where funeral rights were held. Marcus Aurelius used the opportunity back in Rome to deal with the extreme financial cost of raising the troops necessary to go on the offensive. The Antonine

Plague killed so many that the empire came up short on tax revenue, and the high mortality rate in the army reduced troop levels below their typical numbers. To address this, Marcus offered freedom to slaves in exchange for military service. Mercenaries were increasingly hired, and a unit called the Compliant was composed of gladiators. To avoid raising taxes on a population struggling to recover, Aurelius auctioned off imperial possessions in the Forum of Trajan. Over the course of two months, the emperor's household offered jewels, clothing, and ornate household goods to raise the money necessary to finance the Marcomannic War. The auction was an apparent success; and after the war's completion, Marcus bought back what he could but did not resent anyone who opted to keep the royal possessions.[48]

At the end of 169 CE, Marcus Aurelius returned to the northern frontier, anticipating a successful invasion of enemy territory the following year. However, fortune was not on Rome's side. While Roman legions crossed the Danube River, barbarian tribes surged into the empire at two locations. The Jazyges and other unspecified Germanic tribes defeated and killed the Roman senator and consul Claudius Fronto in Upper Moesia in 170 CE. Also in the Balkan Peninsula, a tribe called the Costoboci swept down through Macedonia and Achaea, where they destroyed the ancient shrine at Eleusius.

The Romans had not expected the barbarians to be so bold. While both defeats were terrible, the most damaging and unprecedented blow came in northern Italy. Alexander of Abonutichus, the oracle who offered a charm verse against the Antonine Plague, made the pronouncement of a great victory for Rome if the army threw two lions into the Danube River as a sacrifice. The lions survived their ordeal and swam to the other side, where they were beaten to death by the clubs of the Marcomanni and Quadi. The barbarians then crossed the river, killed 20,000 Roman troops, and destroyed the town of Opitergium. The victorious invaders also surrounded Aquileia, Marcus's former base of operations, but the Romans managed to hold on to it.[49] The retaining of Aquileia was a hollow success. Wherever the emperor and his legions were in 170 CE, they experienced similar losses.

Marcus Aurelius knew an offensive strategy must wait until Rome had pushed the invaders out of Roman lands. The two commanders chosen for this task were Pompeianus, a politician, general, and son-in-law of Aurelius, and Pertinax, a future emperor. The military command was moved to the Pannonian city of Carnuntum, on the Danube River in modern-day Austria. In 171 CE, Rome repelled the invaders, ended the occupation of northern Italy, and regained lost plunder. The empire celebrated the victory.

Marcus stayed in Pannonia to negotiate with any tribe willing to show their submission to Rome. The terms appear to have been different for each tribe or group of tribes. One confederation, led by a 12-year-old named Battarius, agreed to help defend Roman territories against Tarbus, the leader of another tribe. The Quadi offered livestock and 13,000 captives, and they agreed to sever their alliance with the Marcomanni and the Jazyges. In Dacia, a northern Balkan province, the Astingi and Lacringi each entered into agreements with Rome, but with mixed success. A tribe with Celtic origins, the Cotini, betrayed the peace that was arranged for them. Other tribes were granted land in various provinces and conscripted into the Roman army to replace losses. These last policies helped to address the shortage of troops caused by the Antonine Plague; and if some of the accounts of the epidemic are correct, the civilian population needed replenishment as well.[50]

Having manipulated the balance of power on the frontier to his satisfaction, Marcus Aurelius was prepared to invade in 172 CE. Cassius Dio's history describes the defeat of the prefect Vindex at the hands of the Marcomanni and also records Marcus's ultimate victory against them.[51] The emperor received credit for two miracles that year. The first took place during a battle, where his prayers caused lightning to strike a "war-engine" belonging to the enemy. The second happened after a tribe managed to trap the Romans, intending to let them die slowly rather than attacking outright. Badly injured, many Roman soldiers had no access to water, "when suddenly many clouds gathered and a mighty rain, not without divine interposition, burst upon them." The rain was so plentiful that the Romans were able to fill their helmets and provide spare water for their horses. Hail and lightning followed the rain, but the Romans were reportedly immune to both. This miracle appears in several sources, though the details sometimes vary. Some accounts attributed the rain to the god Mercury, and others credited the prayers of Christians, depending on who was writing. The historical record is also unclear as to the tribe involved (either the Cotini or the Quadi, both who broke their peace with Rome) or which Roman commander was present.[52] The victories of that campaign season, however, secured for Marcus the title "Germanicus."[53]

The Marcomannic War was wrapped up over the course of the next three years. One reason for the delay was the Quadi's betrayal of the peace agreement, which came to a head in 174 CE. The peace fell apart in three ways. The Quadi realigned themselves with the Marcomanni and Jazyges shortly after the conflict. They also refused to return Roman captives. Additionally, the Quadi deposed the pro-Roman leader, Furtius, in favor of Ariogaesus, who was not inclined to yield to Marcus Aurelius. By the end of the year, however, Rome had captured Ariogaesus and exiled him to Alexandria. After a decisive defeat on the banks of the Danube, the Jazyges attempted to make peace, but the emperor no longer trusted them in light of so many prior broken agreements. He finally accepted a second offer of peace, even though Marcus preferred to simply eliminate the Jazyges and take their territory as new provinces. A revolt on Cassius in Syria drove this decision, as the toll of war and disease meant he could not afford further distractions or division of his increasingly limited military forces. The general peace terms for all the tribes included requiring them to hand over remaining captives and remove themselves beyond the Danube River. By 175 CE, the Marcomannic War was declared a success.[54]

Combined Impact of the Antonine Plague and War on Rome

Amid these Marcomannic Wars, the realities of the ongoing plague took their toll, though it is difficult to detail the impact on the population in the heart of Rome, which spanned only 10 kilometers but was home to over 1 million Roman citizens. Approximately 95 percent of the population lived in poverty and had substandard diets.[55] Combined with the constant trade with other regions and interactions with Rome by its military leaders and forces, the city not surprisingly experienced thousands of deaths per day during the height of the Antonine Plague. This death toll played out in the lower production of food and goods, trade, and the inability to collect taxes and recruit soldiers.

Fears generated by the plague also took their toll. Marcus, who experienced long-term health issues, became extremely ill in 175 CE and was reported to have died, presumably by the plague. Rumors of his death reached Avidius Cassius, Aurelius's general in Egypt, who assumed the worst and accepted election by his own military forces as the new emperor. But Marcus Aurelius recovered and continued to rule another five years before he finally succumbed to a weeklong illness of unknown origin.[56]

It is often the case that epidemics and conflict go hand in hand. History is filled with examples of invading forces carrying infectious diseases with them to virgin populations and military forces being afflicted themselves during warfare. Similarly, the long-term impacts of epidemics on population and resources sometimes make wars difficult or impossible to win. The Antonine Plague is a rare example of how an epidemic affected both the invading forces and the general population. The war between the Roman and Parthian Empires in the second century CE gave the disease access to a population that lacked both immunity and any understanding of how to treat it. Whatever the mortality rate, enough people died to affect Rome's policies and economy, domestically and internationally. The raging epidemic within the army and population hampered Rome's abilities to prosecute further hostilities on the northern frontier immediately following of the Parthian war. Nonetheless, chroniclers of Marcus Aurelius praised him for his success in the Marcomannic War, particularly his ability to raise the necessary troops in the face of spreading disease and the conditions of war.

It is also possible that the epidemic influenced the emperor's peace agreements. Marcus, rather than forbidding the defeated frontier tribes entry to Roman territory, granted many the right to settle within the empire's boundaries to replace those who had died from war or disease. Certainly, the quote attributed to Commodus shortly after his father's death, and his own decision to negotiate peace and withdraw from the frontier, indicates the extent of the plague's impact on Rome. Commodus reportedly said, "Tasks can be completed by a man in good health, if only gradually; a dead man can complete nothing."[57] The years of attrition on Rome's army, the necessity of auctioning off the imperial family valuables to raise funds to recruit forces, and Aurelius's own caution to Commodus to remain at a distance during his illness for fear of his son contracting the disease all indicate the strain and fear associated with the Antonine Plague. It is possible Commodus had already contracted the plague and was successfully treated by Galen, an experience that would have heightened fears of a little understood disease.[58] These fears played themselves out in traditional fashion, with the creation of scapegoats in society. An example of such backlash during both Marcus Aurelius's and Commodus's reigns was the increased persecution of Christians. Accused of black magic, Christians were blamed for angering the Roman deities by their blasphemous monotheistic beliefs that denied the existence of local gods.[59]

This influence, restricted to one-half of one century, may be seen by some as immaterial. However, the epidemic played an important role in these two wars, even if historians still debate which disease raged through the military ranks and how long the epidemic influenced the empire. The disease is credited with increasing the persecution of Christians and changing the demographic structure of the Roman armies. The Antonine Plague exemplifies how disease can change—and be changed—by human conflict.

NOTES

1.   B. G. Niebuhr, "Lectures on the History of Rome, from the Earliest Times to the Fall of the Western Empire," ed. Leonhard Schmitz, 2nd ed., Vol. III (1849), 251.
2.   William H. McNeill, *Plagues and Peoples* (New York: Doubleday Press, 1977), 135.
3.   Cheston B. Cunha and Burke A. Cunha, "Great Plagues of the Past and Remaining Questions," in *Paleomicrobiology: Past Human Infections*, ed. Didier Raoult and Michel Drancourt (Berlin: Springer-Verlag, 2008), 1–3.
4.   J. F. Gilliam, "The Plague under Marcus Aurelius," *American Journal of Philology* 82 no. 3 (July 1961): 227–228.
5.   R. J. Littman and M. L. Littman, "Galen and the Antonine Plague," *American Journal of Philology* 94 no. 3 (Autumn 1973), 246–248.
6.   Barthold Georg Niebuhr, *Nieburh's Lectures on Roman History* (London: Chatto & Windus, Piccadilly, 1875), 251.
7.   H. M. D. Parker, *A History of the Roman World from A.D. 138 to 337* (London: Methuen & Co. Ltd., 1958), 20.
8.   Gilliam, "The Plague under Marcus Aurelius," 227.
9.   August Hirsch, *Handbook of Geographical and Historical Pathology*, vol. 1, *Acute Infective Diseases*, trans. Charles Creighton, MD (London: J. B. Adlard, Bartholomew Close, 1883), 126.
10.   Cartwright, *Disease and History*, 13–14.
11.   McNeill, 130–131.
12.   Abu Becr Mohammed ibn Zacariya ar-Razi, *A Treatise on the Smallpox and Measles*, trans. William Alexander Greenhill, MD (London: C. and J. Adlard, 1848), 1.1.
13.   Arturo Castiglioni, *A History of Medicine*, trans. E. B. Krumbhaar (New York: Jason Aronson, Inc., 1975), 244.
14.   Littman and Littman, "Galen and the Antonine Plague," 244–245.
15.   Littman and Littman, "Galen and the Antonine Plague," 245–252.
16.   Littman and Littman, "Galen and the Antonine Plague," 252–255.
17.   Cunha and Cunha, "Great Plagues of the Past," 10–12.
18.   Yuki Furuse, Akira Suzuki, and Hitoshi Oshitani, "Origin of Measles Virus: Divergence from Rinderpest Virus between the 11th and 12th Centuries," *Virology Journal* 7 (2010): 52; and Jennifer Manley, "Measles and Ancient Plagues: A Note on New Scientific Evidence," *Classical World* 107 no. 3 (Spring 2014): 395.

19. McNeill, *Plagues and Peoples*, 69, 124–130; and Igor V. Babkin and Irina N. Babkina, "The Origin of the Variola Virus," *Viruses* 7 (2015): 1102.

20. Cassius Dio, *Roman History*, trans. Earnest Cary, PhD (London: William Heinemann LTD, 1927), Book LXXI, 1; David Magie, trans., "Marcus Aurelius Antoninus," in *Scriptores Historia Augustae* (Cambridge, MA: Harvard University Press, 1991), 8; Lucian of Samosata, "The Way to Write History," in *The Works of Lucian of Samosata*, trans. H. W. Fowler and F. G. Fowler, vol. 2 (Oxford: Clarendon Press, 1905), 21; and Anthony Birley, *Marcus Aurelius: A Biography* (New Haven: Yale University Press, 1987), 121–123.

21. Magie, "Lucius Verus," 6.

22. Lucian, "The Way to Write History," 29; Magie, "Marcus Aurelius Antoninus," 9; and Birley, *Marcus Aurelius*, 123, 128–130.

23. Birley, *Marcus Aurelius*, 131, 140.

24. Lucian, "The Way to Write History," 19.

25. Cassius Dio, *Roman History*, Book LXXI, 2; Magie, "Lucius Verus," 8; Lucian, "The Way to Write History," 20, 28; and Birley, *Marcus Aurelius*, 140.

26. Lucian, "The Way to Write History," 15. Lucian referenced a lost history by Crepereius Calpurnianus, which supposedly covered the entire Roman-Parthian Wars of the second century CE.

27. Magie, "Lucius Verus," 8.

28. Ammianus Marcellinus, *The Roman History of Ammianus Marcellinus during the Reigns of the Emperors Constantius, Julian, Jovianus, Valentinian, and Valens*, trans. C. D. Yonge, MA (London: George Bell & Sons, 1902), XXIII 6.24.

29. Magie, "Lucius Verus," 8; and Marcellinus, *Roman History*, XXIII 6.24.

30. Dragos Mitrofan, "The Antonine Plague in Dacia and Moesia Inferior," *Journal of Ancient History and Archeology* no. 1.2 (2014): 10, 12.

31. Orosius, *Seven Books of History against the Pagans: The Apology of Paulus Orosius*, trans. Irving Woodworth Raymond (New York: Columbia University Press, 1936), VII 15.

32. P. Aelius Aristides, *The Complete Works: Volume II, Orations XVII-LIII*, trans. Charles A. Behr (Leiden: E. J. Brill, 1981), XLVIII, 38–45.

33. Marcus Aurelius, *Meditations*, trans. Meric Casaubon (Auckland, NZ: The Floating Press, 2011), 9.2.

34. Birley, *Marcus Aurelius*, 150–151.

35. Magie, "Marcus Aurelius Antoninus," 13; Frank McLynn, *Marcus Aurelius: A Life* (Cambridge, MA: De Capo Press, 2009), 462.

36. Lucian, "Alexander, the Oracle-Monger, the False Prophet," *The Works of Lucian of Samosata*, trans. H. W. Fowler and F. G. Fowler (Oxford: Clarendon Press, 1905), 36.

37. Magie, "Marcus Aurelius Antoninus," 13.

38. Magie, "Marcus Aurelius Antoninus," 28.

39. Cassius Dio, *Roman History*, Book LXXII, 14.

40. Herodian, *History*, trans. C. R. Whittaker (Cambridge, MA: Harvard University Press, 1969), I.12.

41. Cassius Dio, *Roman History*, Book LXXI, 1a; Birley, *Marcus Aurelius*, 149.

42. Orosius, *Seven Books of History against the Pagans*, VII, 15.

43. Magie, "Marcus Aurelius Antoninus," 17; and Eutropius, *Abridgement of Roman History* trans. Rev. John Selby Watson, MA (London: Henry G. Bohn, 1853), VIII, 12.

44. *Epitome de Caesaribus*, trans. Thomas M. Banchich (Buffalo: Canisius College, 2009), 16.2–3.

45. Arthur E. R. Boak, *Manpower Shortage and the Fall of the Roman Empire in the West* (Ann Arbor: University of Michigan Press, 1955), 19, 113.

46. Magie, "Marcus Aurelius Antoninus," 14; Birley, *Marcus Aurelius*, 155–156.

47. Magie, "Marcus Aurelius Antoninus," 14; Magie, "Lucius Verus," 9; and Birley, *Marcus Aurelius*, 156–158.

48. Eutropius, *Abridgement of Roman History*, VIII, 13; Magie, "Marcus Aurelius Antoninus," 17, 21; Birley, *Marcus Aurelius*, 159–160.

49. Lucian, "Alexander," 48; Marcellinus, *Roman History*, XXIX 6.1; and Birley, *Marcus Aurelius*, 163–165.

50. Cassius Dio, *Roman History*, Book LXXI, 3, 11–12; Eutropius, *Abridgement of Roman History*, VIII, 13; Magie, "Marcus Aurelius Antoninus," 21–22; and Birley, *Marcus Aurelius*, 165–171.

51. Dio, *Roman History*, Book LXXI, 3.5.

52. Dio, *Roman History*, Book LXXI, 8–10, 13; Birley, *Marcus Aurelius*, 171–174.

53. Dio, *Roman History*, Book LXXI, 3.5.

54. Dio, *Roman History*, Book LXXI, 7, 13–14, 8, 16–17; and Birley, *Marcus Aurelius*, 176–179, 189, 197.

55. Eriny Hanna, "The Route to Crisis: Cities, Trade, and Epidemics in the Roman Empire," *Vanderbilt Undergraduate Research Journal* 10 (Fall 2015): 2.

56. Birley, *Marcus Aurelius*, 185–186.

57. Marcel van Ackeren, *A Companion to Marcus Aurelius* (Oxford, UK: John Wiley & Sons, 2012), 235.

58. Birley, *Marcus Aurelius*, 209–210.

59. McLynn, *Marcus Aurelius*, 462.

Chapter 3

English Sweating Sickness and the Battle of Bosworth: Misfortune or Retribution, 1485 CE

Edwin Wollert

> It used to be said that the disease [sweating sickness] broke out when Henry landed at Milford Haven on August 6, 1485; but from contemporary evidence the disease seems to have appeared first in London sometime after the battle [Bosworth Field], when Henry's Norman mercenaries were swarming in the capital.[1]
>
> —E. Ashworth Underwood

Studying diseases in a historical context is often frustrating. When records of diseases provide little in the way of identification, historians attempt to piece together information from primary sources to outline probable culprits. Fortunately, for the era of the Battle of Bosworth, historians benefit from various primary sources. Unfortunately, those primary sources related to the sickness and Bosworth rarely overlap. Indeed, the most frequently cited resources on the sweating sickness, or the sweat, originate from the 16th century, rather than the late 15th century when the Battle of Bosworth occurred. Consequently, part of the historical task entails considering both elements of research in relative isolation and then comparing them.

Problems with Retrospective Diagnoses

The study of the English sweating sickness presents the typical problems associated with retrospective diagnosis. Although biological diagnosis may be possible, the ability to ensure uncontaminated specimens is unlikely and complicated by legal issues connected with disinterring victims from the past. Societal impacts from the disease are also hard to determine, as they must be considered in the context of the time. Missing and disconnected documentation makes understanding societal impacts harder to determine; this includes the sweat's impact with regard to the Battle of Bosworth Field and the rise of the Tudor monarchy. While certainty of the source of the disease remains elusive and debated by medical scholars and historians, other questions regarding the disease's impact have generated much interest and study. Key among these is the role the sweat played in Thomas Stanley and his family's decision to eventually side with Henry VII. As a result of that shift in loyalty, the question arises of what influence the sweat had upon the continued struggles of the new Tudor dynasty to hold power in a fractious and fearful English society.

To answer these questions requires examination of the disease, its presentation in English society in the late 15th to early 16th centuries, and the uncertainty and fear it spread over several decades. Some background is necessary to place the era in context for the Battle of Bosworth Field and the emergence of the sweating sickness. After years of conflict between the Yorks and Lancasters, Richard III (the king and a York) and Henry Tudor (the Earl of Richmond and the senior surviving male heir to the Lancaster claim) were the remaining royal contenders to the crown. A distant claimant to the throne, Henry nonetheless had supporters, even among Yorkists. To avoid capture and execution in 1471, Henry fled to Brittany, where he was befriended and protected by the French Duke of Brittany, Francis II. With support and troops provided by the French, and more raised in Wales and from Lancaster strongholds, Henry set out in 1485 to defeat Richard III. Unbeknownst to him, some of his foreign forces carried other unwelcome guests, namely a variety of diseases.

One possible origin of the English sweating sickness includes the probability that some of Henry's mercenaries had carried the seeds of this epidemic with them. However, records indicate the forces raised in the north to support Richard III had also been besieged by the epidemic in the summer of 1485, delaying and reducing the amount of support Richard could use in his defense of the Yorks' claim to the throne. Among other versions of the disease's origins is the oft-repeated belief that it was sent as a punishment for the English, a version that continued to undermine Tudor authority in the next several decades as the sweat sporadically reemerged.

The academic literature about the sweat utilizes the process of retrospective diagnoses. It also considers the availability of evidence and the level of medicine generally known during the Tudor dynasty. When used collectively, these approaches create numerous disputes and ambiguities. What emerges is a mixture of possibilities of the agent in question, most falling under the categories of bacterial and viral.

Historical Debates Regarding the Cause and Identity of the "Sweat"

When considering early historical works, several authors contemporary to the 1551 epidemic are most often referenced. A key commentator was Italian physician Girolamo Fracastoro. His work is often noted for the natural philosophy known as *atomism*, with his claim that tiny "spores" could infect living creatures, even over distances and through minimal contact. This perspective was remarkable for someone without access to microscopes or knowledge of germ theory, and at a time when medical explanations were based on miasma or humors. Fracastoro's work is most important for his revelations about the sweating sickness. Part of his interest arose from studying his home of Verona, which had been struck by plague in 1510 and typhus in 1528. As for Britain, Fracastoro wrote, "In the island Britain . . . there is a kind of pestilent and contagious fever, which apparently must be classed among ephemeral fevers, because, in a single day, it either kills its victim or lets him escape."[2] Fracastoro asserted that prevention was crucial, but once infected, "no food must be given: it is a question whether any drug should be administered, or whether they act wisely in Britain where they give no remedy and only keep the patients in bed and lying down, to make them sweat."[3]

Fracastoro recommended a possible medical treatment, though it seemed more a desperate panacea, an example of spagyric medicine, within alchemy. Above all, Fracastoro stressed abstaining from wine, as he believed it made fevers worse. Although this was not a means of reducing fever, his recommended treatment prevented further dehydration in patients already experiencing water loss from fevers.

Historian Polydore Vergil, a contemporary of Fracastoro, served as a humanist scholar and church official. Vergil arrived in England in 1502, where he became the archdeacon of Wells Cathedral. His impressive *Anglica Historia*, an account of the first half of the Tudor period, included the first historical analysis of the sweating sickness.[4] Like Fracastoro, he returned to the earliest Tudor years:

> In the same year . . . a new kind of disease swept the whole country; . . . one which no previous age had experienced. A sudden deadly sweating attacked the body and at the same time head and stomach were in pain from the violence of the fever. . . . Some were unable to bear the heat and removed the bedclothes or undressed themselves; others slaked their thirst with cold drinks; yet others endured the heat and the stench and by adding more bedclothes provoked more sweating. But all alike died.[5]

Vergil maintained that no resistance or immunity seemed to confer to survivors. Vergil even suggested a higher fatality rate than the plague. He advocated encouraging the patient to sweat as much as possible and that the most direct way to accomplish such was to wrap a patient in as many clothes and as much bedding as possible. Similarly, patients were to be kept awake by any means. If these precautions did not work, the disease was often comprehended as an omen foreshadowing the harshness of the monarch.[6]

Another writer to emerge during the mid-16th century was Englishman Edward Hall. In his coverage of the second year of Henry VII's reign, Hall described how a new sickness had suddenly appeared in the region with the king's arrival and that it was more painful than any known prior to that time:

> For sodenly a dedly & burnyng sweate inuaded their bodyes & vexed their bloud with a most ardēt heat, infested the stomack & the head greuously: . . . beyng not hable to suffre the importunate heat, they cast away the shetes & all the clothes liyng on the bed.[7]

This account is noteworthy for two reasons: (1) the amount of detail surpasses that of the earlier primary accounts, and (2) this account also comes from someone with no training in medicine, apothecary knowledge, or surgery. Not even John

Caius, the most prolific physician to document the sweat, offers so specific an account. The same can be said of other contemporary physicians: Andrew Boorde dealt with the sweat, as did Henry VIII's later personal physician, William Butts. Hall's account is familiar, including the common desire of sufferers to feel cooler and escape heat. Of special interest in Hall's description is the recognition of the same affliction that presented itself for different patients in varying ways.[8]

The terrifying realization of this unknown disease was not just due to the apparently high fatality rate. The potential treatments varied, from commonsensical approaches to those with little or no effect. Yet, despite fears of high fatality rates, many survived. Some contemporaries viewed the sweat as divine judgment, a common explanation for illness as long as humans have reported their afflictions. Epidemics of the bubonic plague almost certainly took more lives, but at least the plague was more of a known factor by this time. Fleeing the plague or any known disease outbreak was perceived as the best course of action. While some Tudors still decried the plague as God's wrath upon a sinful populace, at least there was some perceived predictability of when and where it might occur, how it affected victims, and theories on how to avoid it in the first place. But the sweat was much less certain, and therefore more frightening. Questions emerged about who was most vulnerable, where the disease came from, and whether some were more susceptible than others; but few if any answers were forthcoming.

Some commentators used reason to approach the issue. The main work of Andrew Boorde focused on various aspects of health care, a "Dyetary," and observed that the common response was to flee "from the contagious and infectious ayre."[9] He indicated the rapid onset, stating some were "mery at diner and dedde at supper."[10] The second part of this passage has acquired a certain infamy about the sweat. Caius emphasized that "this disease is not a Sweat onely . . . but a feuer."[11] He also maintained that "it lasteth but the time of xxiiii houres."[12] This marks the start of the tradition that if a person could survive the crucial first day, then recovery was likely.

Other commentators deferred to less rationale explanations. Similar to Thucydides's assertion about the selectivity of the Plague of Athens affecting only Athenians, Caius provided a clue to the fear of the disease's appearance in that "this disease is almoste peculiar vnto vs Englishe men, and not common to all men."[13] The illness not only developed into something mysterious, but it appeared to prefer certain victims. Indeed, no reports of the sweat appear in Welsh or Scottish accounts. Divine judgment had plenty of tradition by the Tudor period, but the conflicting symptoms and treatments must have given strength to fears and assertions of divine retribution.

The plethora of primary accounts of the sweat that focus on the 16th-century outbreaks, not those from the late 15th century, have shaped the focus and interpretations of later secondary works. An excellent example is historian Danae Tankard, who summarized the overall influence of the disease, taking her cue from the last outbreak in 1551. By then, England had endured four epidemics, and there existed some evolution in thought about the illness. Realization finally hit that "the sweating sickness did not lead to the kind of crisis mortality associated with severe outbreaks of bubonic plague,"[14] as Tankard indicated. Still, "the swiftness with which it killed combined with exceptionally high levels of morbidity [relative incidence of a disease] ensured that its passage was marked for posterity."[15]

Tankard and other secondary historians relied heavily on the best records of the sweat, including a collection of family letters documenting the 1551 epidemic. These "Johnson Papers," named for John Johnson and his wife, Sabine, new members of the gentry involved in the booming textile industry, provide historians with an impressive collection of letters by a number of parties. The collection reveals that "the usual response was to try to avoid all contact with [the sweat], if possible by vacating the area of infection."[16] Tankard summarized the general symptomology discussed in the collection, noting how "death or recovery would occur within eight or ten hours,"[17] and that its swiftness may have increased from earlier epidemics. Young King Edward VI "noted the sweat's arrival in his journal on 9 July, commenting that it was 'more vehement than the old sweat'"[18] that afflicted the realms of his father and grandfather.

Using primary documents, later historians pieced together the practices that essentially constituted the best knowledge of dealing with the disease at the time. "They keep the patient wrapped up, to give them very little to drink, and most of all to prevent them from sleeping."[19] This hardly differs from Charles Creighton's summary in the 19th century, who wrote that one should not permit the sufferer "during the fit, any cold drink, or to allow a draught of air to reach the drenching skin; the covering should be rather more ample than usual, but there was danger in heaping too many bed-clothes on the patient."[20] Frederick Homes noted that the enema treatment for dehydration, offered by Thomas More, was an example of "a lawyer saving his dying daughter with a physiologically sound treatment prescribed by God: surely a unique event in the annals of medicine, theology, and law."[21] Creighton offered his own frustration about the sweat's subsequent historiography, as it "presents to the student of epidemics much that is paradoxical although not without parallel, and much that his research can never rescue from uncertainty."[22]

Part of offering a "retrospective diagnosis" typically entails a logical process of elimination. The sweating sickness is a curious example of how such a retrospective diagnosis might, in some circumstances, become more popular than an apparently stronger, and even empirical, diagnosis. There are notable problems with such an idealistic approach. Andrew Cunningham, a historian of medicine, acknowledged the tendency for modern interpretations to find diseases and their identities to be rather constant over time when studied without the benefit of cultural and social processes. Cunningham asserted the presumption that modern analyses are superior to earlier medical interpretations begs the question of whether the current analyses incorporates relevant and reliable information and whether the current scientific models for diagnosis are accurate.[23]

It is essential to point out that 16th-century commentators understood that the sweat was something different. Part of their trepidation appears to have arisen from the knowledge that sweating sickness was clearly not plague, nor leprosy, nor anything else known, thus introducing a palpable fear of the unknown. More recent efforts to identify the source of the sweat tended to offer academic optimism, even though the retroactive approach questions the outcome. Recent analysis of potential causes for the sweat, based on available historiography, considers a wide spectrum of diseases. Historians contributing to these analyses included a mix of specialties. At one end of the spectrum is epidemiologist Paul Heyman and parasitologists Leopold Simons and Christel Cochez. Together, these scientists considered various potential offenders before arguing largely in favor of the more recently identified hantavirus. Prior to such work, historian Robert Gottfried contended that the most probable culprit was influenza, and he showed how historiography of the sweat has benefited from particular types of primary sources in the form of legal documents, particularly wills, as they tended to be amended in the case of the deaths of family members from whatever causes, including diseases. John A. H. Wylie (pathologist and theologian) and Leslie H. Collier (professor of virology) offered the original move away from bacteria into viruses generally, and they argued for arboviruses. Another decade passed before Paul Hunter, a professor of health protection, offered an early summary of research up to that point. His work outlined various possibilities, but he admitted that the English sweating sickness remained "as mysterious today as it has been for more than 500 years."[24]

Recent Historical Revelations—Bacteria or Virus?

Recent literature includes the utility of parish records listing causes of mortality (pored over by historian Alan Dyer) and a report inspired by current events of the possibility of anthrax. Microbiologist Edward McSweegan found anthrax a possible cause of the sweat. Terrorist attempts to use anthrax as a weapon in 2001 helped reveal that inhalational anthrax is transferred via its spores and is no longer considered contagious. While this appears to contradict the historical perception that the sweat was quite contagious, McSweegan postulates that wool and other animal hair provided a common method of transporting the spores to humans. This supposition corresponds to the occurrence of sweat among rural males.[25] However, this retrospective diagnosis does not account for the reports of the disease among the armies that prepared to fight at Bosworth or among the nobility who contracted the disease in late summer. Additionally, this diagnosis does not account for the failure of the disease to spread among wool workers later with the industrialization of wool production.

As for rheumatic fever, Adam Patrick made a brief reference to the possibility of inflammatory rheumatic fever. He referred to the support of J. F. C. Hecker and F. von Niemeyer for an inflammatory rheumatic fever diagnosis, but he then focused attention on the sudden onset of the sweat, comparing it with similar phenomena regarding modern outbreaks of food poisoning.[26] Paul R. Hunter, who studied epidemiology and microbiology of infectious diseases, shifted the emphasis from rheumatic fever to enteroviruses.[27] Citing a fever, sweating, muscle pains, and meningitis as common symptoms with the sweat, Hunter argued that entero-viruses typically spread in the late summer and early fall. He postulated that these highly infectious viruses could be spread directly or through the contamination of food and water, making a connection with Patrick's theory. However, Hunter pre-ferred the likes of *Neisseria meningitidis*, mentioned by Wylie and Collier, though that is another bacterium.[28]

Wylie and Collier led the transition in research by historical and medical schol-ars from bacteria to viruses. They preferred arboviruses, those requiring arthro-pod carriers (ticks and other insects), giving examples such as dengue fever and encephalitis. They noted how fear of the sweat affected the judgment of some military leaders in the buildup to the Battle of Bosworth, but they indicated that the sweat "exerted only a marginal influence upon national or provincial demog-raphy."[29] Wylie and Collier asserted that the "suddenness" with which the vari-ous sweat epidemics ended suggested "that an unidentified rodent reservoir of the virus was susceptible to an epizootic and was killed off,"[30] essentially in the early autumn; these assertions are bolstered by the rapidity of the epidemics and how outbreak years "were wet, warm, or both." To their credit, Wylie and Collier con-sidered major virus families in turn, accounting for explosive rates of infection in each year the sweat was known to strike. They explained away a counterargument, namely the lack of historical reference to signs of hemorrhage (expected in victims of arboviruses). They contended that fear of the disease likely resulted in superfi-cial examinations of patients on the part of physicians and that the significance of such hemorrhagic spots was not understood until the 1890s.[31]

Historian Alan Dyer built upon Wylie and Collier's theory, explaining that the rapid spread of the sweat required the ability for an arbovirus to be transmitted from human to human, which was an unlikely process, though not impossible. A year later, Guy Thwaites, Mark Taviner, and Vanya Gant (historian and biomedical scientists) pushed the theory that hantaviruses (the genus of arboviruses) were the source of the sweat. Thwaites and others in the 1990s reviewed the same sympto-mology from primary sources and applied their own scientific specialties based on the scant information offered by such reports. "Viral hemorrhagic fever therefore seems most unlikely,"[32] as Thwaites, Taviner, and Gant initially concluded. This put them at odds with the conclusions of scientists Paul Heyman, Leopold Simons, and Christel Cochez, who specifically looked into an "older" form of hantavirus, HFRS (a hantavirus in the form of hemorrhagic fever with an accompanying renal issue).

Two issues are worth noting here. First, these two teams agreed on hantavirus but disagreed on its exact form. Second, disagreement over the final working ver-sion of the disease left room for both of these teams to share a link with the work of Dyer, who emphasized diffusion of the disease along British roadways, at least in the case of the 1551 outbreak. This idea of "a viral disease with a rodent vector"[33] seems reinforced, even with Dyer's continued stress on the importance of further researching parish records. As Thwaites and his colleagues asserted, these "might equally be interpreted as reflecting a simultaneous clustering of infected and small mammal populations."[34] Ultimately, for Thwaites, Taviner, and Gant, the causal agent of the disease likely included "human-to-human contact as well as initial transmission through a zoonosis or an environmental vector."[35]

Virologists James Carlson and Peter Hammond favored a viral explanation, noting that the rapid dissemination of the disease during all outbreaks, including in 1485, "was attributed to travelers."[36] They concluded the disease was highly contagious and of short duration but high intensity. Based on their detailed summarized criteria and symptomology, they argue for Crimean-Congo hemorrhagic fever (CCHF), a member of the *Nairovirus* genus, itself part of the larger Bunyaviridae family. These are arboviruses, not hantaviruses, that require insect vectors, in this case ticks. Person-to-person transmission of arboviruses is rare, but CCHF is one of just four known versions that transmit more easily among human victims and has also "been shown to produce epidemic outbreaks that are brief and violent."[37] CCHF infection has an incubation of just a few days and a list of signs and symptoms that closely match sweating sickness. CCHF overlaps with other diseases as well, but the hemorrhagic state of CCHF has the most specific similarities and commonly results in death.

Scientists Paul Heyman, Leopold Simons, and Christel Cochez argued against the "newer" hantavirus favored by Thwaites and his colleagues, citing a lack of reports on isolated cases over time.[38] Heyman's team ruled out diseases known to Tudor England as well as some of those suggested by more recent secondary reports. The "speed with which the symptoms appeared and the extremely short course of the disease"[39] ruled out typhus. Influenza was disqualified due to "the absence of any respiratory symptoms or secondary causes of pneumonia."[40] Heyman's team remained collectively neutral with the ideas of McSweegan, though they consider that his approach may warrant further study. They indicated that arboviruses have a certain plausibility based on limited climatic information, but the theory lacked sufficient argumentative strength. Interestingly, they refer to other research not otherwise considered, such as the fungus *Claviceps purpurae*, which affects grasses and cereal crops and provides an explanation more in accord with Patrick's food poisoning theory, though this is the only reference to any fungi in the literature.

Finally, Heyman's team recognized the need to account for the strange sporadic nature of the outbreaks, suggesting that the irregular intervals indicated "an ecological or meteorological trigger."[41] The older hantavirus explanation helps account for this. As such, they maintain that the early modern virulence "cannot be explained by genetic variation in present-day hantaviruses,"[42] prompting them to consider this "Old World" variant instead. The only notable issue remaining is that there is no known evidence of any type of hantavirus in the British Isles.[43]

The team of microbiologist Colleen Jonsson, virologist Luiz Figueiredo, and infectious disease specialist Olli Vapalahti pointed out the flaw in the Heyman team's Old World theory. Jonsson's team focused on hantaviruses generally, but with regard to the disease under review, and observed that "a review of these epidemics suggested that HPS [Hantavirus Pulmonary Syndrome] does not match the English sweating sickness completely."[44]

Another viral contender comes from Robert Gottfried, a historian who employed the use of diverse primary resources and interdisciplinary research. Gottfried assessed whether an increase in human fertility may have affected "secular trends of growth from the 1470s,"[45] knowing that 1485 marked the first documented outbreak of the sweat. His called for "testamentary demographic analysis" entailed studying wills, as wills "are first and foremost a reliable account of mortality."[46] Despite his effort to use more statistical measures, his own conclusion of influenza as the likeliest culprit runs counter to his own argument: influenza often spreads and continues killing throughout the winter, but historical records indicate that, like plague, the sweat did not last from season to season. This confusion between older diseases and influenza was a general mistake of 20th-century historiography following efforts to understand the global influenza epidemic. Still, the key feature worth pursuing from Gottfried's article was his emphasis on a particular type of source material, as wills are often ignored from the perspective of disease research.

A major dilemma in studying the epidemic includes how to know whether the source of the sweat was viral or bacterial. Viruses are supported in recent historiography because the primary sources uniformly describe very rapid onset; bacteria and other microbes, such as fungi, typically do not cause illness in host organisms so quickly. A possible solution is to exhume human remains that exist for known sufferers of the disease and attempt to analyze a tissue or other organic sample. McSweegan is the only writer to suggest this as an option. As indicated in his work, anthrax spores have tremendous longevity, and they do not require "an insect or rodent accomplice."[47] The potential problem is that anthrax is not viral; it is bacterial, caused by *Bacillus anthracis*, and therefore not as rapid in its spread and onset. Additionally, regardless of the true nature of the illness, the politics involved with exhumations is fraught with barriers. Nonetheless, some counties maintained thorough enough records that known sufferers and victims could be identified and, if approval was granted, could have their remains tested.

Impact of the Sweat on Events in the War of the Roses

Having examined the historiography regarding the sweating sickness in English history, the next questions concern the impact on events of the time. Did the sweat affect the Battle of Bosworth Field and the rise of the Tudor monarchy? If so, what extent did the epidemic play in English Tudor history? It would be inaccurate and overly simplistic to assert Richard III lost his crown to the man who became Henry VII because of a disease. Even if such a case could be argued, support for the argument would quickly collapse because certain knowledge of the source of the sweating sickness remains undetermined. To better understand this disease requires contextualization; namely, contemporary fears about this disease appear to have played a notable part in who actually showed up at Bosworth and even under what circumstances and with what loyalties.

The shifting loyalties and tenuous family ties involved in the battle are worth considering. Historian Alfred Rowse noted the strange politics of how the first husband of Lady Margaret Beaufort "died when she was only a girl of thirteen, leaving her pregnant with Henry, later Henry VII. She married twice more, Henry Stafford and then Thomas Stanley, the 1st Earl of Derby."[48] Consequently, Henry Tudor was actually the stepson of Thomas Stanley, a Yorkist and supporter of Richard III. Dynastic family ties notwithstanding, recent historian Michael Jones confirmed that "the Stanleys were a rising force . . . determined to protect their landed estates and influence."[49] Even more tellingly, the family pursued a policy of self-interest, backing both sides in various conflicts.[50] As Jones indicated, "The extraordinary juggling act was to complicate the forthcoming battle. . . . The prevarication of the Stanleys shows us how difficult it is to interpret Bosworth simply on moral grounds."[51] This dilemma includes the assessment of Richard and Henry.

Shortly after Henry and his forces landed in southwest Wales, William Stanley (Thomas's younger brother and Henry's step-uncle) permitted them to pass through his lands.[52] Alarmed, Richard summoned Stanley to explain this unnecessary kindness and apparent dereliction of duty, but "Stanley replied that he was ill of the sweating sickness."[53] It is unknown whether Stanley really contracted the illness and, if he did, whether he had contracted it from Henry's forces. Nonetheless, historian Gladys Temperley asserted, "Stanley, who had allowed Henry to march through Wales unopposed, was proclaimed a traitor."[54]

A key part of the answer might lie in a secret meeting at the village of Atherstone, Warwickshire, on August 21, the day before the battle. Rowse described this meeting, stating, "Richard sent a message to Lord Thomas Stanley ordering him to join in against the enemy without delay,"[55] and he threatened to kill Stanley's son, who was being held hostage by Richard. Henry, meanwhile, "was also kept in anxiety as to what Lord Stanley would do," though "after the conference at Atherstone, Henry was in better heart,"[56] even if he received a more dubious reply the morning of the battle. According to Temperley, Henry received assurances at the secret meeting of Stanley's support in the impending battle. More recent scholarship by Michael Jones indicates that "the most likely member of the family to take positive steps in Tudor's support was Stanley's younger brother Sir William, but following a tense meeting at Atherstone[,] . . . neither man committed himself directly."[57] Still, even with the somewhat unreliable aid of Thomas Stanley, Richard came close to winning. These historians seem to agree with Jones that, "as it was so hard to comprehend the battle's outcome, the only explanation some could find was one of treachery. Sir William Stanley's intervention could rightly be seen as a betrayal of Richard III by that powerful, self-interested family" in support of one of their own lineage.[58]

Temperley confirmed that the Stanleys "preferred not committing themselves to either party until they saw how things were going."[59] If the family had truly remained ambiguous in its loyalties until the midst of the battle, what had swayed them, or at least Sir William, to support Henry Tudor? Did the sweating sickness really play any part in Stanley's decision to forgo his loyalty and thereby switch sides? Rowse clearly described Henry's arrival in London after the battle, implying a connection: "As soon as he could Henry dismissed his foreign mercenaries. He made his ceremonial entry into the City on 3 September 1485, though an outbreak of sweating sickness postponed the coronation till 30 October."[60] This is Rowse's final mention of the disease, though it seems quite telling. These were the same mercenaries who may have unwittingly brought the disease with them from France and through the English countryside. Temperley confirmed this scenario, describing how Henry "was busy preparing for his coronation when the 'sweating sickness,' hitherto unknown in England, appeared in London. The disease was very virulent,"[61] killing but then vanishing by October. More telling, Temperley revealed the epidemic "was popularly regarded as an omen of a stern rule and trouble[d] reign."[62]

Biographer Sean Cunningham offered a succinct yet powerful explanation. "Unfortunately for Henry," Cunningham asserted, "his army carried a virulent new disease, known at the time as 'sweating sickness,' which began to kill hundreds of Londoners within a month of Bosworth."[63] Cunningham pointed out how Henry was blamed for the epidemic. "The violent change of ruler and the outbreak of disease were linked as an omen of disaster,"[64] with some likely questioning whose side had received divine favor after all. The outbreak "tested the organisational and propaganda skills of the fledgling king,"[65] who worked to censor public news about this aspect of his very new reign. Certainly, Henry was not alone in receiving blame for unfortunate events associated with the Divine Will regarding the monarchy. Mary Ann Lund, in her coverage of Richard III, observed how his physique and character were also distorted in relation to events of the time.[66]

Despite all the possible influences of diseases in general and of the sweat in particular, part of understanding the ensuing drama of Bosworth Field and its correlation to the sweating sickness lies in knowing that the Stanleys perceived themselves as kingmakers. Thomas Stanley and his brother William both played key roles in determining the outcome of the Battle of Bosworth Field. Earl Thomas Stanley of Derby also received credit from literary researchers Aisling Byrne and Victoria Flood for his help in thwarting the royal designs of pretender Lambert Simnel and for playing a "crucial role" at the Battle of Flodden in 1513 during Henry VIII's first military excursion to France. Even alleged kingmakers could falter, though: William Stanley was "executed in 1495 for supporting Perkin Warbeck,"[67] another impostor to the throne, this one falsely taking on the role of the Duke of York.

The contributing factors for the Stanleys' decisions to betray Richard III and support Henry remain uncertain. Were the claims of illness by the sweat responsible for delays in support? Did the sweat impact William Stanley's forces to such an extent that he could not give the support needed? If the sweat had a significant impact, did he and his men contract the sweat from Henry's forces as they were allowed to pass through Wales? Had Stanley's long-term Yorkist sympathies waned in favor of his step-nephew Henry? Or was the sweat an excuse to delay until he could determine which contender to side with in the conflict that would determine the monarchy?

Combined Impact of the Sweat and the Battle of Bosworth on England

Definitive answers continue to confound historians and medical researchers. Those who historically wrote about the sweat or the Battle of Bosworth typically fall into one of two categories: they either described the disease and mentioned the battle in passing or not at all, or they addressed the battle and mentioned the disease in passing or not at all. The lack of detailed documents and historic evidence supporting a particular diagnosis continues to elude medical researchers. While the location of victims of the sweat are known, the legalities of disinterring the bodies and realization that evidence contained within has likely become contaminated with time continues to block medical examination. Understanding that retrospective diagnosis is not complete for this disease, medical and historical researchers should return to the admonition of Wylie and Collier, who noted three obstacles to arriving at a working etiology of sweat epidemics: "first, their remoteness in time; second, the nonspecific nature of the signs and symptoms; and third, the well-known tendency of infectious diseases to change their characteristics."[68]

Even if a direct connection between the epidemic and the battle cannot be proven, the perception of fear surrounding the disease was enough to warrant its use as an excuse to disobey the ruling monarch. Additionally, fear of the unknown sweating sickness combined with general shock over the militant overthrow of Richard III to taint the initial rise of Henry VII to power. The continued intermittent and random outbreaks of the sweat for the next several decades contributed to assertions that the rise of the Tudors was illegitimate and an evil omen of the future. One can argue that the sweating sickness derived at least some of its power and mystique through its very name. This is not to suggest that some new horrific illness was somehow foretold in British mysticism. Rather, like the name Bosworth, which has come to denote a reference to a major English dynastic change, so too has the "sweat" been used to terrify or justify during the same period of English history.

NOTES

1. E. Ashworth Underwood, "Milestones in Medicine: 11, The Sweating Sickness," *Health Education Journal* 8 (1950): 127.
2. Girolamo Fracastoro (Hieronymus Fracastorius), *De Contagione et Contagiosis Morbis et eorum Curatione*, ed. and trans. William C. Wright (1546; repr., New York: G. P. Putnam's Sons, 1930), 96.
3. Fracastoro, *De Contagione et Contagiosis Morbis*, 240.
4. The first person to publish anything on the sweat was Thomas Le Forestier, a French physician who was present in England during the 1485 epidemic.
5. Polydore Vergil, *Anglica Historia*, ed. and trans. Denys Hat (1513, 1537; repr., London: Offices of the Royal Historical Society, 1950), 6.
6. Vergil, *Anglica Historia*, 142.
7. Edward Hall, *The Vnion of the Two Noble and Illustre Femelies of Lancastre & Yorke, Beeying Long in Continual Discension for the Croune of this Noble Realme, with all the Actes done*

in bothe the Tymes of the Princes, bothe of the One Linage and of the Other, Beginnyng at the Tyme of Kyng Henry the Fowerth, the First Aucthor of this Deuision, and so Successiuely Proceadyng to the Reigne of the High and Prudent Prince Kyng Henry the Eight, the Vndubitate Flower and very Heire of both the Sayd Linages. 1548 (1548, 1809; repr., New York: AMS Press, 1965), 425.

8. Hall, *The Vnion of the Two Noble and Illustre Femelies*, 425.

9. Andrew Boorde, *The Fyrst Boke of the Introduction of Knowledge: A Compendious Regyment, or, a Dyetary of Helth Made in Mountpyllier. Barnes in the Defence of the Berde* (1542, 1870; repr., London: Adamant Media, 2001), 289.

10. Boorde, *The Fyrst Boke of the Introduction of Knowledge*, 351.

11. John Caius, *The Sweating Sickness: A Boke or Counseill against the Disease Commonly Called the Sweate or Sweatying Sicknesse* (1552; repr., Memphis, TN: General Books, 2010), 7.

12. Caius, *The Sweating Sickness*, 6.

13. Caius, *The Sweating Sickness*, 5.

14. Danae Tankard, "Protestantism, the Johnson Family and the 1551 Sweat in London," *London Journal* 29, no. 2 (2004): 1.

15. Tankard, "Protestantism," 1.

16. Tankard, "Protestantism," 4.

17. Tankard, "Protestantism."

18. Tankard, "Protestantism," 8.

19. Tankard, "Protestantism."

20. Charles Creighton, *A History of Epidemics in Britain* (Cambridge: Cambridge University Press, 1894), 246.

21. Frederick F. Holmes, "Anne Boleyn, the Sweating Sickness, and the Hantavirus: A Review of an Old Disease with a Modern Interpretation," *Journal of Medical Biography* 6, no. 1 (February 1998): 43.

22. Creighton, *A History of Epidemics in Britain*, 265.

23. Andrew Cunningham, "Identifying Disease in the Past: Cutting the Gordian Knot," *Asclepio* 54, no. 1 (2002): 14.

24. Paul R. Hunter, "The English Sweating Sickness, with Particular Reference to the 1551 Outbreak in Chester," *Reviews of Infectious Diseases* 13, no. 2 (March–April 1991): 306.

25. Edward McSweegan, "Anthrax and the Etiology of the English Sweating Sickness," *Medical Hypotheses* 62, no. 1 (2004): 156.

26. Adam Patrick, "A Consideration of the Nature of the English Sweating Sickness," *Medical History* 9, no. 3 (July 1965): 274, 277.

27. These viruses are named for their transmission through the intestinal tract of humans.

28. Hunter, "The English Sweating Sickness," 303, 305.

29. John A. H. Wylie and Leslie H. Collier, "The English Sweating Sickness (Sudor Anglicus): A Reappraisal," *Journal of the History of Medicine and Allied Sciences* 36, no. 4 (1981): 432.

30. Wylie and Collier, "The English Sweating Sickness," 433.

31. Wylie and Collier, "The English Sweating Sickness," 445.

32. Guy Thwaites, Mark Taviner, and Vanya Gant, "The English Sweating Sickness, 1485 to 1551," *New England Journal of Medicine* 336, no. 8 (February 1997): 581.

33. Guy Thwaites, Mark Taviner, and Vanya Gant, "The English Sweating Sickness, 1485–1551: A Viral Pulmonary Disease?," *Medical History* 42 (1998): 98.

34. Thwaites, Taviner, and Gant, "The English Sweating Sickness, 1485–1551: A Viral Pulmonary Disease?," 98.

35. Thwaites, Taviner, and Gant, "The English Sweating Sickness, 1485–1551: A Viral Pulmonary Disease?," 96.

36. James R. Carlson and Peter W. Hammond, "The English Sweating Sickness (1485–c. 1551): A New Perspective on Disease Etiology," *Journal of the History of Medicine and Allied Sciences* 54, no. 1 (1999): 32.

37. Carlson and Hammond, "The English Sweating Sickness," 36.

38. Paul Heyman, Leopold Simons, and Christel Cochez, "Were the English Sweating Sickness and the Picardy Sweat Caused by Hantaviruses?," *Viruses* 6 (2014): 160.

39. Heyman, Simons, and Cochez, "Were the English Sweating Sickness," 159.

40. Heyman, Simons, and Cochez, "Were the English Sweating Sickness."

41. Heyman, Simons, and Cochez, "Were the English Sweating Sickness," 153.

42. Heyman, Simons, and Cochez, "Were the English Sweating Sickness," 160.

43. Colleen B. Jonsson, Luiz Tadeu Moraes Figueiredo, and Olli Vapalahti, "A Global Perspective on Hantavirus Ecology, Epidemiology, and Disease," *Clinical Microbiology Reviews* 23, no. 2 (2010): 423.

44. Jonsson, Figueiredo, and Vapalahti, "A Global Perspective," 424.

45. R. S. Gottfried, "Population, Plague, and the Sweating Sickness: Demographic Movements in Late Fifteenth-Century England." *Journal of British Studies* 17, no. 1 (Fall 1977): 13.

46. Gottfried, "Population, Plague, and the Sweating Sickness," 16.

47. Edward McSweegan, "Anthrax and the Etiology of the English Sweating Sickness," *Medical Hypotheses* 62 (2004): 156.

48. Alfred L. Rowse, *Bosworth Field: From Medieval to Tudor England* (Garden City, NY: Doubleday & Company, 1966), 118.

49. Michael Jones, *Bosworth, 1485: The Battle That Transformed England* (2002; repr., New York: Pegasus Books, 2015), 24.

50. Jones, *Bosworth, 1485*, 25.

51. Jones, *Bosworth, 1485*, 167.

52. Rowse, *Bosworth Field*, 216.

53. Rowse, *Bosworth Field*, 11.

54. Gladys Temperley, *Henry VII* (1914; repr., Westport, CT: Greenwood Press, 1971), 18.

55. Rowse, *Bosworth Field*, 219.

56. Rowse, *Bosworth Field*.

57. Jones, *Bosworth, 1485*, 166.

58. Jones, *Bosworth, 1485*, 203–204.

59. Temperley, *Henry VII*, 17.

60. Rowse, *Bosworth Field*, 229.

61. Temperley, *Henry VII*, 39.

62. Temperley, *Henry VII*, 40.

63. Sean Cunningham, *Henry VII* (London: Routledge, 2007), 233.

64. Cunningham, *Henry VII*, 234.

65. Cunningham, *Henry VII*.

66. Mary Ann Lund, "Richard's Back: Death, Scoliosis, and Myth Making," *Medical Humanities* 41, no. 2 (December 2015): 91.

67. Aisling Byrne and Victoria Flood, "The Romance of the Stanleys: Regional and National Imaginings in the Percy Folio," *Viator* 46, no. 1 (2015): 333.

68. Wylie and Collier, "The English Sweating Sickness," 437.

Part II

Bacterial Epidemics in the Context of Wars: Introduction

Rebecca M. Seaman

In time of war, soldiers, however sensible, care a great deal more on some
occasions about slaking their thirst than about the danger of enteric fever.[1]
—Winston Churchill

Wars and epidemics have occurred throughout history, and bacterial infections
have plagued each in turn. But what is a bacterial infection, and how do epidemics
that spread via bacteria differ from other contagious outbreaks? These questions
are crucial to understanding the chapters selected in this section and assist the
reader in more fully understanding the process and impact of the individual epidemics selected.

Bacteria are unicellular organisms that replicate autonomously. They are small
and rather primitive in structure. Yet, bacteria are alive and capable of rapid asex-
ual reproduction through cellular division. Unlike viruses, bacteria have both DNA
and RNA. Some bacteria depend on elements outside of their cellular walls for
mobility, and others are independently motile. These latter bacteria possess whip-
like appendages, or flagella, that rotate and move them through liquids. Other
bacteria boast hairlike structures that assist them in adhering to surfaces.[2]

The growth rate, and therefore spread, of bacteria varies based on the species
as well as the physical environment and necessary nutrients. Bacteria are found in
almost every environment in the world, which makes bacterial infections a common problem for militaries, especially those military forces relocated to new environments with unknown bacteria. Each species of bacteria has specific preferred
parameters that facilitate or hinder its growth: nutrition, temperature, light, acidity,
humidity, and atmosphere, to name a few.[3] The absence of any bacterial epidemic
during a particular war is an indicator that the bacteria present were not harmful,
that the military personnel built up a resistance to the bacteria, or that the parameters needed for propagation were not met in the environment.

The bacterial infections discussed in part II are quite diverse. Two chapters deal
with bacteria conveyed to human hosts by way of ectoparasites that serve as disease vectors. Typhus, associated with Napoleon's invasion of Russia in 1812, is

commonly conveyed through body lice, though ticks can also convey these bacteria. The bubonic plague that ravaged Europe in the late Middle Ages is often associated with rats, but it was in fact spread through infected fleas. The infection was often passed on through a direct bite. However, fecal matter deposited by the ectoparasite also entered the host's system through scratching or open wounds or abrasions.

The bacterial infections for cholera and typhoid fever were most often the result of drinking water or eating foods that had become contaminated with infected fecal matter. In both cases, the bacteria (*Vibrio cholerae* and *Salmonella typhimurium*, respectively) entered the body and became attached to the mucosal tissues of the intestinal wall. Once attached, the bacteria produced toxins that caused the body to release liquids in an effort to purge the intestinal tract. The severity of the toxins and purging process varied, from short periods of diarrhea to extreme diarrhea and vomiting. Extreme dehydration, sepsis, and perforation of the intestine could occur, and the host often died if effective treatments were not provided. The wars associated with cholera (Crimean War) and typhoid fever (Spanish-American War) both occurred in the 19th century, at the time medical progress was being made in identifying these bacteria. Unfortunately, cholera was not clearly identified nor treatment determined until after the Crimean War. In the case of typhoid fever, the bacteria were discovered almost two decades before the outbreak of hostilities between Spain and America in the late 1890s. However, the exigencies of war and mobilization resulted in the circumvention of precautions against typhoid fever until epidemics broke out in recruitment camps and deployment sites.

Diphtheria is another bacteria studied in part II. It is associated with World War II and the Tajikistan Civil War. The cause of the disease in these conflicts, *Corynebacterium diptheriae*, attached itself to the mucosal membranes of a host's throat or nasal passages, but it was also found in cutaneous or skin lesions. Spread through contact or through coughing and sneezing, the disease had been identified and antitoxins developed by the advent of World War II. However, the conditions of war prevented access to such countermeasures. This was most obvious during the Bataan Death March and subsequent imprisonment of thousands in the Philippines during World War II. Four decades later, the disruptions of civil war and the ensuing poverty and corruption caused a lack of medical supplies for the Tajik population. The resulting diphtheria epidemic spread throughout the country and was carried by refugees into neighboring countries. This chapter provides an example of how epidemics thrive in disruption created during wartime despite medical advances.

Each chapter in this section is associated with a distinctly different period in history, from the Middle Ages to the turn of the 21st century. Conditions and causes of epidemic outbreaks, and subsequent impacts on societies, also differ for each war. Through this diversity, the chapters in part II demonstrate the wide disparity in bacterial infections and how they affect or are affected by periods of war.

NOTES

1. Winston Churchill, "Parliamentary Debate" (March 21, 1902), quoted in *Churchill by Himself: The Definitive Collection of Quotations*, ed. Richard Lanworth (New York, Public Affairs, 2008), 469.
2. Sheila C. Grossman and Carol Mattson Porth, *Porth's Pathophysiology: Concepts of Altered Health States*, 9th ed. (Philadelphia: Wolters Kluwer Health, Lippincott Williams and Wilkins, 2014), 256–258.
3. Grossman and Porth, *Porth's Pathophysiology*, 258.

Chapter 4

The Black Death and Nation-State Wars of the 14th Century: Environment, Epigenetics, Excess, and Expiation, 1346–1450

Sarah Douglas

Some say that it descended upon the human race through the influence of the heavenly bodies, others that it was a punishment signifying God's righteous anger at our iniquitous way of life.[1]

—Giovanni Boccaccio

While the English and French vied for territories and the French throne and Italian merchants contested trade rights and territories, an unprecedented human pandemic emerged in Eurasia's continental interior.[2] This "Great Pestilence" broke out in Asia in the 1330s, traveled to the Black Sea in 1346, and then was carried into the Mediterranean by merchants in 1348. After reaching Italy, it spread across the continent, killing an estimated 50 percent of the European population by 1351.[3]

Characteristics of the *Yersinia pestis* Bacteria

Yersinia pestis, or the Black Death, was a soil bacterium typically carried by fleas.[4] The outbreak in the 1330s spread via the Mongol army as it conquered territory west along the Silk Road. Once it reached the Black Sea, it spread to European merchants, who carried it back to Italy.[5] From there it swept through both urban and rural areas alike. This journey was facilitated by wars of conquest and trade in Asia, Asia Minor, and across Europe.

Understanding the devastation of the Black Death pandemic requires examining the identity and diffusion of this ecological disaster. It also requires one to study the effects of the disease on both trade and some of the largest wars of the medieval period, including the Hundred Years' War. The plague relied on more than just patterns of normal contagious diffusion; it also spread through a hierarchical pattern dependent on travel and the movement of trade goods. It was the competition for those trade goods, power, land, and food in general during an extended period of climatic change and famine that helped prompt the wars that rippled across the Eurasian continent in the 14th century. It was not until the 20th century that historians turned their attention to the plague's possible impact and examined why England in particular adapted to the disaster with marked efficiency while France and other European nation-states did not. This adaptability contributed to the comparative success of the English over the French in the early phase of the Hundred Years' War and prompted internal reforms that positioned England for economic and political expansion in the future.

Yersinia pestis is a nonmotile oval-shaped bacterium that evolved from the soil-dwelling bacillus *Yersinia pseudotuberculosis*.[6] It is made up of a single chromosome and has 4,600,755 base pairs in its DNA strand. The bacterium has three types (or biovars): *antiqua*, which is found in Africa; *mediaevalia*, which is from Central Asia; and *orientalis*, which is found in East Asia and elsewhere. *Y. pestis* thrives in warm temperatures and is contracted by infected fleas. The fleas transmit the bacterium by biting indigenous mammalian populations.[7] Recent research indicates the Asian gerbil was responsible for the initial outbreak, as opposed to the rat, which likely served only as an intermediary host along trade routes west.[8]

Forms of the Plague—Methods of Contagion

Once contracted, the infection took one of three forms: bubonic, pneumonic or septicemic. These forms were not different strains of the *Y. pestis* bacterium. Instead, they provided an indication of the infection site and how it spread from host to host. Bubonic plague infected the lymph nodes and was named for the black swellings that formed in those locations on the body. Bubonic plague was transmitted through fleabites or exposure to bodily fluids of infected individuals. Pneumonic plague involved an infection of the respiratory system and spread when an infected host released microscopic mucus into the air through sneezing or coughing. Septicemic plague, the rarest of the infections, involved the spread of the bacterium into the bloodstream after exposure to a fleabite or to infected bodily fluids. This form of the plague was often a secondary consequence of the spread of the bubonic or pneumonic plague throughout the body.[9]

Whatever form the plague presented itself through, the infection incubated in the human host for less than a week after exposure (two to six days for bubonic and one to three days for pneumonic). During this incubation period, the bacterium replicated enough to cause visible symptoms.[10] Symptoms mimicked influenza or pneumonia, including fevers, muscle aches, and fatigue. If the lymph nodes were infected, large black lumps called buboes formed on the groin, neck, or underarms. These buboes, which were 1 centimeter to 10 centimeters in diameter, gave this infection its name.[11] Sometimes infected hosts died before indicators occurred, as in the case of septicemic infection, which caused more severe influenza or pneumonia symptoms, including fevers, vomiting, diarrhea, an enlarged liver, and shock. Pneumonic plague's "airborne" nature, short incubation period, and deceptive similarity to severe influenza or pneumonia made it the most lethal for those who contracted this form.[12] Left untreated, bubonic plague had a mortality rate of 50–75 percent, and septicemic and pneumonic plague mortality rates were at 100 percent.[13]

Historical Waves of the Black Death

Three confirmed *Y. pestis* outbreaks or waves appear in historical records: the earlier Justinian Plague (540–750 CE); the Black Death of the Middle Ages; and the Manchurian/Asian wave (1855–1896). The Black Death, referred to as "the Great Pestilence,"[14] first appeared in Central Asia and then moved into the Crimea in 1346 before spreading to Europe. This wave appeared to die out in 1351, but it reappeared at least 15 more times before the 16th century.[15] Microbiologist Alexandre Yersin identified the bacterium named after him during the last Manchurian/Asian wave.[16] Four years later, French physician and biologist Paul-Louis Simond discovered that the plague was transferred from rats to humans, with fleas serving as the vector of transmission.[17] Historians who compared this relatively modern outbreak to the accounts of the Black Death during the Middle Ages concluded that the two diseases were the same. The identity of the Black Death, long a mystery, was apparently discovered.

Not all researchers are in agreement, however, on this discovery. Some remains from identified victims of the Black Death outbreak showed no signs of *Y. pestis*. A comparison through recent studies of the mortality rates and symptoms for the three waves of plague further muddied the waters. Historian Samuel K. Cohn, a leading opponent of the idea of a single strain of the *Y. pestis* for the three waves, argued that the medieval plague was either a more virulent mutation of the modern *Y. pestis* strain, a combination of known diseases, or a disease yet unknown to modern medical science.[18] His claims received support from scientific studies released in subsequent years. In 2007, researchers examining skeletal remains in England and Denmark found that the disease was "selective with respect to frailty."[19] A subsequent 2010 article by Mark Welford and Brian H. Bossak titled "Revisiting the Medieval Black Death of 1347–1351" claimed that the Black Death could not have been caused by a bacterium due to the complexities and virulence of the outbreak. Instead, they posited that a virus was likely to blame.[20]

Discoveries and Changing Historical Debates

In 2010, another study located the presence of *Y. pestis* in medieval plague victims.[21] The study identified protein signatures specific to *Y. pestis* in mass graves from northern, central, and southern Europe known to be Black Death burials.[22] Research revealed the Black Death was due to two biovars of *Y. pestis*, *mediaevalia* and *orientalis*, indicating that plague waves from both Central and East Asia reached Europe at the same time. In 2011, a study addressed Cohn's claims directly, arguing that the medieval plague was caused by a variant of *Y. pestis* that was different from modern strains, thus explaining the differences in virulence, symptomology, and mortality. A subsequent study, focused specifically on plague victims found in

London, identified no mutations present in the reconstructed *Y. pestis* DNA that would differentiate it from modern outbreaks. Instead, the authors urged researchers to instead "consider factors like environment, vector dynamics, and host susceptibility" to explain differences in outbreak.[23]

New contributions from the scientific community have occurred in rapid succession. Most notably, in 2013, during the digging of a pit for a new cross-rail project in London, 25 skeletons were found alongside mid-14th century pottery.[24] When 12 of the bodies were later analyzed, *Y. pestis* was located, and the reconstructed DNA was nearly identical to that identified during the subsequent 2014 outbreak of bubonic plague in Madagascar.[25]

The consensus of most recent research contends that the Black Death was the work of *Y. pestis*. Researchers currently study the plague in relation to the social, biological, and environmental circumstances that surrounded it. The study of this potential expression and DNA's interaction with an individual's internal environment is referred to as *epigenetics*.[26] The theory asserts that although the recovered DNA strands of *Y. pestis* could be identical, their epigenetic contexts could affect humans in entirely different ways. This may explain why *Y. pestis* affected medieval people of varying degrees of frailty differently and why outbreaks following 1348–1351 had increasingly lower mortality rates. The fact that two out of three *Y. pestis* biovars were endemic to Asia helped bolster the argument that the modern plague was far less virulent in that region of the world due to an epigenetic immunity present in Asian populations frequently exposed to the disease.

Impacts of Health and Environment on Virulence of the Plague

Evidence indicates that health and physical environment both played a role in the virulence of the Black Death. Some historians theorized that famines throughout Europe, due to overpopulation and climate depression in the first half of the 14th century, created a population ill-equipped to fight off such a deadly bacterial infection. Most Europeans at the outbreak of the plague suffered from chronic shortages of protein, calcium, and vitamin B12.[27] Environmental historian Philip Slavin argued that the epizootic that killed many European animal species in the first half of the century specifically contributed to the calcium and protein deficiencies.[28] Examination of the London cross-rail plague victims bolstered such claims, as a majority of the skeletons possessed the physical markers of malnutrition, 16 percent had rickets, and many showed obvious signs of prolonged and physically damaging heavy labor.[29]

So far, scientists have examined the bones or teeth of less than 100 Black Death victims. However, even with the increased discovery of bodies, improved diagnostic tools, and the expanding medical knowledge of DNA, epigenetic factors, and the role of nutrition, conclusive answers are unlikely. Medical historian Andrew Cunningham warned against assuming that the modern understandings and identification of historic epidemics are correct due to the use of "superior" modern tools and knowledge. The methods of recording past symptoms and diagnoses throw doubt upon certain historical records.[30] Making broad assumptions about the nature of the plague based on 667-year-old reconstructed DNA strands from a small sampling is problematic. Yet, dismissal of *Y. pestis* based solely on symptomology, especially when records of symptoms were documented for reasons other than diagnoses, ignores the highly complex and still largely mysterious relationship between the human body, diseases affecting it, and its interaction with the surrounding environment pre- and postmortem.

Historical discussions, while informative and intriguing, are secondary to the real issue: namely, that the plague "killed an awful lot of people."[31] Many believed the pestilence was a punishment from God for various violations of good Christian order, for which humans of all ranks in society must undergo expiation to ensure salvation. One English account referred to church officials as mere hirelings, "motivated by the desire for money. Such workers deserve to come to some grief."[32] Another blamed children, indicating that because they had dishonored their parents, "God is slaying children by pestilence."[33] Others credited the alignment of planets and eclipses.[34] Some looked toward mortal culprits to blame for the plague. A Spanish account claimed that "many beggars and mendicants of various countries" were guilty of poisoning rivers, houses, churches, and food, and a German account noted that bags full of poison were found in many wells and springs.[35] In Germany, it was commonly believed that Jews were to blame; upon capture, they "confessed as much under torture that they had bred spiders and toads in pots and pans, and had obtained poison from overseas."[36] Jews, popular scapegoats for a wide variety of public ills, were arrested and interrogated throughout Europe as a consequence to this theory, and those who did not convert through force were burned.[37]

Tracking the Plague's Diffusion

Most chroniclers agreed that plague spread to Europe when the Mongol army besieged Caffa, in the Crimea, using catapults to fling plague-ridden bodies over the city walls.[38] Caffa and the neighboring Italian enclave of Tana exchanged hands repeatedly between Mongol and Italian merchants. However, the 1346 siege had a lasting impact. Italian chronicler Gabrielle de Mussis stated that Genoese merchants inside the twice-walled city of Caffa were safe until the attacking Mongols contracted a devastating plague that "overran the Tartars and killed thousands upon thousands every day." Mussis referred to mountains of disfigured bodies that were launched by the Mongols into the walled city. The Genoese that attempted to escape the carnage carried the pestilence to Constantinople in the spring of 1347 and then back to Italy by the spring of 1348. "We Genoese and Venetians bear the responsibility for revealing the judgment of God," he wrote in his *Historia de Morbo*. "Alas, once our ships had brought us to port we went to our homes. . . . But, to our anguish, we were carrying the darts of death."[39] The Italians who fled Caffa took the plague with them, to Genoa, Venice, and other coastal cities. Strategically, the siege of Caffa was ineffective, as the Mongols fled and the Italians continued to lay claim to the city.[40] However, as the disease spread farther westward, it had a dramatic effect on the subcontinent of Europe.

Chroniclers agreed that the death toll was catastrophic. In Venice, where merchants from Caffa had fled, it killed more than 70 percent of the people and 83 percent of the physicians.[41] In Florence, where the greatest banking families resided and competed for economic influence, people attempted to purify themselves from the "evil," isolated themselves, or even fled from the disease.[42] Nonetheless, almost 60 percent of the population died within a year. The Florence economy, already in turmoil when King Edward III of England defaulted on loans from the Bardi and Peruzzi banking families, failed and left the city bankrupt and war-torn for the next 35 years.[43]

From Italy, the plague swept through Western Europe, killing close to 90 percent of the population in the region around Avignon.[44] By summer, it had reached the English Channel and then spread to Britain.[45] The plague moved through the south, killing "innumerable people in Dorset, Devon, and Somerset."[46] It then turned north, leaving a path of death so that "there was such a shortage of people that there were hardly enough living to look after the sick and bury the dead."[47]

Historians have traditionally estimated the death toll of the plague to be one-third of the European population, but recent studies have estimated it was 50 percent.[48] The plague was preceded by successive famines in the first two decades of the century and an animal panzootic that had emerged in Bohemia between 1314 and 1316 before moving west.[49] Both emerged during a time of environmental stress referred to as the Dantean Anomaly, which involved markedly lower temperatures throughout Europe. Thirty years later, the plague occurred during another anomaly that affected the entire globe and caused the coldest years of the millennia, 1348–1350.[50] The confluence of Little Ice Age, disease, wars, and famine led some to assert that people of the 14th century were "the victims of a joint physical and biological conspiracy of Nature, deadly in its collective human impact, and profound in its short-, medium- and long-term economic consequences."[51]

The Events and Context of the Hundred Years' War

The Black Death occurred during one of the largest and most significant European wars of the medieval period: the Hundred Years' War. Lasting longer than 100 years, the war included bouts of temporary peace and shifting alliances that turned with Europe's internal political tide. The conflict involved disputed rights to both French duchies and the monarchy itself. The English king Edward III's dynastic claim to the French crown set the stage for the conflict and was compounded by French prompting of Scottish aggressions in England and English intervention in Flanders and Brittany.

The French objected to Edward's English claim and instead turned to a parallel royal line from the House of Capet, in the person of Philip of Valois.[52] Philip VI, a court outsider, was nonetheless born in France. The two monarchs disagreed over feudal dues and control over the very profitable woolen trade with Flanders immediately after Edward III became king of England.[53] In 1338, Edward refused to pay homage to Philip, interfered in Flemish politics, proclaimed he was the rightful king of France, and declared war.

The war did not start well for either side. Philip VI hired Genoese ships to periodically raid the English coast. The English victory at the naval Battle of Sluys, in 1340, was Edward's only success during the initial years of the war due to his inability to establish steady financial support.[54] Between 1337 and 1340, Edward used wool customs to pay his mounting debts and then turned to granting wool export tax collection rights (the wool staple) to his Italian super-company allies, the Bardi and Peruzzi families, in return for sizeable cash advances.[55] His magnates also provided him with loans by pledging their own possessions as collateral and then despoiled monasteries for any ornaments fit to sell for cash.[56] Edward even pawned the English Crown Jewels on two separate occasions. These efforts were in vain, and he was barely solvent as he marched into France in 1340.[57] After the lengthy and costly siege of Tournai, Edward's excesses in fighting the war threatened to undermine any hope of victory, and he was essentially a prisoner to his many creditors.

Edward's insufficient financing and limited manpower at Tournai prompted him to increase his forces for the Battle of Crecy and the subsequent Siege of Calais, spending more than £300,000 in related costs.[58] Most of the weaponry, foodstuffs, and 60 percent of the soldiers were gathered in a process somewhat analogous to a modern draft called *array*, with towns, villages, and merchants given a specified number of soldiers, supplies, or weaponry to provide.[59] The rest of the soldiers were part of private retinues raised by Edward III, his son Edward the Black Prince, and prominent English magnates. Although some of the cash came from kingdom-wide taxation and commodity revenues, Italian super-companies provided the majority. This entire campaign constituted a massive capital-extensive effort. In other words, Edward III gathered the manpower and resources needed to overwhelm his enemy either in combat or in siege.

English success at this stage of the war was due in part to French internal tensions. Philip VI relied on feudal military service owed to him by his vassals when he chose to call upon them.[60] Although he paid for their services by the time that the Hundred Years' War began, Philip could demand the considerable support of the duchies of Brittany, Guyene, Normandy, the county of Flanders, and, in 1346, the king of Bohemia. This service was supplemented by the *arrière ban* system, which was composed of urban militias and supplies provided by their rural counterparts. With these systems working in concert, the French Crown could theoretically summon the largest army in Europe.[61]

In practice, however, the French system was unstable. French urban militias were poorly trained, and lords were unwilling or unable to support the king, especially during the Hundred Years' War. The French Crown dealt with these problems by hiring mercenaries, either French knights or even foreign mercenaries commanded by their own captains. Nonetheless, the French went into the Battle of Crecy with around 30,000 soldiers, compared to the 14,000 on the English side.[62]

The battle did not go well for the French and left King Philip VI injured. This and the loss of Calais to the English the next summer won Philip no favors with the nobility or the French people.[63] The king's council was liquidated, Italian moneylenders were expelled, and several Crown financial ministers were imprisoned. None of this pacified an increasingly dissatisfied French people, and Philip eventually met with Crown ministers to plan for an expedition to defend the kingdom.[64] The Black Death soon interrupted his plans.

War and Nations Disrupted by Ravages of the Black Death

Already fragmented and decentralized by the time the plague arrived, France's first noted outbreak of the disease occurred in November 1347 in Marsailles.[65] From this southern population center, the disease spread first to surrounding urban centers and then across the countryside. Avignon was hit in November, where Pope Clement attempted to organize religious processions and medical care for the infected before leaving the city himself.[66] By spring, the plague had spread to Lyon, Rouen, and Bordeaux, reaching Burgundy by the end of 1348 and Paris by the summer of 1349.[67]

Most historians have recently settled on a European mortality rate of 50 percent; yet, Ole J. Benedictow has argued that nearly 60 percent of the French population died in the outbreak.[68] On top of these heavy losses due to the plague, the French monarchy was in crisis at the time due to military defeats at the hands of the English. Inflation was rampant, and in December of 1349, Philip VI's wife, Queen Joan of Burgundy, died of the plague. A month later, Philip married his son John's fiancée, alienating him from his son and the nobility. Philip died in August the following year, leaving John to inherit a troubled French Crown and fragmented kingdom.[69]

In England, the plague's short-term impact was catastrophic. The plague raced across England from the spring into the fall, reaching London in October in 1348. Edward III, like many English Crown officials and London inhabitants, abandoned the city to escape the disease. The plague so devastated Europe that, in November, Edward III and Philip VI agreed to extend the Anglo-French truce of the Hundred Years' War until the end of 1349, and in January, as the plague moved north, Parliament adjourned without sitting.[70] The Great Pestilence killed 2.5 million English subjects, and national and local administration ground to a halt. Prices for grain, livestock, and labor fluctuated wildly, reflecting the unstable workforce and market in a society turned upside down. With temperatures colder than any in the entire millennium; near-constant warfare between the English, French, Flemish, and Scottish; widespread animal disease; and the introduction of the Black Death, it is no surprise that many believed "it is from divine wrath that the mortality of these years proceeds."[71]

In contrast to France, the English government quickly adapted to this seemingly insurmountable biological disaster. Although many royal officials fled London, they continued to meet at alternate locations. The Privy Seal office continued operations, moving its headquarters from Westminster to Woodstock. Although the King's Bench in the capital ceased operations, those in York and Lincoln continued to hear cases. By August 1349, most offices had returned to Westminster, and by the fall, the English Crown was operating at full capacity. The Crown was stubbornly determined to "sit out the period of disruption and ensure that proprietary interests survived intact once the temporary emergency had passed."[72]

Many positions, vacated by casualties to the plague, were replaced to ensure successful operations. Chancellor Offord, 12 Chancery clerks, two high-ranking officials in the Exchequer, the clerk of pleas, and the royal chamberlain in Receipt died from the plague. Many royal attorneys in the King's Bench along with 9 clerks of Commons Pleas, 10 clerks of the Bench, and several tax collectors perished as well. These deaths prompted Edward III to appoint a range of new officials to the various offices so the English Crown could continue its normal operations.[73]

Economic stability was quickly reestablished. Although commodity, livestock, and labor prices did fluctuate during the plague's height, they soon stabilized. Inflation did occur, but the unpredictable fluctuations ceased. Wheat, considered a luxury cereal, suffered the greatest cost increase in the years after the plague due to its labor-intensive harvest, but prices never reached the heights achieved during the famines of the early 14th century.[74] Livestock prices functioned similarly, and cart horses saw the most drastic price increase, perhaps due to their utility as a labor-saving device.[75]

With heightened competition for a vastly contracted labor pool, wages increased markedly as the plague faded. Like elsewhere in Europe, unskilled heavy laborers were in the highest demand, and the ability of the peasantry to command higher wages created notable tension within English society. Unlike elsewhere, the English Crown attempted to resolve this tension by instituting the 1349 Ordinance of Laborers and then the 1351 Statute of Laborers, which demanded workers create standard working contracts with those hiring them. Most importantly, the statutes dictated that workers not be paid higher wages than before the crisis.

Though ultimately unsuccessful, the ordinance set a legal precedent for the intervention of the Crown into societal affairs. It was an early instance of a government attempting to establish and then enforce the status quo.[76] The legal concept behind the statute was groundbreaking, and because labor wages increased on pace with foodstuffs, the ordinance was actually rather effective in its efforts to curb wage inflation.[77] Of critical importance was the elevated competition for labor, particularly unskilled labor, which affected how the English Crown raised troops for war.

It was the combination of calamities, the plague (with prior climatic shifts, epizootic and famine), and the military upheavals that contributed to the extensive death toll in Europe. The first examination of these twin disasters appeared in Barbara Tuchman's *A Distant Mirror*, which covered the Black Death and the Hundred Years' War.[78] This century was one of the most unsettled in European history. For three years, the plague ravaged Europe. Just as society began to recover after the Black Death, military concerns for English or French supremacy swiftly reemerged.

When word reached Edward in December that French noble Geoffrey de Charny was prepared to launch an attack on Calais, Edward raised a small force of retainers and secretly sailed to France in January 1350, reviving the conflict and ending the truce. Once in Calais, he repelled the French offensive, thus reviving "Edward's general appetite for war."[79] Philip VI died in August of 1350, leaving Edward to press his hereditary rights with Philip's son John II.[80]

Edward III was confronted with new problems during the continuation of war that had not been encountered before the plague. The English population was much smaller; prices for labor, livestock, and commodities had risen; and significant debts lingered from the Crécy-Calais campaign. The campaigns amply demonstrated that these funds were not enough to support a major military expedition overseas. Moreover, the plague had deprived the English Crown of a crucial source of supplementary income. Edward III could no longer rely on Italian super-companies, as they had been bankrupted by the combination of Edward's failure to repay his loans and the impact of the plague in Florence. Even English merchants were unable to provide him with the necessary loans. The Black Death had halted trade, and as a consequence, the Bardi, Peruzzi, and several major English merchant conglomerates had been financially ruined.[81]

Again, the English government adapted effectively. In addition to enacting the aforementioned ordinance, to minimize inflation, the English Crown passed the Statute of Purveyors in 1352, which promised to end currency devaluation and increase its bullion supply. It also required foreign merchants to pay custom fees in bullion.[82] Additionally, the Exchequer attempted to establish "comprehensive and definitive records of royal expenditure."[83] With no established budget and no organized attempt to monitor, let alone regulate, royal expenditures, the "colossal debts incurred by the king's wars" compelled Exchequer treasurer William Edington to control revenues and expenditures.[84] He created the Protecolla Rolls to centralize the financial obligations of the English Crown, thus allowing Edward III to overcome his financial hardships and effectively prosecute the war for the rest of the decade, despite population decline and labor shortages due to the plague.

The corrupt and inefficient wool staple was additionally reformed. The old system had practically invited regular corruption or evasion by woolen merchants. Consequently, prior to the Black Death, the average customs yield was approximately £22,650.[85] In 1352, the loss of labor and soldiers due to the plague necessitated a change. The King's Council banned English wool merchants from exporting their wool, moved the wool staple back to England, outlawed wool export by foreign merchants living in England, and forced foreign merchants to come to England to purchase wool.[86] The King's Council instituted "a clean sweep of personnel of the customs, in an attempt to eradicate the connexions [sic] and influences which had built up while the farmers had held control of appointment at the ports."[87] These officials cracked down on smuggling through a specially appointed council and collected 50 shillings on every sack of wool exported.[88] The system was so effective that the customs yield increased to an average of £75,000 between 1351 and 1360.[89]

This significant increase in revenue helped restore the English economy and allowed the king to discharge many debts lingering from before the plague.[90] He also spent nearly £200,000 on building and defensive works for Wales, Calais, and Gascony.[91] More importantly, Edward III used these funds to continue his war effort on the Continent. With more funds and less available manpower, he shifted from the capital-extensive methods used before the plague to capital-intensive methods. He abandoned the large armies and methods of campaigning of the 1340s and adopted military forces that were nearly all volunteers, paid for directly by the Exchequer. The Black Death forced this shift because it created an intense competition for labor that made the old array system impractical. A "landmark" 1352 statute only enforced this change by outlawing the conscription of soldiers based on property and wealth assessments.[92] Soldiering progressively became a sustainable, paid occupation, which increased the "professional" nature of the English military.

The French adopted no such changes. French monarchs had less power to alter the infrastructure of royal administration than their English cousins. France also had a large population base from which to conscript soldiers despite the losses experienced from the plague. The dissention within the nobility and French monarchy prevented financial reforms. Indeed, the general dissatisfaction with the monarchy lingered from before the plague and helped explain why, when John II was captured at the Battle of Poitier in 1356, his own son, Charles, did not pay his ransom.[93] In addition to Charles's political intrigues, the Jacquerie, or peasant revolt, broke out in France, further dividing the people and undermining French royal authority.[94]

Hoping to take advantage of the turmoil in France, Edward III began to prepare for yet another operation on the continent.[95] The 1359–1360 Reims campaign was Edward III's next, and ultimately last, military expedition, and it demonstrated the full effects of the Black Death on logistical organization. The English Crown was forced to almost exclusively use contracted retinues on this campaign, as the old array system was incapable of providing the necessary number of soldiers required. The decrease in population after the Black Death and rising wages for labor meant that the Crown became yet another contender in the labor market. The only soldiers arrayed for the 1359–1360 Reims campaign were archers, and most were raised in Wales.[96] The English Crown also did not bother collecting supplies for the expedition, instead using tax revenue to purchase what it needed once in France.

Edward III shipped his 8,000-man army to the continent in six separate crossings between August and October.[97] This time-consuming process was due to a lack of available ships. Just as the Black Death had forced a change in how the Crown gathered soldiers, it also made locating sailors difficult. Smaller ships had to be used to transport the army because relatively small crews could operate them.[98] Once in France, a northern countryside devastated by plague, civil unrest, and decades of war had resulted in a scarcity of needed supplies. Unseasonably cold weather and the fact that the French would not engage the English in battle forced Edward to abandon the siege of Reims and the subsequent planned siege of Paris.[99]

Although Edward had to settle for terms, his considerable show of force led to a favorable peace agreement. The methods England employed to accomplish these early successes under Edward III were in part the result of the Black Death and its impact on the population and economy during the ongoing Hundred Years' War.

Combined Impact of the Plague and War on Society

The Black Death, or the "Great Pestilence," had a marked effect on European society, trade, and conflicts, especially through the early phases of the largest war in medieval Europe, the Hundred Years' War. The demographic impact created labor shortages across the continent and drove religious perceptions of divine punishment and expiation that affected Christians and non-Christians alike. The plague's impact on trade and banking shifted the economics of society and the ability of kings, nobles, and banks to raise funds for war. The English were forced to change how they prepared for and waged war, which led to a shift from capital-extensive to capital-intensive methods of preparation. These methods included the hiring of soldiers with professional contracts, which paved the way for the emergence of the professional soldier in late medieval England and success in the early phases of the Hundred Years' War. The environment also affected the epidemic and Hundred Years' War, with the Dantean Anomaly and the Little Ice Age contributing to the famines and poor health of European populations at a time when two divergent types of the plague, *mediaevalia* and *orientalis*, had converged on Europe at the same time. The resulting devastation of the Black Death had a profound effect upon the war. In concert, the war and plague helped shape the late medieval and early modern world.

NOTES

1. Giovanni Boccaccio, *Decameron*, quoted in *The Black Death*, ed. and trans. Rosemary Horrox (Manchester and New York: Manchester University Press, 1994), 26.
2. Bruce M. S. Campbell, "Physical Shocks, Biological Hazards, and Human Impacts: The Crisis of the Fourteenth Century Revisited," in *Economic and Biological Interactions in Pre-Industrial Europe from the 13th to the 18th Centuries*, ed. S. Cavaciocchi (Florence, Italy: Firenze University Press, 2010), 13.
3. Samuel K. Cohn, "The Black Death: End of a Paradigm," *American Historical Review* 107, no. 3 (2002): 703–738. The estimates of those killed by the plague vary from 20 percent to as high as 70 percent. The stated 50 percent appears to be the most reliable estimate.
4. Philip Ziegler, *The Black Death* (Stroud, Gloucestershire: Sutton Publishing Ltd., 1969), 14.
5. David Herlihy, *The Black Death and the Transformation of the West* (Cambridge, MA: Harvard University Press, 1997), 24–25.
6. Kirsten I. Bos et al., "A Draft of *Yersinia pestis* from Victims of the Black Death," *Nature* 478 (October 27, 2011): 506; and Patrick S. G. Chain et al., "Complete Genome Sequence of *Yersinia pestis* Strains Antiqua and Nepal516: Evidence of Gene Reduction in an Emerging Pathogen," *Journal of Bacteriology* 188, no. 12 (June 2006): 4453–4463.

7. Ryan T. Jones, Sara M. Vetter, and Kenneth L. Gage, "Exposing Laboratory-Reared Fleas to Soil and Wild Flea Feces Increases Transmission of *Yersinia pestis*," *American Journal of Tropical Medicine and Hygiene* 89, no. 4 (October 9, 2013): 784–787. This study indicates that 50 percent of the rodents exposed to infected fleas contract *Y. pestis*. B. J. Hinnenbusch et al., "Role of Yersinia Murine Toxin in Survival of *Yersinia pestis* in the Midgut of the Flea Vector," *Science* 296, no. 5568 (April 2002): 733–735.

8. Boris V. Schmid et al., "Climate-Driven Introduction of the Black Death and Successive Plague Reintroductions in Europe," *Proceedings of the National Academy of Sciences of the United States of America* 112, no. 10 (January 2015): 3020–3025. This study also finds that contrary to traditional assumptions, the plague did not lay dormant in indigenous rat populations within Europe between each subsequent outbreak of the disease, but rather was brought into Europe through contact with Central and East Asia.

9. Joseph P. Byrne, *The Black Death* (Westport, CT: Greenwood Press, 2004), 20.

10. Division of Vector-Borne Diseases, "Plague," Centers for Disease Control and Prevention, accessed September 2, 2017, http://www.cdc.gov/plague.

11. Byrne, *The Black Death*, 19; "Boubon" is Greek for "groin"; and Paul Bugl, "History of Epidemics and Plagues," accessed September 2, 2017, http://uhavax.hartford.edu /bugl/histepi.htm#plague.

12. Michael B. Prentice and L. Rahalison, "Plague," *The Lancet* 369, no. 9568 (April 7, 2007): 1196–1207.

13. Bugl, "History of Epidemics."

14. Aberth, *The Black Death*, 1.

15. In addition to an outbreak in 1360–1363, Byrne identified 1379–1383, 1389–1393, 1400, 1405–1407, 1413, 1420, 1427, 1433–1434, 1438–1439, 1457–1458, 1463–1464, 1467, 1471, 1479–1480, and 1485 (Byrne, *The Black Death*, 60).

16. Byrne, *The Black Death*, 16.

17. H. H. Mollaret, "The Discovery by Paul-Louis Simond of the Role of the Flea in the Transmission of the Plague," *Bulletin de la Société de pathologie exotique* 92, no. 5, pt. 2 (December 1999): 383–387.

18. Cohn, "The Black Death," 57.

19. Sharon N. DeWitte and James W. Wood, "Selectivity of Black Death Mortality with Respect to Preexisting Health," *Proceedings of the National Academy of Sciences of the United States of America* 105, no. 5 (November 13, 2007): 1436–1441.

20. Mark Welford and Brian J. Bossak, "Revisiting the Medieval Black Death of 1347–1351: Spatiotemporal Dynamics Suggestive of an Alternate Causation," *Geography Compass* 4, no. 6 (June 2010): 561–575.

21. Stephanie Haensch et al., "Distinct Clones of *Yersinia pestis* Caused the Black Death," *PLoS Pathogens* 6, no. 10 (October 2010): 2.

22. Haensch, "Distinct Clones."

23. Verena J. Schuenemanna et al., "Targeted Enrichment of Ancient Pathogens Yielding pPCP1 Plasmid of *Yersinia pestis* from Victims of the Black Death," *PNAS* 108, no. 38 (September 20, 2011): 15673–15674; and Kristen I. Bos et al., "A Draft Genome of *Yersinia pestis* from Victims of the Black Death," *Nature* 478 (October 27, 2011): 506–510.

24. James Morgan, "Black Death Skeletons Unearthed by Crossrail Project," *BBC News: Science & Environment* (March 30, 2014), accessed December 11, 2017, http://www .bbc.com/news/science-environment-26770334.

25. Vanessa Thorpe, "Black Death Skeletons Reveal Pitiful Life of 14th-Century Londoners," *The Observer* (March 29, 2014); and World Health Organization, "Plague—Madagascar" (November 21, 2014), accessed September 2, 2017, http://www.who.int/csr/don/21-november-2014-plague/en/.

26. Josep Casadesus and David Low, "Epigenetic Gene Regulation in the Bacterial World," *Microbiology and Molecular Biology Reviews* (September 2006): 830–856.

27. Sharon DeWitte and Philip Slavin, "Between Famine and Death: England on the Eve of the Black Death—Evidence from Paleoepidemiology and Manorial Accounts," *Journal of Interdisciplinary History* 44, no. 1 (Summer 2013): 37–60.

28. Philip Slavin, "The Great Bovine Pestilence and Its Economic and Environmental Consequences in England and Wales, 1318–50," *EcHR* 65, no. 4 (2012): 1239–1266.

29. Morgan, "Black Death Skeletons."

30. Andrew Cunningham, "Identifying Disease in the Past: Cutting the Gordian Knot," *Asclepio* 54, no. 1 (2002): 15, 22.

31. Aberth, *The Black Death*, 16.

32. Thomas Wright, ed., *Political Poems and Songs*, Vol. 1 (London: Longman, Green, Longman and Roberts, 1859): 280.

33. Harleian Manuscript 2398, fos. 93-94, in Horrox, *The Black Death*, 134.

34. Rosemary Horrox, trans. and ed., *The Black Death* (Manchester, UK: Manchester University Press, 1994), 159.

35. Jaime Villanueva, *Viage Literario a las Iglesias de Espana XI Viage a Gerona,* in Horrox, *The Black Death*, 223; and Herman Gigas, *Hermanni Gygantis, ordinis fratrum minorum, Flores Temporum seu Chronicon Universale ad Orbe condito ad annum Christi MCCCXLIX,* in Horrox, *The Black Death*, 207.

36. Gigas, *Hermanni Gygantis*, 207.

37. Samuel K. Cohn, "The Black Death and the Burning of Jews," *Past & Present* 196, no. 1 (August 2007): 3–36.

38. Aberth, *The Black Death*, 15.

39. Gabriele de' Mussis, *Historia de Morbo*, in Horrox, *The Black Death*, 19.

40. Mark Wheelis, "Biological Warfare at the 1346 Siege of Caffa," *Emerging Infectious Diseases* 8, no. 9 (September 2002): 971–974, accessed September 2, 2017, https://wwwnc.cdc.gov/eid/article/8/9/pdfs/01-0536.pdf.

41. de' Mussis, *Historia de Morbo*, 20.

42. Boccaccio, *Decameron*, 30.

43. Bill Gilbert, "The Italian City-States of the Renaissance," accessed September 2, 2017, http://vlib.iue.it/carrie/texts/carrie_books/gilbert/03.html.

44. Rudolf Higden, "Polychronicon," in Horrox, *The Black Death*, 62.

45. Antonia Gransden, ed., "A Fourteenth-Century Chronicle from the Grey Friars Lynn," *English Historical Review* 72 (1957): 274.

46. F. S. Haydon, ed., *Eulogium Historiarum sive Temporis*, Vol. 3 (London: Longman, Green, Longman and Roberts, 1863): 213–214.

47. Haydon, *Eulogium Historiarum*, 214.

48. John Aberth, for example, is a proponent of this death toll (Abert, *The First Horseman*; and Aberth, *The Black Death*).

49. Campbell, "Physical Shocks," 13.

50. Campbell, "Physical Shocks," 13–15; and Christian Pfister, Rudolf Brazdul, and Mariano Barriendos, "Reconstructing Past Climate and Natural Disasters in Europe Using Documentary Evidence," *PAGES Past Global Changes News* 10, no. 3 (December 2002): 7.

51. Campbell, "Physical Shocks," 14.

52. Jonathan Sumption, *The Hundred Years War I: Trial by Battle* (Philadelphia: University of Pennsylvania Press, 1990), 103–112.

53. David Nicholas, *Medieval Flanders* (London: Longman, 1992); David Nicholas, *Town and Countryside: Social, Economic, and Political Tensions in Fourteenth-Century Flanders* (Brugge: De Tempel, 1971); and John H. A. Munro, *Wool, Cloth, and Gold: The Struggle for Bullion in Anglo-Burgundian Trade, 1340–1478* (Toronto: The University of Toronto Press, 1972).

54. Sumption, *The Hundred Years War I*, 260–265.

55. For example, see *Calendar of Close Rolls (CCR), 1339–1341*, 11; and Ephraim Russell, "The Societies of the Bardi and the Peruzzi and Their Dealings with Edward III," in *Finance and Trade under Edward III*, ed. George Unwin (Manchester, UK: Manchester University Press, 1918), 93–135.

56. Henry Knighton, *Knighton's Chronicle*, ed. and trans. G. H. Martin (Oxford: Clarendon Press, 1995), 6.

57. Edward's credit was so dismal that most of those to whom he owed money refused commodities for payment and insisted on the discharge of his debts with cash.

58. Andrew Ayton, "The English Army at Crécy," in *The Battle of Crécy, 1346*, eds. Andrew Ayton and Philip Preston (Rochester, NY: Boydell & Brewer, Ltd., 2005), 189; Craig L. Lambert, *Shipping the Medieval Military: English Maritime Logistics in the Fourteenth Century* (Rochester, NY: The Boydell Press, 2011), 139; Craig L. Lambert, "Taking the War to Scotland and France: The Supply and Transportation of English Armies by Sea, 1320–60" (PhD diss., University of Hull, 2009), 207; James Field Willard, *Parliamentary Taxes on Personal Property 1290 to 1334* (Cambridge, MA: The Medieval Academy of America, 1934), 5–6; and Russell, "The Societies of the Bardi and the Peruzzi," 129–131.

59. For the best analysis of how the English government gathered soldiers, consult H. J. Hewitt, *The Organization of War under Edward III* (Manchester, UK: Manchester University Press, 1966).

60. Bertrand Schnerb, "Vassals, Allies and Mercenaries: The French Army before and after 1346," in Ayton and Preston, *The Battle of Crécy*, 265.

61. Schnerb, "Vassals, Allies and Mercenaries," 266.

62. Andrew Ayton, "The English Army at Crécy," 423.

63. Françoise Autrand, "The Battle of Crecy: A Hard Blow for the Monarchy of France," in Ayton and Preston, *The Battle of Crécy*, 274.

64. Autrand, "The Battle of Crecy," 277–281.

65. Ole J. Benedictow, *The Black Death 1346–1353: A Complete History* (Woodbridge, Suffolk: Boydell Press, 2004), 96.

66. Ziegler, *The Black Death*, 67.

67. Benedictow, *The Black Death 1346–1353*, 97–107.

68. Benedictow, *The Black Death 1346–1353*, 337. Because France was so heavily populated at the time, it was easier for the plague to spread; therefore, the percentage of those killed was likely higher than in other regions.

69. Autrand, "The Battle of Crecy," 280–281.

70. W. Mark Ormrod, "The English Government and the Black Death of 1348–49," in *England in the Fourteenth Century: Proceedings of the 1985 Harlaxton Symposium*, ed. W. Mark Ormrod (Rochester, NY: Boydell Press, 1986), 175; and W. Mark Ormrod, *Edward III* (New Haven, CT: Yale University Press, 2011), 323–324.

71. Karl Sudhoff, "Pestschriften aus den ersten 150 Jahren nach der Epidemie des 'schwarzen Todes' 1348." *Archiv für Geschichte der Medizin (AGM)* 5 (1912): 47.

72. Ormrod, "The English Government," 175–177.

73. Ormrod, "The English Government," 177–178.

74. David Farmer, "Prices and Wages, 1041–1350," in *The Agrarian History of England and Wales*, Vol. 2: *1042–1350*, ed. Joan Thirsk (Cambridge: Cambridge University Press, 1988), 734; and David Farmer, "Prices and Wages, 1350–1500" in *The Agrarian History of England and Wales*, Vol. 3: 1350–1500, ed. Edward Miller (Cambridge: Cambridge University Press, 1988), 444.

75. William Henry Beveridge, "Prices and Wages, 1100–1800," Vol. 1 (London: Longmans Green & Co., 1939), 248; and Farmer, "Prices and Wages," Vol. 3, 457.

76. Robert C. Palmer, *English Law in the Age of the Black Death* (Chapel Hill: University of North Carolina Press, 2001), 5.

77. Ormrod, "The English Government," 178–179.

78. Barbara Tuchman, *A Distant Mirror: The Calamitous 14th Century* (New York: Ballantine Press, 1978).

79. Ormrod, *Edward III*, 324, 327.

80. Ormrod, *Edward III*, 327.

81. Ormrod, *Edward III*, 369.

82. Munro, *Wool, Cloth, and Gold*, 35.

83. W. Mark Ormrod, "The Protecolla Rolls and English Government Finance, 1353–1364," *English Historical Review* 102, no. 404 (July 1987): 622.

84. G. L. Harriss, "Budgeting at the Medieval Exchequer," in *War, Government and Aristocracy in the British Isles, c. 1150–1500: Essays in Honour of Michael Prestwich*, ed. Chris Given-Wilson, Ann Kettle, and Len Scales (Rochester, NY: The Boydell Press, 2008), 179–196; and Ormrod, "The Protecolla Rolls," 627.

85. James H. Ramsay, *A History of the Revenues of the Kings of England 1066–1399*, Vol. 2 (Oxford: Clarendon Press, 1925), 292.

86. Ormrod, *Edward III*, 369.

87. W. Mark Ormrod, "The English Crown and the Customs, 1349–63," *EcHR*, New Series 40, no. 1 (February 1987), 29.

88. Ormrod, "The English Crown," 28–29. After a high yield due to the resumption of trade in 1351, the revenue jump in 1352 is likely due to the increase in efficiency from this reform alone.

89. Ormrod, "The English Crown"; and Ramsay, *A History of the Revenues*, 292.

90. T. F. Tout, *Chapters in Administrative History*, Vol. 4 (Manchester, UK: Manchester University Press, 1928), 111–112.

91. R. A. Brown and H. M. Colvin, "The King's Works 1272–1485," in *The History of the King's Works*, Vol. 1, ed. H. M. Colvin (London: Her Majesty's Stationary Office, 1963), 228; and H. M. Colvin, "Calais," in, *The History of the King's Works*, Vol. 1 (1963), 431; Harriss, "Budgeting at the Medieval Exchequer," 330.

92. Ormrod, *Edward III*, 342.

93. Neil Murphy, *The Captivity of John II, 1356–60: The Royal Image in Later Medieval England and France* (New York: Palgrave MacMillan, 2016), 12.

94. Jonathan Sumption, *The Hundred Years War II: Trial by Fire* (Philadelphia: University of Pennsylvania Press, 1999), 294–302, 314–315, 317–337.

95. Ormrod, *Edward III*, 396.

96. Jim Bradbury, *The Medieval Archer* (New York: St. Martin's Press, 1985).

97. National Archives (TNA), E101/393/11, mm. 81, 82d, 84, 85-85d; Lambert, *Shipping the Medieval Military*, 148. For army size, see Andrew Ayton, *Knights and Warhorses: Military Service and the English Aristocracy under Edward III* (Rochester, NY: The Boydell Press, 1994), 268. TNA, E101/393/11, m.115d.

98. Sir Thomas Gray, "Scalacronica 1271–1363," in *The Publications of the Surtees Society*, vol. 209, ed. and trans. Andy King (Rochester, NY: The Boydell Press, 2005), 171; and Lambert, *Shipping the Medieval Military*.

99. Ormrod, *Edward III*, 403.

Chapter 5

Typhus: Napoleon's Tragic Invasion of Russia, the War of 1812

John Jennings White III

If Tchaikovsky wanted to accurately record the sound of Napoleon's defeat, one would only hear the soft, quiet sound of lice munching on human flesh.[1]
—Joe Knight

In 2001, construction workers in Vilnius uncovered what appeared to be a mass grave, with thousands of bodies, under an old Soviet KGB barracks. It was at first assumed that the construction crews had uncovered a pit holding the bodies of KGB victims or even casualties from the Nazi extermination squads of World War II. It was not until they discovered regimental buttons and French brocade that they realized the bodies were remains from Napoleon's Grande Armée that had invaded Russia in 1812. Through forensic analysis and a sampling of nitrogen isotopes, the archeologists were able to discern several facts about the bones found in Vilnius. The isotopes helped identify the country and region of origin of the skeletons, their diet, and what had caused their deaths. In this instance, archeologists found the skeletons had extremely high traces of nitrogen, almost as if their bodies had lacked the proteins needed to survive. Archeologists surmised that more than a quarter of the 3,000 soldiers had perished from louse-borne typhus, an illness that increases the loss of bodily fluids through urine, sweat, and diarrhea.

With their source unknown, illnesses such as typhus forced generals to take into account casualties from a variety of infections and diseases as part of the attrition expected on extended campaigns. Still debated is how a small bacterium took down the Grande Armée, the largest military force the world had seen up to that point. To find the answer, one needs to explore the infection, the symptoms, and the diffusion of typhus. The influence of the infection on past conflicts also provides insights into the effects of typhus on the disastrous Napoleonic invasion of Russia.

Understanding the Bacteria That Causes Typhus

Typhus fever comes from the Greek word *typhos*, which means a "stupor caused by fever."[2] The literal translation for the word is "smoke." Both translations of the word are extremely appropriate when describing epidemic typhus. Typhus also has many names, such as jail fever, spotted fever, and camp fever. The title "typhus" was first used in its modern sense in 1760; this originally described any fever that was characterized by a stupor. It was not until 1829 that doctors were able to tell the difference between typhus fever and typhoid fever, and it was not until 1916 that the bacteria *Rickettsia prowazekii* was identified as the causal agent of typhus. There are different strains of the *Rickettsia* microbe responsible for the infection. These strains cause different versions of the typhus infection, such as spotted fever and scrub typhus. The strain that is the focus of the Napoleonic Wars is *Rickettsia prowazekii*, which is carried by, but not limited to, the human body louse. Ticks as well as the ectoparasites that live on the flying squirrel can also serve as delivery methods for the infection.[3]

The cause of typhus fever results from a human host coming into contact under appropriate conditions with a parasite that has been infected with a strain of a bacillus bacterium from a rickettsial microbial. The transfer of disease from infected host to louse occurs through the sucking of the host's blood. Subsequent contamination of a noninfected human from the louse occurs from louse fecal matter entering the bloodstream via its human host scratching at lice or through an open wound.

Symptoms of Typhus Fever

Once the host is infected, the disease usually has an incubation period that generally lasts one to two weeks. After the incubation period, the onset of symptoms is very quick. General symptoms include chills, fever, and severe headache. The headache is usually generalized, intense, and without any respite. Because of the fever, the patient also becomes severely dehydrated. Toward the end of the first week after the incubation period, the patient experiences a rash of small pink macules, which typically first appear on the upper torso. This rash then spreads to rapidly cover the torso, and it finally spreads to the hands and feet. These macules become darker over time and then become maculopapular.[4] This swelling or rising of the rash is one of the unique peculiarities of the illness. Another characteristic of the disease is an extremely high fever, sometimes as high as 105 degrees Fahrenheit. An additional physical characteristic includes bloodshot eyes and generally marks the beginning of the infection.

These are the overt physical symptoms of the disease; what lies under the skin is far more sinister and deadly. Once the infection enters the bloodstream, it begins to attack the cells that line the small arteries and veins. These cells are the endothelial cells, which cover the surface of the insides of the blood vessels and lymphatic vessels, called the *endothelium*. The endothelium is what provides a connection between either blood circulating through vessels or lymph through the lumen. The infection attacks these cells in the smaller veins of the skin, lungs, brain, and gastrointestinal tract. The rickettsial microbes attach to the endothelial cells, causing the cells to grow in mass and swell. This causes the infected blood vessels to become blocked. The blocked blood vessels eventually rupture, causing the infection to spread and kill off more cells in the body. The resulting attempts of the immune system to prevent infection inadvertently cause more damage to the body by trying to fight off the infection. The rupturing of cells and blocking of blood flow, if not addressed, results in gangrene that starts at the extremities, toes, fingers, ear lobes, nose, and genitals. Gangrene is common for typhus infection in extreme cases. In addition to the potential for gangrene, typhus produces lesions to the brain that cause the patient to go into a stupor. Patients can also become delirious, begin to hallucinate, gain sensitivity to light, and become easily excitable.[5]

Simultaneous to the blood vessels swelling and the rash becoming maculopapular, the patient begins to vomit, causing further dehydration. Loss of appetite follows, along with constipation, insomnia, and the tongue drying out. Once the vessels in the lungs are infected, the patient develops a cough, and pneumonia often sets in. The final blow is dealt by renal and vascular system failures, which are often accompanied by coma. The final stages of the disease occur between the second and third weeks of the infection. For those patients who recover from the fever after the first week, a full recovery still takes about two to three months, during which time the soldier is incapable of keeping up with the demands of a military campaign. The rash disappears with recovery and does not leave any scarring. However, those who contract typhus fever often experience mild relapses of the disease, further incapacitating their military service. This recurrence is called Brill-Zinsser disease. Although not fatal, this reappearance of typhus can cause the patient to become a carrier for the fever while in relapse.[6]

Diffusion and Disease Vectors for Typhus

What truly made typhus such a devastating infection to armies of bygone eras was that human beings are the breeding ground for the disease's vectors. Typhus was usually spread by small insects, fleas, ticks, mites, and body lice that had fed on the blood of other organisms that were infected with the *Rickettsia* microbes.[7] Usually, the point of infection was a bite that was scratched or massaged by the host, thereby spreading the infection into the bloodstream. In the past, armies were for the most part considered a great unwashed horde. They made camps in crowded conditions, and multiple soldiers often shared a shelter or tent; a bedding of straw only made matters worse.

By itself, the common body louse is not a very capable method of infection. The common body louse cannot fly; it has no wings and so is limited to a crawl. However, common soldiery on a campaign rarely practiced proper hygiene; not bathing and not changing uniforms for days, weeks, or even months were the norm. Conditions were made especially worse in winter, when it was even more difficult to bathe and the close proximity for sleeping was encouraged to maintain warmth. This lack of hygiene and the closeness allowed infected lice to spread by moving between hosts' bodies and their clothes, especially in colder climates.

The French Grande Armée, approximately 600,000 men and about 50,000 camp followers of every range and walk of life, traveled the route to Russia for

Napoleon's invasion of 1812. As the journey progressed across Europe, tents were discarded as being too much for the baggage train to carry. Without proper shelters, soldiers were forced to bivouac in the open or sleep in houses with civilians as they marched from town to town.[8] Thus, people huddled together in the wet and cold and shared far more than just warmth. Constantly moving lice prompted their human hosts to scratch with irritation. This response infected the host and simultaneously caused the lice to move from location to location, on the same body or from one host to another. The common body louse was also extremely sensitive to temperature and constantly sought warmth. Once a host died, the louse quickly left the cadaver in search of a new host, and the cycle of infection continued. Army field hospitals, when available, became ideal breeding grounds for the common body louse.

The presence of lice did not ensure the conveyance of typhus infection in human hosts, even if the louse was infected. The other component to disease susceptibility was malnourishment. During Napoleon's march into Russia, the size of the campaign made it impossible to ensure enough supplies, especially as the distance lengthened between Napoleonic-controlled Europe and the invasion forces. Additionally, the Russians practiced a scorched-earth policy, destroying provisions that might be used to feed the invading forces. Napoleon's military resorted to living off the land and local populations, but such a strategy did not provide the amount of food necessary for the men and camp followers. The standard for rations was 24 ounces of wheat bread, one pound of meat, and usually a pint of wine or even two pints of beer daily. However, during the invasion, spirits were often reserved for when the meat was less than fresh. Cavalrymen, considered the elite forces, were given more food as a general rule. In many cases, officers sold rations to the men at a greater price than the soldiers could afford.[9] These combined factors left the invading French forces poorly fed and in ill health.

Beyond malnourishment, general health standards and hygiene conditions affected the ability of the human host to fight off the contagion. The standing militaries in Europe started to see some reforms in food rationing, clothing, and medical care in the late 18th century. Doctors and surgeons, along with their assistants, were imbedded within regiments to care for the wounded and the ill. Also, part of the regimental surgeon's job was to look out for the soldiers' physical well-being and hygiene. Yet, outside of accompanying medical officers and assistants, the Napoleonic forces lacked the other structural reforms necessary to protect the health of its soldiers. Long after the 1812 invasion, even into the 1860s and beyond, soldiers resorted to foraging or stealing to provide food during campaigns into enemy territory.[10]

History of Typhus in Wars of the Past

It is not surprising that one disease consistently associated with war is typhus. Some historians have even considered it as a "siege disease" because it creeps up in areas that are depleted of provisions but rife with sickness and death. Sieges are especially brutal operations that militaries perform from time to time, and they usually involve all of the necessary conditions for the spread of disease and illness. The instances where typhus fever shows up in conjunction with military sieges and invasions are usually costly in terms of both fighting men and civilians. Because the discovery of the bacterium that causes typhus was still 17 years beyond the French invasion into Russia, there are few records available that use the term *typhus fever*. Instead, most of the historical references by doctors and assistants utilize the reported symptoms to determine the diseases presence.

Early records show that the disease was probably present at the siege of Belgrade in 1456. There, the Hungarian army, under the command of John Hunyadi, was able to defeat the army of Mohammed the Second. The Turkish army that followed Mohammed the Second possibly carried typhus with them from Anatolia. Following the siege, a plague descended on Belgrade shortly after the Muslims were driven off, killing many Hungarians, including King Hunyadi.

In 1489, with the siege of Granada in Spain, the Spanish lost more than a third of their main fighting forces to a mysterious malady whose symptoms strongly resemble typhus. Some figures put their casualties in the range of 17,000. This created a major problem because siege doctrine recommended that attacking forces outnumber their foes by a ratio of three to one. Seriously depleted in numbers by the epidemic, those that did not die of the disease fled, only to spread the contagion to the remainder of Spain. The Spanish were eventually able to fill their ranks and conquer the city of Granada, but they were not able to force the Muslims from Spain until January 1492. Despite the Spanish victory, the reconquest of Spain was delayed for four years by typhus fever, or "El Tabarillo," as the Spanish called it. In the process of retaking the peninsula, they lost almost a third of their total fighting strength to illness. The Spaniards believed that mercenary soldiers probably brought the disease into their ranks from Cyprus. The physician Hans Zinsser correlated this conjecture to the evidence available at the time. His records provided historians with the first documentation of typhus fever as a recognizable disease rather than just a general plague in European history.[11]

The next time typhus showed up in military history was in the 1529 siege of Naples during the Italian Wars, or Renaissance Wars. The Renaissance Wars were a series of conflicts that started in 1492 and continued off and on until 1559. For his part, Holy Roman Emperor Charles V (Charles I of Spain) was victorious for the majority of the conflicts in Italy. The siege of Naples started in 1527 with the sack of Rome by Charles V. With the removal of Pope Clement the VII, the French signed the treaty of Westminster with the English to join the League of Cognac against Spain. Thus, the French renewed attacks into Italy, placing Charles V in a real bind, contending simultaneously with the French, the English, the Vatican, the Duchy of Milan and the Republics of Venice and Florence. By 1527, the League of Cognac had destroyed the Spanish navy, and the French had surrounded the Spanish army in Naples, laying siege to the city and kingdom with 35,000 soldiers. After a month of laying siege to Naples, almost three-quarters of the French forces had perished from typhus. Taking advantage of the depletion of enemy siege forces, the Spanish routed the French and destroyed them. The defeat of the French forces at Naples combined with Francis I's defeat at the Battle of Landriano, thus ending any hope the French had in Italy. In 1529, Francis I sought peace with Spain and signed the treaty of Cambrai. The treaty removed France from the war, in essence defeated, in part, by typhus.[12]

During the Middle Ages, plagues were a constant part of life. For Charles V, the typhus plague saved his forces at the siege of Naples in 1529; yet, in 1552, a plague of similar description turned against his forces. In 1552, Charles V, in an attempt to bring Protestants to heel in Germany and Northern Europe, laid siege to the town of Metz with a force of 220,000 fighting men. The opposing force of 6,000 defenders was under the command of the Duke of Guise. The siege size was not the deciding factor in this instance; instead, it was illness that determined the outcome. Extremely outnumbered, the Duke of Guise made a constant effort during the siege to keep his men healthy and to prevent the outbreak of disease that often depleted military ranks during this period in history. He made sure the men were properly fed, and physicians were hired to oversee the distribution and ensure the quality of rations provided. Waste was disposed of over the city walls. Special groups of soldiers, called pioneers, were created to sweep the streets of the city. Water was constantly under guard and checked to make sure it was not poisoned or brackish. Finally, not one person was allowed to eat meat from wild game out of a fear that it could be tainted. Guise was rewarded with disease-free forces during his defense. Meanwhile, Charles V's large force was compelled to live off the land. Unable to maintain any level of hygiene or sanitary water under siege conditions, he lost 26,000 men to typhus and other illnesses.[13]

During the Thirty Years' War, typhus, in concert with plague and malnutrition, killed about 10 million people from 1618 to 1648. By comparison, about 350,000 men died in combat. Historians have concluded that most of the damage caused by typhus occurred before 1632. It was in 1632 that typhus accidentally prevented a battle from occurring near Nuremburg, Germany. The armies under King Gustav Adolphus of Sweden and Baron von Wallenstein met at Nuremburg. Von Wallenstein laid siege to the city, trapping the Swedish army inside. However, typhus broke out in both armies, killing around 18,000 men. After 11 weeks, both forces withdrew from Nuremburg. The battle had no other real significance to the Thirty Years' War except to show that typhus was truly an indiscriminate killer.[14]

A hundred years after Napoleon's failed invasion of France, typhus appeared once again during World War I, primarily on the Eastern and Balkan Fronts. The Serbians had suffered deaths at epidemic levels by the second year of the war. Large numbers of troops succumbed to typhus, with figures varying from 150,000 to 200,000. Another 30,000 Austro-Hungarian prisoners died of typhus in Serbian prison camps. This epidemic was in large part due to the swarm of refugees that had headed to the southern part of Serbia in advance of the Austro-Hungarian army's offensive. Of the 400 physicians and doctors that practiced in Serbia, 126 of them perished while trying to treat patients. The epidemic was so bad that the Austrian forces, which had been pushed out of Serbia by an earlier Serbian counteroffensive, refused to move back into the country once the epidemic began, despite being reinforced by the German military.

The Germans, too, made no move to enter Serbia, despite strategic goals to secure the oil fields of Ploesti and obtain supplies from Russia. It took six months for the epidemic to abate. The delay slowed the German advance into Russia, which in turn delayed Germany's ability to force Russia to accept a peace agreement. Exposed to typhus by outbreaks of the disease among their Russian foes, the German's eventual withdrawal from the Eastern Front became a drawn-out process because of the need to delouse soldiers before sending them to the Western Front to defend against the new Allied push of 1917–1918. Consequently, German reinforcements took too long to arrive and failed to shore up the Western Front against the Allies.[15]

During World War II, the city of Naples again saw an epidemic of typhus begin to spread. The German commander Albert Kesselring decided to land at Salerno and Taranto to create a defensive south of Rome. He abandoned everything south of the Volturno River and established two defensive lines, Volturno and Barbara. The city of Naples had been abandoned and ransacked by the retreating Germans. Allied bombing raids furthered the destruction to the city. The citizens of Naples were forced to live in bomb shelters. The crowded and unsanitary conditions in the shelters provided the perfect breeding ground for the infected lice. By January of 1944, at least 700 citizens had fallen victim to typhus. When the Allies occupied the city, they immediately focused on treating the illness with newly developed techniques. This was the first time that typhus was stopped in the middle of a winter campaign.

Napoleon's 1812 Invasion into Russia

In the 18th century, typhus was already the bane of human existence for militaries. When the Napoleonic Wars began, the louse-born infection was already a reality of war that soldiers accepted as a part of everyday life. In 1812, Emperor Napoleon Bonaparte I set out on a course to restore France to its former glory by invading Russia. The main objective was to pass through Russia and then swing south into Asia Minor. Napoleon's ultimate objective was to defeat the Russians and, if possible, wrest control of the British Empire's crown jewel, India.

Napoleon undertook this venture against the advice of his most trusted aides and generals. He believed the Grande Armée was impervious to anything that Russia or Europe could put in its way. Napoleon was warned that his forces were not equipped properly for the Russian winter and should delay the planned invasion until the following spring. Furthermore, to accomplish the task, the Grande Armée had to defeat the Russians under General Mikhail Kutuzov with an army of about 800,000 soldiers. That estimate did not include the approximately 500,000 garrisoned forces and partisans that constantly threatened Napoleon's perimeters.

Napoleon understood that this undertaking required some preventative measures to ensure that his men survived the invasion march into Russia. He established field hospitals in Germany to receive wounded from the campaign. He set about issuing edicts and orders to preserve cleanliness as well as to maintain the overall effectiveness of his combat formations. Despite the measures taken by the emperor, medicine had made only limited progress by this time. Doctors still practiced the theory of disease caused by humors, proposed and taught by Hippocrates in the fifth century BCE.[16] If one of these humors became imbalanced, through poor diet or exhaustion, then the host became ill. To add to the problems of limited medical knowledge of the time, there were a multitude of superstitious and unproven theories imbedded with this outdated humor doctrine. Doctors had developed prescriptions of leeching, cupping, and bleeding. While some proved useful, others were barbaric and exacerbated injuries and illnesses. Physical injuries, like those from sabers or bullets, were painful, but patients often survived as long as the wounds were cleaned properly.[17] In the environment of Napoleon's invasion into Russia and the ensuing flight back to Europe, such cleanliness was not to be found.

Napoleon started the campaign of 1812 with anywhere from 400,000 to 600,000 soldiers in his Grande Armée. The numbers vary because they are based on the accounts of various French officials. The chief surgeon, Dominique Jean Larrey, reported an army of 400,000, while Napoleon's personal aide, the Duke of Vicenza, reported that the emperor had marched into Russia with 500,000 soldiers at his command. Historical records estimate close to 600,000 combined forces by the time the Grande Armée reached Russia. Regardless of the number, problems began for Napoleon almost immediately. When the Grande Armée crossed the Niemen River into Poland, the French supply train broke down and subsequently fell behind the main body of the army. This forced soldiers to start foraging for supplies and even raiding for food, which inevitably brought them into contact with the Polish population. By this time, Poland was already dealing with an epidemic of typhus. Foraging soldiers returned to camp with body lice and typhus.

In June, the army already showed signs of illness. By the time the army reached Vilna, around 5,000 soldiers a day were being lost to disease. Soldiers fell out of formation, unable to keep up with the pace of the main force. The nunnery and monasteries in Vilna were converted into hospitals for the sick and dying. Close to 30,000 ailing soldiers were crammed into every available space. By the first of August, dysentery affected another 80,000 soldiers and caused the hospitals to run out of the supplies needed to keep the men clean. Furthermore, another 30,000 soldiers had deserted. All told, by the time Napoleon reached Vilna, he had lost almost 25 percent of his total fighting force.

Yet, Napoleon continued onward into Russia. The descriptions of what the French soldiers met on the road to Moscow can only be described as the living embodiment of the nine circles of hell described by Dante Alighieri in his book *Inferno*. Soldiers were drenched in rain. French field guns had to be dragged through the mud. Bloated corpses of dead horses lined the roads where they had fallen from eating unripe grain. Later, men who fell out of formation due to exhaustion or disease were left to die. However, none of these sights matched the horrors yet to come on the march out of Russia. The size of the army and its inability to sustain supply lines caused it to resemble a swarm of locusts as the men desperately sought provisions from the countryside. Whole villages and farms were stripped bare of meat and grain within a matter of hours. Undeterred, Napoleon advanced with his army, even though he was losing men at an alarming rate. Meanwhile, the Russian forces kept drawing the French farther into Russia and away from the army's supply lines.

As the French advanced, the Russians kept retreating, and because of the illness within the Grande Armée, many French commanders were unable to keep the Russians from escaping. One such example occurred in July 1812, when the French engaged the Russians near the Dnieper River in the Battle of Mogilev. Marshal Davout set out to stop the Russian general Bagration from moving farther into Russia toward Smolensk. Davout entered the battle with about 17,000 soldiers, though he had started the campaign with about 70,000. Davout's corps had lost 76 percent of its troops due to disease. This was not only unacceptable; it left the unit ineffective for combat. A few days into August, the Russian armies slipped away from the French at Mogilev and linked up in the town of Smolensk. The French drove the Russians out of Smolensk 16 days later, burning the city in the process.[18] Though considered a French victory, the Russians had again escaped, and the invasion continued.

Riddled with illness, the French set up multiple field hospitals across the city to treat the wounded and the ill. Unfortunately, they made a grievous error. Because of the large number of convalescing soldiers, they were made to lie close together without any food or medical supplies to treat them. Some medical historians have blamed the hospitals for the spread of typhus at this point in the campaign. The doctors forced physically injured soldiers, Russian and French alike, to lie in close proximity to soldiers who were infected with typhus or dysentery, thus spreading the diseases even further among those unable to fight off illnesses.[19] By the time Napoleon left Smolensk, he was under 50 percent of his original fighting strength.

Food supplies at this point were already the lowest yet experienced and getting worse. The stores of Smolensk had burned along with all the medical supplies, leaving nothing for the wounded or the uninjured. To make matters worse, the Russians had taken to using their now famous scorched-earth tactic. As they retreated, they burnt villages and towns to keep supplies out of the hands of the French.[20] The shortages of food continued to plague the Grande Armée the farther it progressed into Russia. The morale of the soldiers was so low that most of Napoleon's army gave up on any attempts at personal hygiene. The lack of food forced the French soldiers to loot and pillage, and their lack of morale and subsequent declining discipline resulted in the rape of the Russian countryside as they continued toward Moscow. The French commissariat was largely ineffectual at keeping the soldiers in line, even though they had orders to prevent looting. By the time the French took the town of Smolensk from the Russians, the supply lines were thin and vulnerable. The sick men deserted in droves, scattering all over Lithuania and Belorussia.[21] This caused even more problems for the French troops, as the Russian peasants began to revolt against the invading French.

Before Napoleon reached Moscow, he had fought the bloodiest battle of the campaign, the Battle of Borodino. Borodino provided another opportunity for typhus to spread even further. The French combat losses were about 28,000 to 30,000, and the Russians lost more men, approximately 44,000. Again, field hospitals were set up, and wounds were treated as best they could; the ill were looked after once the battle injuries were seen. With far more casualties than beds, injured and sick solders were laid upon beds of straw. Lice infested the straw bedding and spread from dead to living hosts, carrying typhus to wounded soldiers. One French soldier recalled his experience at a hospital after being carried from Borodino. What he described can only be compared to a charnel house; corpses were piled indoors, and the sickeningly sweet fragrance of death mixed with the final bodily functions prevailed throughout the hospital.[22]

In September 1812, the Grande Armée marched into Moscow, some shoeless and all hungry from days without food. They were greeted with a city set ablaze by the retreating Russians. Napoleon, in a letter sent to Czar Alexander I, insinuated that it was not his forces but those of the retreating Russians that had started the fires in Moscow.[23] Furthermore, Napoleon had arrived in the city with only 90,000 effective soldiers able to fight, out of an original force of 600,000 from the beginning of the campaign. After the city burned, French soldiers spent days combing the city for anything of value, fighting with each other, or pillaging. Meanwhile, Napoleon hoped that the loss of Moscow would provoke the Russian people to revolt against Czar Alexander and force Russia to surrender.

Ironically, while in Moscow, Napoleon spent his time reading about Charles XII of Sweden and his equally disastrous invasion of Russia in 1708. Charles XII had decided to winter in the Ukraine and lost the majority of his army to cold, hunger, and sickness. It was reportedly so cold that elk were found frozen to death standing up. Consequently, Charles XII's army was destroyed after the winter, and he was forced to flee to Turkey. He lived there for about five years before signing a peace with Russia.[24]

The lessons of the past were lost upon Napoleon; he continued to wait for Czar Alexander to make a move as winter rapidly approached. The Russians used this time to reinforce and reorganize. It was after the French defeat at the Battle of Tarutino that Napoleon decided to retreat from Russia. By this time, his forces had been reduced to a little over 75,000 soldiers. On the march out of Russia, French soldiers discarded their muskets to carry more loot. Upon their return to Borodino, they found the field littered with armor, weapons, and about 30,000 half-eaten corpses gnawed by wolves.[25] Meanwhile, peasant partisans placed a bounty on the heads of French soldiers. The Frenchmen, fearful of angry Russian peasants and Cossacks, avoided traveling in small groups.

Sick and wounded soldiers were carried in heavy carts. The cart drivers often passed over rough terrain to try to dump the ill and injured in the back of the cart onto the road to lighten the load for the journey home. Those who fell were often left to die on the side of the road. Once back in Smolensk, Napoleon lost even more of his army. Ailing and wounded soldiers unsuccessfully sought beds in the overcrowded hospitals, so large numbers ended up frozen to death in the streets.[26]

Napoleon abandoned the army in December 1812. In the same month, Marshal Kutuzov arrived in Vilna to find frozen corpses littering the ground or hanging from burnt trees. Typhus-ridden men drifted through the streets, seeking shelter, food, and warmth, only to die in the doorways of Russian citizens. The Russians had the Imperial Guard artillery transport many of the cadavers to the city walls to await burial or burning later, once the ground had thawed out from the winter. It was reported that almost half of the men assigned to this duty also contracted typhus. The Russian hospitals were like scenes from a horror film. Czar Alexander reported one scene, where corpses had been stacked as a high as the walls of a vaulted room.[27]

By the time Napoleon's retreating army arrived back in France, only 3,000 men of the original 600,000 soldiers had survived the long trek into and out of Russia. Had it not been for the efforts of the Imperial Guard, it is likely that the Grande Armée may not have made it out of Russia at all. As a final insult, the French army brought typhus out of Russia with them, spreading it across much of the rest of Europe. In Germany, civilians were afraid to house soldiers for fear of catching typhus. When the disease spread, German doctors confined patients to an isolated section of the hospital. However, these facilities had to be cleaned and disinfected daily, and doctors wore special cloaks and washed after leaving the isolated areas. The Russians claimed they had to bury or dispose of approximately 250,000 bodies that had perished from the disease. Typhus and cold weather had utterly destroyed the French army as well as its myth of invincibility. Furthermore, the typhus-ridden army had left a lasting mark on Europe, killing whole swathes of people by disease. The total losses for the Russian campaign have been estimated in the millions for the French, French allies, Russians, and civilians.

The loss of his army in Russia forced Napoleon to recruit and quickly train an entirely new army. To do that, he was forced to turn to the nobility to fill the ranks. This strategy did not bode well for the emperor. While Napoleon was able to raise another army before the Battle of Leipzig in 1813, the men were new recruits that lacked the strength and ability of the army that had been lost to typhus and the Russian winter. Because of this, Napoleon was unable to match the numbers of the Sixth Coalition that opposed him at Leipzig. Prussia was emboldened and joined an alliance with Russia. The allies Napoleon had previously depended on for support abandoned and turned on him, joining the coalition forces. So, in 1814, Paris fell, and Napoleon abdicated in favor of the Bourbon line. Ultimately, his defeat in Russia led to the downfall of the French Empire and his initial banishment to Elba.

Lessons Learned?

Napoleon's failed offensive into Russia served as a cautionary tale for future military commanders. It forced officers to consider the cost of foraging for food, the effect of weather on morale, and, further, the effect of morale upon field hygiene. However, it did not deter Hitler from making the same mistake in 1941, more than a hundred years later. Medicine has greatly improved since the Napoleonic Wars;

yet to this day, commanders must practice proper field sanitation to prevent the spread of disease. Prepackaged field rations cut down on the likelihood of dysentery, properly dug latrines help deter typhoid, and bathing allows soldiers to operate in the field with less fear of typhus. Operating in the field is stressful enough without adding the presence of disease to the situation.

It is argued that one of the many reasons for the failed Russian invasion was that Napoleon's subordinates misinformed him regarding the condition of his army. This was due to the fear of the punishments Napoleon handed out to subordinates that he found lacking. Others argue that the emperor was not in his right mind. One incident that has been considered to corroborate this theory occurred as Napoleon traveled back to Paris with his aide, the Duke of Vicenza, Armand-Augustin-Louis de Caulaincourt. In his recollections, the Duke of Vicenza reported that Napoleon was never afraid of what might happen to him, nor was he worried about his ability to turn this massive defeat into a future victory.[28] Larrey believed Napoleon saw himself as the liberator, the conquering hero of legend.[29] Adding to the rationales for the failed offense was knowledge that the emperor often failed to take advice from others around him. Many aides and confidants had argued that entering Russia was vainglorious and did not further the agenda of the empire; nonetheless, the campaign took place.

Combined Impact of War and Typhus on Napoleon's Invasion

Whatever Napoleon's mental state, the results of the gamble speak for themselves. For the majority of the campaign, the Russian army eluded the French, who tired themselves out in the pursuit of a fixed battle. In the end, the combination of harsh weather, the elusive Russians, the Pyrrhic victory at Borodino, and the lack of supplies all worked against the Grande Armée. Morale was eroded, and coupled with the constant pressure to advance, the hygiene of the army was abandoned along with men and camp followers ailing from injuries, exhaustion, and disease. In the memoirs of the chief surgeon, Baron Larrey, it was revealed that exposure to the cold and wet, as well as drinking pillaged liquor, resulted in the loss of more than 500,000 soldiers. At the same time, he recorded the signature symptoms of typhus in the troops. Larrey recognized the stupor, fatigue, delirium, and even the gangrene that signaled a typhus epidemic. Other surgeons of the time also blamed liquor, describing an incident in which three patients died in six hours from ingesting several bottles of liquor.[30] However, it was typhus, transmitted by a small parasite, that put the nails in the coffins of so many Napoleonic soldiers.

The French were not prepared for the Russian winter or Russian tactics of retreat and scorched-earth policies. The seeming success of their advance simultaneously separated them from their own supplies and forced them to live off an increasingly bleak landscape. In scavenging for supplies and seeking the warmth of comrades in the cold, they unwittingly facilitated the movement of lice and, consequently, the spread of typhus. The French were also unprepared for the ferocity and speed of the disease, especially in conditions extremely ideal to the spread of body lice, which moved among the malnourished and unwashed men as they treaded across Europe. In the end, the vast majority of Napoleon's great army fell victim to this tiny combatant as it spread the typhus virus among the once great French military forces.

NOTES

1. Joe Knight, "Napoleon Wasn't Defeated by the Russians," *Health and Science: Pandemics* (December 11, 2012), accessed September 2, 2017, http://www.slate.com/articles /health_and_science/pandemics/2012/12/napoleon_march_to_russia_in_1812_typhus _spread_by_lice_was_more_powerful.html.
2. Douglas Harper, "Typhus," Dictionary.com, Online Etymology Dictionary, accessed September 2, 2017, http://www.etymonline.com.
3. Jennifer McQuiston, "Infectious Diseases Related to Travel," Center for Disease Control and Prevention, accessed September 2, 2017, https://wwwnc.cdc.gov/travel /yellowbook/2016/infectious-diseases-related-to-travel/rickettsial-spotted-typhus -fevers-related-infections-anaplasmosis-ehrlichiosis.
4. William A. Petri, "Epidemic Typhus", *Merck Manual*, accessed September 2, 2017, www.merckmanuals.com/professional/infectious-diseases/rickettsiae-and-related -organisms/epidemic-typhus.
5. Ethne Barnes, *Diseases and Human Evolution* (Albuquerque: University of New Mexico Press, 2007), 254.
6. Barnes, *Diseases and Human Evolution*, 256.
7. Barnes, *Diseases and Human Evolution*, 254.
8. Digby Smith, *An Illustrated Encyclopedia of Uniforms of the Napoleonic Wars* (London: Lorenz Books, 2008), 19.
9. Charles Heizmann, "Military Sanitation in the 16th, 17th, and 18th Centuries," in *Journal of the Military Service Institution of the United States*, eds. William Huskin and James Bush (Governor's Island, NY: Military Service Institution, 1893), 717.
10. Heizmann, "Military Sanitation."
11. Joseph M. Conlon, *The Historical Impact of Epidemic Typhus*, Montana University, accessed September 2, 2017, www.montana.edu/historybug/documents/TYPHUS-Conlon.pdf.
12. Conlon, *Historical Impact*.
13. Heizmann, "Military Sanitation," 713–717.
14. Hans Zinsser, *Rats, Lice, and History* (Boston: Little, Brown and Company, 1963), 159.
15. Conlon, *Historical Impact*.
16. This early medical doctrine explained that bile, phlegm, and blood were linked and balanced within the body.
17. Louis Alexandre Hippolyte Leroy-Dupre, *Memoir of Baron Larrey: Surgeon-in-Chief of the Grande Armée, from the French* (London: Henry Henshaw, 1861), 111.
18. Stephan Talty, *The Illustrious Dead: The Terrifying Story of How Typhus Killed Napoleon's Greatest Army* (New York: Crown Publishers, 2009), 91.
19. Talty, *The Illustrious Dead*, 91.
20. Talty, *The Illustrious Dead*, 119.
21. Dominic Lieven, *The True Story of the Campaigns of War and Peace: Russia against Napoleon* (New York: Penguin Group, 2010), 170.

22. Rory Muir, *Tactics and the Experience of Battle in the Age of Napoleon* (New Haven, CT: Yale University Press, 1998), 262.

23. David Chandler, *The Campaigns of Napoleon* (New York: The MacMillan Company, 1966), 813.

24. Richard Hilley, *A Compendium of European Geography and History* (London: Spottiswoode and Co., 1870), 102.

25. Chandler, *The Campaigns of Napoleon*, 823.

26. Talty, *The Illustrious Dead*, 233.

27. Lieven, *The True Story*, 286.

28. Eilleaux (Countess) Armand Augustin Louis de Caulaincourt, *Recollections of Caulaincourt, Duke of Vicenza* (London: Henry Colburn Publisher, 1838), 85–86.

29. Leroy-Dupre, *Memoir of Baron Larrey*, 117.

30. Talty, *The Illustrious Dead*, 206.

Chapter 6

Cholera: Dread Disease of the Crimean War, 1854–1855

Rebecca M. Seaman

The Crimean campaign taught a lesson that I trust will never be forgotten by the nation, that unless the medical department of the army is made efficient, and supplied with its proper complement of officers and ambulance during peace, it cannot be expected to do its duty efficiently during war.[1]
—Lt. Col. Ed. M. Wrench

Cholera has a history as a dread disease. Its sudden and horrific impacts on victims caused terror in societies beset by cholera epidemics. The cholera epidemic of the Crimean War is such a case. Competitions of imperializing countries helped spread the disease through the harvesting of natural resources and then in the trade of those same goods. The economic competition among these nations was complicated by political jealousies, religious tensions, and nationalism. Imperial powers that vied for control or influence over the waning Ottoman Empire not only created a disastrous war, but they also helped create the perfect conditions to perpetuate the already spreading cholera pandemic of the 1850s.

The Crimean War's extensive death toll from cholera and other diseases caused public upheaval back home in the imperializing nations and their colonies. The resulting reforms, from the nursing profession to urban sanitation standards, helped improve public health, if not actually eliminate cholera. This chapter examines cholera and its method of spread and impact on humans. It also explores how the Asiatic cholera epidemic made its way from India to various 19th-century imperial countries and specifically how it impacted the Crimean War, where imperial powers competed for growing political and economic influence over the declining Ottoman Empire. Importantly, the lasting impact of reforms in medicine and the nursing professional are examined in the historical context of the time.

Understanding the Historical Origins of the Bacteria *Vibrio cholerae*

Cholera is a disease that is caused by the bacteria *Vibrio cholerae*. One of numerous diarrhea diseases, cholera is particularly virulent, spreading rapidly among previously unexposed populations. The very form of the disease facilitated its spread in the 19th century, as victims experienced a sudden onset of symptoms that usually included extreme, uncontrollable diarrhea and vomiting. The suddenness and the watery uncontrolled excrement contaminated clothing, bedding, water supplies, food, and the entire surrounding environment. During this century, when sanitation features were either nonexistent or overwhelmed by the ballooning populations in industrial societies and their associated colonial cities, the waste of society quickly spread into public cesspits, polluted streets, flowed into rivers, and seeped into aquifers and wells. Unbeknownst to the people of the era, *V. cholera* spread with the waste, infecting people from all walks of life.

The disease has historically been referred to by two names: European cholera and Asiatic cholera. The former is a reference to diarrheic diseases, including dysentery, that had been common to Europe for centuries. While references to European cholera were mistakenly associated with the more severe Asiatic cholera by J. McPherson in his 1872 work, *Annals of Cholera from the Earliest Period to the Year 1817*, later historians perpetuated this confusion in their own works.[2] Asiatic cholera references a bacterial infection that causes sudden and devastating diarrhea, vomiting, dehydration, and often death. It is this disease that is the focus of this chapter.

Historically, Asiatic cholera was found in the tidal waters of the Bay of Bengal and the brackish waters that reached inland. Largely unpopulated until the influences of British imperialism compelled indigenous peoples to relocate for purposes of harvesting desired timbers and planting cash crops, the riverine and delta regions of the Indian subcontinent were the primary locations of initial localized outbreaks. With few people exposed to the bacteria, cholera rarely reached the contagious level to even be classified as a local epidemic. This changed in 1817 with the increased peopling of the region, allowing for the bacteria[3] to spillover from its natural host of the copepods in the brackish waters to human hosts. Within 50 years, the region went from unpopulated wetlands with mangrove forests and mudflats to almost 800 square miles of deforested farmland and colonial settlements.

The spillover process included the shift in *V. cholerae* to produce toxins that attacked host systems. The bacteria lodged itself in the intestines of its human hosts and produced toxins to purge the intestines of competing bacteria, resulting in the intestines reversing their natural processes of absorbing fluids to instead extracting fluids from the body.[4] Called "the Purge" by many societies because of the rapid onset of related symptoms, Asiatic cholera quickly spread among large populations without previous exposure. The warm, humid climate of the Bay of Bengal, with its monsoonal conditions and poor drainage, facilitated the spread of the disease, as watery human excrement contaminated the rivers and groundwater. But the epidemic remained largely endemic to the Indian subcontinent until the 19th century, when trade, transportation, and wars transferred it to surrounding regions and even to the imperializing countries that had inadvertently caused the emergence of the disease in the first place.[5]

Context of Cholera Epidemics during a Period of Imperialistic Competition

Many epidemic diseases have ancient pasts, typically erupting in overpopulated regions, precipitated by periods of upheaval, and then spread through wars and trade. The perception emerged that traumatic epidemic diseases were no longer threats to societies as scientific discoveries occurred and treatments and cures were postulated. Nothing could be further from the truth. Scientific advances also impacted the rise of industries, increased the number of inventions, and encouraged rapid urbanization as new commercial opportunities outpaced the economic investments of agricultural ventures. People, left underemployed or landless from declining agriculture opportunities, heeded the calls of cities with their promise of employment and adventure. This prompted migration patterns that have continued to current times. The industrial revolution also improved the means of transportation for goods and people, thereby creating a means for transporting bacterial diseases such as cholera at rates that ensured its spread from a regional epidemic to a continental and transcontinental pandemic.[6]

Hopes of opportunities and consistent improvements in new industrial regions such as Europe and America were dashed as the overpopulated and industrialized urban areas failed to keep pace with the escalating needs of shelter, food, and sanitation.[7] Single-family homes were converted into tenement housing. Sanitation systems were rudimentary and often composed of privies out back and the dumping of "night soil"[8] into streets and cesspits. The cities smelled like sewage and teemed with masses of people housed in cramped quarters. The food and water sources were increasingly unfit for human consumption. The stage was set for a modern catastrophe in the form of dangerous microbes, bacteria, or viruses.

Transportation improvements added to the advancements in this industrial age, transferring goods at lower prices but also relocating diseases. Faster sailing vessels, propelled by steam and streamlined for speed, facilitated the transfer of deadly, often short-lived diseases, thereby allowing the spread of deadly epidemics far beyond the previous limits of the bacterial life spans. Railroads were built that facilitated faster overland travel. They also accelerated the migration of disease through the transport of material goods, food, and drinking water barrels—some containing contaminated water. Even the ship ballasts that helped stabilize ocean-going vessels were filled with contaminated waters that were released at distant ports, spreading cholera bacteria in the process. Bacteria, often unseen and sometimes deadly, were spread through advanced means of transportation from region to region around the globe.

As the 19th century progressed, the spread of the bacterial epidemic cholera emerged numerous times, laying waste vast populations in India, the Middle East, Russia, Europe, and even America, traceable by overland and seagoing transport routes. The first pandemic began in Calcutta, India, where Britain had located its central control of the British East India Company. Beginning in 1817 and lasting until 1823, the disease spread with the British military forces as they put down native rebellions to the north of the Bengal region. From there, the pandemic spread across much of India, north to Nepal, and as far east as Japan. It also reached westward, as far as Syria and even into Astrakhan in Russia.[9]

The second pandemic of cholera began again in India in 1826 and lasted until 1837. Following the trail of the British army throughout India and its neighboring territories, Hindu pilgrims bound for the Kumb festival carried cholera with them, contaminating the Ganges River. Trade routes to Kabul, Tehran, and Astrakhan also transferred the disease and extended it as far north as Moscow, Russia, west to Hamburg, and then on to England. Immigration from Europe then transferred this old-world bacteria to Canada, New York, and New Orleans, and by 1833, it had migrated to Mexico, Cuba, and finally to South America.[10]

The third major pandemic started in India in 1840, and by 1844, it had emerged from the subcontinent along the overland trade routes to Persia, Arabia, the Caucasus, and then into Europe. In the spring of 1848, in conjunction with the Revolution of 1848, the cholera epidemic added to the social and political upheaval in Prussia and elsewhere on the European subcontinent. Britain again felt the impact of cholera, with every county in England experiencing deaths from the outbreak. New York also experienced a new epidemic, despite efforts to quarantine infected passengers on board their ships. The cholera pandemic rapidly spread from this center of trade and immigrated across the continent and along the coastline, following the trail of the California gold rush of 1849. Even the West Indies, until then isolated from the contagion, experienced this third pandemic of cholera from 1850 to 1855.[11] Not surprisingly, the presence of cholera during this pandemic throughout the British Empire and other imperializing nations led to the eventual presence of the disease from 1854 to 1856 at the site of the disastrous war for empire in the Crimea.

The Crimean War was one of the worst such military/epidemic incidents, with numerous competing powers coalescing on a poorly drained piece of land jutting into the Black Sea, the Crimea. Surrounded by the Black Sea and marshlands, the Crimean Peninsula was hard for the invading powers to provision, as the two straits leading into the sea curtailed the shipment of goods during periods of war. The involved parties initially included Britain, France, Russia, and the Ottoman Empire. Other nations joined in the fray, either compelled by alliances or lured by hopes of increased power and influence. The pandemic of cholera did not contain itself to one side of the conflict on the Crimean Peninsula. It was an equal opportunity aggressor, infecting the defeated and victorious armies.

Theories of Cholera in the 19th Century

How the disease spread, or its etiology, was unknown at the time. Theories abounded, including contagion theories, miasma theories, and the then novel germ theory proposed by John Snow of England. The contagion theory was embraced by those who recognized the history of contagion in diseases such as the plague, measles, and smallpox. However, though cholera appeared to follow trade routes and developed at ports and trade centers, there was no explanation for the sudden appearance of cholera great distances from cities where the outbreaks occurred. Likewise, supporters of miasma theories, though predicated on Hippocrates's teachings and correlated to the occurrence of cholera among the poor, who often lived in unkempt environments with human waste and garbage, could not explain why some in these conditions contracted cholera, why others did not, and why those who maintained hygienic lifestyles also contracted the disease. Closely linked to the miasma theory were multiple accounts from numerous cultures and regions of a "cholera cloud" or "mist" phenomena that was reported orally at many pandemic sites but rarely incorporated into scholarly examinations of the disease.[12] Other theories of a less scientific nature included those that asserted one's ethnicity or socioeconomic class increased one's susceptibility to cholera.

Increasingly, the advancement in science and technology allowed for explanations that rejected all or elements of the above theories. John Snow of London and T. Heber Jackson and John Atlee of Pennsylvania postulated the anticontagionist, antimiasma germ theory that microscopic organisms spread cholera. However, Snow's conclusions, based on far more data and quite comprehensive in nature, still struggled with four essential concepts of germ theory: (1) the communicability of certain diseases to spread from person to person, whether directly or indirectly; (2) the causality of cholera coming from microbes that were not yet identified; (3) the concept of these microbes as living creatures that multiplied on their own; and (4) the concept that specific microbes caused specific diseases.[13]

This research was put forth in the midst of the cholera epidemic in London, England, and in Lancaster County, Pennsylvania, (1854) while the cholera epidemic also raged in the Crimea. Nonetheless, governments and military medical staff did not embrace this approach to cholera until Robert Koch's discovery of the bacillus *Vibrio cholerae* in 1883. Instead, it was the predominate theory of miasmas that continued to guide treatment and prevention through the Crimean War period, along with contagionist calls for quarantines.[14] Even the effective actions taken during the conflict in Crimea, of airing out rooms and cleaning up the environment, were largely predicated on the belief that miasmas stemmed from the stench of surrounding conditions, not on germ theory.

Origins of the Crimean War during the 19th Century

The Crimean War, set in the middle of the 19th century's technological, scientific, and nationalistic growth (1853–1856), was the end result of the aforementioned imperialistic expansion and competition. With the waning influence of the "Sick Man of Europe" (the Ottoman Empire), nearby imperial powers sought to extend their own influence or territories. This encroachment on Turkish lands was part of the "Eastern Question" that dominated the Concert of Europe in the 19th century. For Russia, that meant manipulating its Slavic neighbors along the Danube, seeking additional access to warm water ports, and justifying its role as the protector of Christianity in the region. France under Napoleon III desired an alliance or entente with Britain, but it also sought increased influence and profits to pay for its expanding empire and social experiments at home. With France also asserting its own role as protector of Western Christianity in the Eastern Mediterranean, the emotional temperature of diplomatic negotiations quickly rose. Britain, long a supporter of the Ottoman Empire as a means of guaranteeing stability of English trade through the region, had its "place at the table" in the negotiations. The outcome likely would have remained peaceful if not for the direct and indirect influences of other parties, from the Muslim Tatars of the Crimean region[15] to Austrian fears of an expanded Russian presence, and even the role of the Americans in trade with the involved parties.

Czar Nicholas I used old treaties to claim the role of Christian protector while he simultaneously sent his militaries to occupy Turkish lands along the Danube. Abdul Mecid, the Ottoman sultan, struggled with enforcing the rather sectarian reforms of his father, known as the Tanzimat Fermani, without causing a revolt among the conservatives and Muslim governing classes. Nicholas's military actions and assertions of primacy for protecting Christians in the Ottoman Empire forced the sultan's hand, and war was declared in October 1853. Following a successful Russian naval assault at Sinope in late 1853, the French and British declared war against the Russians in March 1854. The rapid movement from jockeying for positions of leverage and influence to war left no time for adequate preparations of wartime necessities.

Military encampments in the Crimean region, especially those erected hastily, facilitated the spread of infectious diseases. As geographers Matthew Smallman-Raynor and Andrew Cliff stated, "The epidemiological hazard is exacerbated by the injudicious selection of campsites and by the deleterious consequences of overcrowding, inadequate or non-existent drainage and sewerage systems, poor or contaminated water supplies, and the failure to institute or to maintain rigid sanitary precautions." This is an apt description of the conditions found in the Crimea from 1854 through 1856. The naval war was fought on the Baltic and Black Seas, and Asiatic cholera was found at both naval fronts. The war was also fought at Varna (modern-day Bulgaria), the Crimea, and in the Caucasus.[16] Soon after the arrival of British and French forces, cholera and other contagious diseases appeared in military reports as increased numbers of cases were admitted to the makeshift hospitals. Russian reports were less clear, as hospitals compiled admissions and deaths due to disease and wounds as casualties under the same category heading.

Using the more detailed records of the French and English, a picture emerges that explains the high incidence of cholera and other diseases. The reports indicated that even early on there was a problem with the lack of provisions. The restrictions of travel through the Bosporus and Dardanelles during wartime were only one explanation for the insufficient supplies. The ability to shut down the straits by the Turks was designed to limit Russian travel, not the travel of the Ottoman allies. However, the large number of ships converging on the region did cause delays that in turn disrupted the provisioning of troops. Corruption and the lack of sufficient security further explain the redirecting of supplies from their intended military destinations to more nefarious recipients. The history of corruption within the quartermaster corps was compounded in the Crimean War by the practice of local populations taking advantage of imported goods, which were oftentimes left stacked along the wharves as transportation or shelter was being arranged.[17] Whatever the cause for delays, the logistics of getting food, medicine, military supplies, and personnel to the Crimea and Bulgaria was a nightmare. Not surprisingly, one of the three major threats reported by the French in the Crimea was scurvy, along with cholera and combat.[18] The insufficient food supplies and unbalanced diets undermined the health of servicemen, increasing the impact of the already virulent Asiatic cholera that sped through camps, ships, and hospitals.

Cholera Makes Its Appearance in the War

The French experienced the first wave of cholera at Varna (Bulgaria) in June 1854. It had been transported there by a troopship out of Marseilles—the only record of cholera spreading from west to east in the Mediterranean Sea.[19] Though the contagion was reported on board, the request for quarantine was declined, as the perceived need for troops outweighed the perceived benefits of quarantine. The epidemic spread rapidly among the French, who reported the loss of 8,084 men, mainly due to cholera, by September 1854, before they had even met the enemy in combat, with 18,073 cases reported at hospitals for care. Turkish troops were simultaneously impacted, though the exact number of casualties is not available.[20]

The first report of cholera among the British in Bulgaria was on June 17, 1854, at Camp Alladyn, from two members of the 19th Regiment. Only occasional reports ensued over the next three weeks. However, by early July, reports of affected soldiers again came from the 19th Regiment, followed by multiple cases from nearby units in the following weeks. The epidemic rapidly spread through British forces at the camps near Varna. High rates of admissions and fatalities in the British section of the hospital at Varna were reported in mid-July, followed by outbreaks in the Crimea soon after.

The first wave of cholera among the British in Varna and the Crimea resulted in 4,630 hospital admissions and 2,717 deaths. The following year, a second wave resulted in an additional 2,228 documented hospital admissions and 1,302 deaths from cholera.[21] However, not everyone contaminated with cholera was admitted to a hospital, as they were overcrowded, understaffed, and undersupplied. Other victims opted for alternative shelters and care, such as the care supplied by volunteers like Mary Seacole, who ran a hotel and dining facility for British and French officers and enlisted personnel while she also provided nursing services at her residence and even in the trenches of the siege works.[22]

Cholera was one of the deadliest killers during the Crimean War, and it was not alone. Reports of malaria, dysentery, typhus, typhoid, and relapsing fevers abounded. Of these, the environmental conditions, including poor drainage, fouled water supplies, sewage, rotting food, and an overabundance of insects that served as vectors were complicit in the diseases. Additionally, the insufficient supply of fresh fruits and vegetables resulted in the aforementioned scurvy. The combination of inadequate food, polluted waters, and insufficient supplies and shelter, along with exposure to the elements and potentially disease-bearing insects, took its toll on the forces arrayed in the Crimean War from the earliest days.

Conditions of War That Facilitated the Spread of Cholera

The geographic features of the camps contributed heavily to the spread of cholera in the Crimean War, especially the low elevations, where streams and rivers fed the still waters of lakes. Consequently, as entire regiments were located along the low-lying tracts of land, waters became muddied and contaminated from their use of streams for washing clothes and bathing and from human waste. A common source of contamination, the characteristics associated with a body of water play a role in the ability of the cholera bacteria to propagate. Fast-flowing streams and rivers, as well as those with high acidity, inhibit cholera production.[23] However, the standing waters around the lower camps facilitated the growth of *V. cholera*. Unfortunately, the British, French, and other combatant forces were heavily reliant upon the local sources for water.

Another geographic attribute that contributed to the spread of cholera was the climate. The cold winters of the region slowed the spread of cholera, causing a disruption of the outbreaks during the coldest of weather. However, the hot, humid summers of the Black Sea region fed the contagion each spring during the war, resulting in waves of cholera that hit in 1854 and again in 1855. The exposure to the bacteria in the first year reduced the number of patients and victims in the second year. However, the constant influx of allied forces into the region provided plenty of previously unexposed people to keep the diffusion of cholera at epidemic levels through much of the war. It also placed higher demands on the need for provisions for the growing number of combatants.

Procurement and delivery of supplies affected all the forces in the Crimea and even their horses. Though the provisions were raised and shipped, the ability to deliver the necessary goods to the camp locations immediately outside of the ports presented a problem. The Crimean commissioners tasked with researching and reporting on the outcome of the war indicated numerous flaws in the process of delivering necessary supplies. One report indicated that English horses for the cavalry "starved within a few miles of Balaklava, while a plentiful store of forage was to be found there."[24] Military personnel complained that they were "all overworked, and the men are in fact dying from fatigue and bad food." Numerous letters insinuated incompetence on the part of the quartermasters, such as Lord Raglan's request for leeches, which were delivered "in stoppered bottles, . . . all dead," and intimations that the director-general had condemned the use of the newly invented chloroform because he thought it was unnecessary. The pressure associated with ensuring that troops reported for duty despite the prevalence of illness is revealed in the following letter:

> Last night in my Brigade we could not muster 900 men out of three Regiments each of which came out 1,000 strong. My duty has been very unpleasant as I often have

to decide whether some 60 men are shamming or really fit to go to their duty. If at home they would all have been in the Hospital weeks ago, but I am often obliged to send them to duty with a harsh word when I feel inclined to cry for the poor fellows—such is War.[25]

The lack of food and military supplies was not the only missing element when the French and British first arrived in Varna and the Crimea. Hospitals were ill-equipped, understaffed, or nonexistent. According to one report on board the ship *Vulcan*, where the wounded and ill were treated in close confines, "there were 300 wounded, and 170 cholera patients, and these were attended to by four surgeons."[26] Another account gave a vivid report of the conditions on board ships:

> Let them imagine a thousand men narrowly caged in a floating box: a heavy sea obliges them to close all the ports; so that, notwithstanding all the appliances of air-sails, the air at night becomes abominably tainted below. Fifty or sixty robust men, in the prime of life, are suddenly, almost in an instant, struck with the death-agony, raving, perhaps, or convulsed, in the midst of this dense mass of sleepers.[27]

Numerous reports indicated a lack of nurses in the initial days, and even late in the war in some locations. Also missing were washing conveniences for the patients, medical staff, and for the clothing and bedding. Documents indicate that wounded soldiers were housed with cholera, dysentery, and fever patients and often lain on the floor for a lack of beds or bedding. Also, the medical staff "were practically without medicines, the supply landed at the commencement of the campaign was exhausted, and the reserve had gone to the bottom of the sea, with the winter clothing (and several surgeons)."[28]

Attempts at Combating Cholera during the Crimean War

The lack of medical staff, including nurses, was a plague for the British until 1855. The turning point occurred with the involvement of Florence Nightingale and her connections. Opinionated about the motives and status of prospective female nurses, Nightingale sought to create a corps of women from the working classes who were diligent and efficient and yet to some extent respectful and deferential. Upon her arrival in Turkey in November 1854, Nightingale found most medical officers at the Scutari hospital hostile at first. She additionally did not welcome the recruits of Mary Stanley, the daughter of the bishop of Norwich, and Elizabeth Herbert, the wife of the secretary of war, whom she thought sought to reinforce the presence of Catholicism in the form of nonprofessional women with noble intents. Nightingale went so far as to assert there was no room for their services, though this was obviously disproved by the overcrowding at the hospital. Indeed, her impression upon first arrival captured the plight of the men and hospitals: "Beggars in the streets of London were at that time leading the lives of princes, compared to the life of our soldiers in the Crimea when I arrived on the scene with thirty-six nurses."[29]

Despite her misgivings about nurses supported by religious orders, Florence Nightingale eventually welcomed some. When two groups of Sisters of the Institute of Our Lady of Mercy were sent from the British War Office, Nightingale accepted the arrival of one group gracefully, including Mother Mary Clare Moore and four other Sisters of Mercy from Bermondsey who had previously worked with her. Yet, relations with the group under the leadership of Mother Mary Frances Brideman of Kinsale, Ireland, were less harmonious. Her personal rejection by the Sisters of Charity in Dublin, when she applied to serve as a religious in their hospital in 1852, prompted reciprocal feelings of rejection by Nightingale toward Irish sisters thereafter. Nightingale's inability to overlook past grievances resulted in her eventual loss of authority over nurses in the Crimea in 1855, except at the hospital in Scutari.[30] Her authority was eventually restored in 1856 at the end of the conflict.

Despite the internal conflicts between leaders of the emerging nursing profession in the Crimea, the services they rendered far exceeded the system previously in place. The recruited nurses, either novices or professionals, quickly sought to clean linens and the facilities, bathe patients, replace bandages, and provide food and comfort to the wounded and ill. Nonetheless, certain hygienic practices were overlooked. Unaware that the common body louse was a vector for typhus, the bedding and clothing of patients, and even the medical staff, were infested with these pests.[31] Additionally, little was yet known about how to successfully treat cholera, though the improved hygiene of the hospitals helped prevent the rampant spread of the bacteria to noninfected patients via contact with fecal residue. The belief that miasmas were responsible for cholera still prompted the nurses to open windows and provide muslin to filter out flies and other flying insects while ensuring fresh air in the hospital wards. This did not eradicate the disease, but it did improve the conditions for patients and medical staff alike.

Other misconceptions of cholera abounded in the Crimean region and elsewhere. The local drink of raki, a strong local spirit, was banned for its deleterious impact on the behavior of soldiers and sailors. Yet, the practice of military personnel imbibing increased quantities of alcohol, though normally considered unhealthy, may have also provided unforeseen benefits in the prevention of cholera, depending on the level of acidity that might counter the growth of the bacteria in human bowels. Local merchants quickly recognized the soldiers' taste for alcohol and produced an inferior version of raki that had been mixed with local water and sold to the soldiers and sailors. The practice of watering down the raki to extend merchant supplies, using contaminated local waters, countered any potential benefits and instead provided additional exposure of military personnel to cholera bacteria. Unwittingly, the aforementioned volunteer, Mrs. Seacole, served cooling drinks at her establishment at the height of the cholera epidemic in 1855, with recipes based on raspberry vinegars.[32] The acidity of these drinks may well have played a beneficial role in the health of many of her more regular guests.

By the end of the Crimean War, the number of casualties had increased to 75,375 French personnel reported dead from disease, or over 24 percent of their effective forces. The British deployed fewer men to the region, approximately one-third the number provided by the French. Not surprisingly, their casualties from disease were lower as well, with upward of 18,000 falling prey to disease, mainly from cholera but also typhus, typhoid, dysentery, and malaria. Sixty-six regiments of British forces that had participated in the conflict reported deaths from cholera.[33] In the brief period from July 14 to August 8, 1854, 7,000 French and 3,000 English died from cholera. One report indicated that 3,000 Zouaves in the French army were lost in three days to cholera.[34] The number of affected personnel was not clearly documented by the Ottoman Turks or the Russians. However, using available data and applying it to the Turkish participants, it is estimated that 25,000 Turks fell prey to disease during the war. Likewise, the projected Russian figures estimate close to 600,000 casualties due to disease and fatigue. The Russian advances to the region were not effectively facilitated by railroads and were marched over extensive distances to reach the fronts of the war, leaving the troops exhausted upon arrival.[35]

The Crimean War came to a close in the spring with the signing of the Treaty of 1856. Russia, by then under the leadership of Czar Alexander II, agreed to the cession of some territories following the siege of Sevastopol. Under this reform-minded ruler, the impacts of the war were mixed for Russia. Failure in the war was blamed on the traditional control of the aristocratic classes and their agricultural focus. In an effort to revitalize the nation's economy, Alexander eventually abolished serfdom, presumably freeing the movement of commoners to migrate to cities and support industries, though initially the migration of serfs was not permitted. The mass exodus of the allied armies from the Crimea, along with the fleeing of the local Tatars, who rightfully feared retaliation by Russians for supporting the allies, greatly diminished the Crimean population and alleviated the unhealthy conditions.[36] Yet, little to no benefit was observed for decades in improved health within the Russian armies or population due to lessons learned during the Crimean War.

Britain's impact from the war was quite different. Immediately following the signing of the peace treaty, medical officers in London founded the Metropolitan Association of Medical Officers of Health (later known as the Society of Medical Officers of Health (SMOH)). The purpose of the organization was "to promote the advancement of public health in every branch, not only by intercourse among the members, but by practical and theoretical study of all questions connected therewithin." Initially focused on general sanitation, the organization eventually targeted preventive medicine to maintain public health.

Four months after the forming of the SMOH, Florence Nightingale turned her energy and focus upon a campaign to reform the medical administration of the British army, thereby initiating permanent reforms in nursing that rippled across the Western world, impacting civilian and military medical structures.[37] Even the peacetime structure of the British military was targeted with calls for reforms. As Lt. Col. Wrench indicated, the army must reform its medical structures and processes in times of peace if it was to be effective during times of war.[38] Unfortunately, the effective implementation of his advice was not employed until after several more wars, including World War I.

Lasting Impacts of Cholera and War on Resulting Reforms

The public calls for reforms to medicine and military structure met with support from individual nations. Though international conferences were hosted and attended only by European nations, in 1881, the United States held a conference on international sanitary issues,[39] partly in response to a series of devastating cholera epidemics that often were initiated at port cities such as New York. However, rapid reforms in medicine addressing the source and containment of cholera were delayed due to continued international competition and distrust. Efforts to establish effective quarantines were only partially enacted, often to preserve the flow of economic trade. Distrust in an era of rising imperialistic and militaristic competition put such medical concerns on hold, especially as improved hygiene and the discovery of the bacillus *Vibrio cholera* led people to erroneously believe that cholera was under control. It took future wars and the recurrence of devastating cholera epidemics before the lessons of the past had more lasting impacts.

NOTES

1. Ed. M. Wrench, "The Lessons of the Crimean War," *British Medical Journal* 2, no. 2012 (July 22, 1899): 205, 206, accessed June 26, 2017, http://www.jstor.org/stable /20261303.
2. Brian Thomas Higgins, "Epidemic Proportions: Cholera in the British West Indies, 1850–1855" (PhD diss., Bowling Green State University, 1993), 30.
3. Ramon Powers and James N. Leiker, "Cholera among the Plains Indians: Perceptions, Causes, Consequences," *Western Historical Quarterly* 29, no. 3 (Autumn 1998): 319.
4. Sonia Shah, *Pandemic: Tracking Contagions, from Cholera to Ebola and Beyond* (New York: Sarah Crichton Books, Farrar, Straus and Giroux, 2016), 17–21.
5. Kelley Lee and Richard Dodgson, "Globalization and Cholera: Implications for Global Governance," *Global Governance* 6, no. 2 (April–June 2000): 218–220, accessed May 14, 2017, http://www.jstor.org/stable/27800260.
6. Jacques M. May, "Map of the World Distribution of Cholera," *Geographical Review* 41, no. 2 (April 1951): 272–273, accessed May 14, 2017, http://www.jstor.org/stable/211023.
7. May, "Map of the World," 220.
8. The term *night soil* has become a euphemism for references to human excrement. The origin of the term comes from the practice of human waste being collected at night from cesspits, privies, and even buckets or chamber pots. The collected fecal matter was then delivered to farms outside of villages and cities or sometimes sold as manure for fertilizer. "Night Soil," *The Phrase Finder*, accessed July 31, 2017, http:// www.phrases.org.uk/meanings/256350.html.
9. Higgins, "Epidemic Proportions," 33–34.
10. Higgins, "Epidemic Proportions," 36–39.
11. Higgins, "Epidemic Proportions," 39–41.
12. Projit Bihari Mukharji, "The 'Cholera Cloud' in the Nineteenth Century 'British World': History of an Object-without-an-Essence," *Bulletin of the History of Medicine* 86, no. 3 (Fall 2012): 303–332, published by John Hopkins University Press, accessed July 12, 2017, doi:https://doi.org/10.1353/bhm.2012.0050.
13. Sunny Y. Auyang, "Reality and Politics in the War on Infectious Diseases," accessed July 12, 2017, http://www.creatingtechnology.org/biomed/germs.pdf.

14. John B. Osborne, "The Lancaster County Cholera Epidemic of 1854 and the Challenge to the Miasma Theory of Disease," *Pennsylvania Magazine of History and Biography* 133, no. 1 (January 2009): 8–11, accessed May 14, 2017, http://www.jstor.org/stable /40543519.

15. Mara Kozelsky, "Casualties of Conflict: Crimean Tatars during the Crimean War," *Slavic Review* 67, no. 4 (Winter 2008): 866–867.

16. Matthew Smallman-Raynor and Andrew D. Cliff, "The Geographical Spread of Cholera in the Crimean War: Epidemic Transmission in the Camp Systems of the British Army," *Journal of Historical Geography* 30 (2004), 33, 35–7.

17. Mary Seacole, *Wonderful Adventures of Mrs. Seacole in Many Lands*, ed. W. J. S., introduction by W. H. Russell (London: James Blackwood, Paternoster Row, 1857), 102–112.

18. "Crimean War, Chapter 1: Loss of Life in Different Ways," *Advocate of Peace,* New Series I, no. 7 (July 1869): 106.

19. Richard J. Evans, "Epidemics and Revolutions: Cholera in Nineteenth-Century Europe," *Past & Present* 120 (August 1988): 134.

20. Smallman-Raynor and Cliff, "The Geographical Spread of Cholera," 42–43.

21. Smallman-Raynor and Cliff, "The Geographical Spread of Cholera," 40–42.

22. Seacole, *Wonderful Adventures*, chapters 15 and 16.

23. Smallman-Raynor and Cliff, "The Geographical Spread of Cholera," 38.

24. William Barwick Hodge, "On the Mortality arising from Military Operations," *Assurance Magazine, and Journal of the Institute of Actuaries* 7, no. 2 (July 1857): 83, accessed June 26, 2017, http://www.jstor.org/stable/41134778.

25. "Letters from the Crimea," *British Medical Journal* 2, no. 4896 (November 6, 1954): 1103, accessed May 14, 2017, http://www.jstor.org/stable/20361410.

26. "Some Sketches from the Present War," *Advocate of Peace* 11, no. 12 (December 1854): 186, accessed September 16, 2017, www.jstor.org/stable/27891349.

27. "Some Sketches."

28. Wrench, "The Lessons of the Crimean War," 1103.

29. Florence Nightingale, "Little Chats with Big People," *The Scrap Book* 5, no. 1 (January 1908), 43.

30. Sister Mary McAuley Gillgannon, "The Sisters of Mercy as Crimean War Nurses" (PhD diss., University of Notre Dame, 1962), I, 42–3.

31. Seacole, *Wonderful Adventures*, 82–91.

32. Seacole, *Wonderful Adventures*, 146–153.

33. Smallman-Raynor and Cliff, "The Geographical Spread of Cholera," 33–34.

34. "Some Sketches," 186.

35. "Crimean War, Chapter 1," 106–107.

36. Hakan Kirimli, "Emigrations from the Crimea to the Ottoman Empire during the Crimean War," *Middle Eastern Studies* 44, no. 5 (2008): 760–764, accessed July 22, 2017, http://dx.doi.org/10.1080/00263200802315778.

37. "A Century of Social Achievement: The Society of Medical Officers of Health," *British Medical Journal* 1, no. 4975 (May 12, 1956): 1102–1104, accessed September 16, 2017, http://www.jstor.org/stable/20335411.

38. Wrench, "The Lessons of the Crimean War," 208.

39. Mark Harrison, "Disease, Diplomacy and International Commerce: The Origins of International Sanitary Regulation in the Nineteenth Century," *Journal of Global History* 1 (2006): 216, accessed September 16, 2017, https://www.cambridge.org/core/terms; and Mark Harrison, *Contagion: How Commerce Has Spread Disease* (New Haven, CT, and London: Yale University Press, 2012), 79.

Chapter 7

Typhoid Fever: Failure in the Midst of Victory in the Spanish-American War, 1898

Hilary Green

Typhoid fever developed in one fifth of all our soldiers in the national encampments during that memorable summer of 1898, and more than eighty per cent. of the total deaths were caused by that disease.[1]
—Henry G. Beyer, MD

The Spanish-American War is noteworthy for a variety of reasons. Victory secured American imperial interests in the Caribbean and the Pacific Ocean. American occupation of Cuba allowed for additional military pursuits throughout Central America, formally and informally.[2] Seen as insignificant in the actual days of combat in the first phase of the war, the United States' greatest enemy proved to be disease. Though the actual number of Spanish-American War dead "paled in comparison to those in the U.S. Civil War," it was the "first major war fought after the establishment of the germ theory of disease and the diagnostic value of X-rays—developments of significant magnitude to alter the course of military medicine and surgery."[3] These realities ushered through significant reforms in terms of overall military organization, design of military encampments, and the upgrade of medical facilities domestically and abroad—all of which had lasting impacts on the wars of the 20th century.

Status of Medical and Military Reforms at the Turn of the Century

Of the various armed branches, the U.S. Army saw the most changes. Several major epidemics were primarily rooted in the army, where unsanitary conditions in the domestic camps and military encampments in Cuba saw the most individuals ravaged by disease. The U.S. Navy and Marine Corps, on the other hand, saw only "sixteen combat deaths and fifty-six deaths from disease" during operations in the Philippines and the Caribbean.[4] Collectively, the military branches' experiences during the Spanish-American War helped facilitate scientific innovation and discovery, but not of new military weaponry; instead, they designed for the ultimate eradication of nonhuman combatants. The wartime establishment of the Typhoid Board allowed for Maj. Walter Reed and his team to systematically study and advance the knowledge of human contact with insects in the spread of typhoid fever, nonsymptomatic human carriers as agents in the spread of infectious diseases, and the elimination of "typhoid-malarial fever as a disease entity."[5] Their work prevented future military engagements from being medical disasters like those observed in Cuba and national encampments during the war. As poignantly argued by scholar Vincent J. Cirillo, the Spanish-American War "had a significant impact on U.S. military medicine" and proved to be "a little war with big consequences."[6]

Prior to the start of the Spanish-American War, military leaders attempted to enact reforms designed to limit the effects of typhoid fever, yellow fever, and malaria. These diseases proved especially crippling in terms of military readiness and effectiveness. According to the Centers for Disease Control and Prevention (CDC), typhoid fever "is a potentially severe and occasionally life-threatening febrile illness caused by the bacterium *Salmonella enterica*."[7] Individuals acquired the illness through the consumption of food or water contaminated by feces. It could also spread through contact with an infected person, convalescent person, or asymptomatic carrier. Typhoid fever symptoms were similar to the other diseases affecting military readiness during the Spanish-American War. They included a rising and sustained high fever, usually accompanied with weakness and lethargy; loss of appetite; and occasionally a pink flat rash. Muscle aches, headaches, and abdominal pains were also common, as was a dry nonproductive cough. If not treated, patients became delirious and fell into a trancelike state; this was usually when complications occurred, such as intestinal hemorrhages. For those who recovered, symptoms often returned. Others became asymptomatic after weeks of recovery but continued to transfer the disease to others in close contact, especially through the sharing of food or contaminated water. Soldiers who contracted typhoid fever were incapable of active service for approximately two to four weeks, remained contagious throughout their illness, and often remained contagious beyond their overt presentation of symptoms.[8]

During the Spanish-American War, like others before it, multiple diseases disrupted troop mobilization and combat despite the best efforts to enact effective medical reforms. New studies focused on the role of insects as vectors of these diseases. Although mosquitoes do not carry typhoid fever, the disease is capable of being transferred through contact with flies and other insects that come in contact with contaminated feces, food, or other items. Unlike typhoid fever, bites from infected mosquitos cause outbreaks of yellow fever and malaria. Specifically, species with the genus *Aedes* or *Haemagogus* result in yellow fever, with *Aedes aegypti* primarily affecting urban mosquitoes.[9] Female mosquitoes of the genus *Anopheles* are responsible for malaria. Both diseases are transmitted through a clear cycle: mosquitoes ingest either the *Flavivirus* or malarial protozoan through feeding on an infected person or animal and then transmit the diseases by biting individuals. Once bitten, high grade fever, fatigue, yellowing of the skin, and other symptoms appear several days later. However, the infected individual can unknowingly transmit both diseases to others.

According to the CDC, individuals who are infected with either yellow fever or malaria "are infectious to mosquitoes (referred to as being 'viremic') shortly before the onset of fever" and up to several days after onset of symptoms.[10] Moreover, these diseases are not limited to rural areas and can spread to urban centers as a result of viremic individuals traveling to urban centers in semitropical and tropical areas. Collectively, these three diseases can be prevented through ensuring clean water supplies, nonconsumption of contaminated foods, and the use of mosquito prevention measures, that is, eliminating standing water and the use of netting. Unfortunately, the conditions of war and the state of the army's medical department hindered the effective use of such preventative measures during the Spanish-American War.

Viewed with little respect at the time, the U.S. Army and its Medical Department were not prepared for the demands of modern warfare in the tropical climates of the Caribbean, Pacific Ocean, and Southeast Asia, specifically in terms of personnel, supplies, and equipment.[11] The rapid downsizing following the Civil War and its limited service over the period between the wars proved to be a liability.[12] Brig. Gen. George M. Sternberg's first official act as surgeon general saw the creation of an Army Medical School on June 24, 1893. Capt. Walter Reed served as a professor of bacteriology and clinical microscopy, Maj. John Shaw Billings as a professor of military hygiene, and Maj. Charles Smart as a professor of military medicine.[13] Initially designed as a four-month course of instruction, the medical school expanded with a strong commitment to scientific research and discovery to reduce combat and noncombat casualties.[14] By the beginning of the war, there were 192 medical officers and roughly 650 contract surgeons.[15]

In terms of scientific knowledge, the U.S. Army had access to the latest medical knowledge about tropical diseases. Surgeon General Sternberg advocated against an invasion during the wet season based on this information. Nonetheless, after consulting with Dr. Juan Guiteras, a Cuban yellow fever expert, Sternberg's and Gen. Miles's concerns were overridden.[16] The medical community was also aware of both the probable cause and effective preventative measures for the diseases that eventually ravaged the military during the Spanish-American War. Civil War army surgeon Joseph J. Woodward's *Outlines of the Chief Camp Diseases of the United States Army* (1863) had advanced the notion of typhomalarial fever as equal to typhoid fever and malaria to the civil-military medical profession. He also introduced infected human feces as the principal cause of the contagious fever.[17]

The research conducted by William Budd and others expanded the notion of germ theory to explain infection and permitted the development of more effective preventative medical measures and procedures.[18] Standard medical textbooks at the start of the war readily distinguished the differences between typhoid fever and malaria. Nonetheless, military culture moved slowly in accepting the new advances in scientific knowledge and ignored protests raised by medical officers and personnel.[19] Although official policy, the medical reforms were neither systematically implemented at the stateside departure encampments along the Gulf Coast nor in the encampments in Cuba. The rapid mobilization of forces, often under the leadership of officers with limited or no training, undermined the employment of these new policies and reform measures. Consequently, poor sanitary conditions contributed to significant health crises that impeded entire military operations from stateside preparations to in-field combat effectiveness.

Status of Gender and Race in Medicine and Military at War's Outset

In this medical structure, gender and racial discrimination also prevailed. Women were not permitted in the ranks as either physicians or nurses, even after the rise of the Red Cross and advances in professional medical training. On the eve of the Spanish-American War, the military slowly began to accept women as volunteer nurses only. Their acceptance of these women as nurses often still required the sway of commanding officers' spouses and an accompanying high volume of patients.[20] Race also regulated the training and usage of black surgeons and nurses, principally in the role of volunteer services. When employed in the field of combat, racial stereotypes often placed black surgeons and volunteers into positions of greater risk for contracting diseases than their white counterparts.[21] For all of the advances made in germ theory by the second half of the 19th century, racial thinking and stereotypes regarding black immunity to typhoid, yellow fever, and malaria contributed to significantly higher death tolls for black soldiers during the war and its aftermath as they were repeatedly placed in harm's way.

Despite the existence of prewar discrimination, African Americans were not deterred from service in regular army military units, which they viewed as part of a broader mission for racial uplift and the defense of black manhood in post-Reconstruction America. They actively sought the "opportunity of providing the world [with their] real bravery, worth and manhood."[22] This bravery was later tested as black units were ordered to serve in hospital wards for those suffering from typhoid, yellow fever, and malaria. Maj. Allen A. Wesley and other black surgeons and physicians endured discrimination within the medical department; yet, they continued to serve.[23] However, unlike the Civil War, black physicians served as contract surgeons, with pay equal to their counterparts.[24] All African American soldiers, including the medical professionals, encountered Jim Crowism and real threats of violence en route to the battlefront. The experience ultimately revealed a national hardening of race relations and attitudes that their military service and heroism could not overcome.[25] Yet, the diseases targeted by physicians, nurses, and volunteers, whether black, white, or brown, did not discriminate in selecting their victims.

Conditions Affecting Diffusion of Typhoid Fever in the Spanish-American War

Disease often began its assault on military personnel before individuals departed for combat in either Cuba or the Philippines. Soldiers mustered at state encampments and then transferred to the national assembly camps for departure to the front.[26] Both the state and national encampments were hastily constructed, often on sites with poor drainage and with limited access to clean water supplies. Unfortunately, the conditions facilitated the spread of contagion in which "sixty-two infected regiments from twenty-nine state camps imported typhoid into the national encampments."[27] Moreover, medical facilities consisted of large tents that lacked proper ventilation and medical equipment and had nonideal sanitary conditions. The facilities were also inadequately staffed and resourced, which significantly contributed to patient mortality rather than recovery. The frontier nature of the encampments also prevented the military from drawing on civilian medical resources in the event of patient overflow or epidemic outbreak.

Camp Miami exemplified the combined effects of poor design, unsanitary stateside departure sites, and disease that impeded military operations. Miami served as a major departure point for soldiers and National Guardsmen en route to Havana. The camp's unsanitary conditions made it prone to exposure to typhoid, malaria, and dysentery. Quickly receiving the moniker "Camp Hell," Camp Miami was hastily constructed in a bad locale. Eleanor (Nellie) Kinzie Gordon, the wife of Brig. Gen. Willie Gordon, assessed Camp Miami's unfortunate location upon her arrival: "This spot is a place—not too hot—but there's no depth in the soil. Tents blow down in high wind. The water is full of lime, disagrees with the men, & gives them dysentery."[28] These conditions were further compounded by the lack of physicians, medical drugs, and spaces for convalescent care.

Reports of illness began almost immediately after the arrival of the 2nd Brigade, 1st Division, 4th Corps, which was commanded by Brig. Gen. Gordon.[29] Gordon's wife further noted in her diary that the drinking water supply "was not from the water works tower, but from the railroad tank, which got its water from two 24 feet wells, located between the two brigades, and into which surface drainage flowed from both brigades."[30] Following several failed attempts to provide clean water, including from the Everglades, Gordon noted in her diary that "orders were given that no water should be used for drinking or cooking unless it had been boiled at least an hour."[31] Within weeks of their arrival, Nellie Gordon proposed a convalescent tent to Maj. Appel, the chief surgeon of the division.[32] Assisted by her daughter, Mrs. Gordon both organized and operated a hospital that had begun as a medical tent. The increasing number of patients and mounting deaths forced Nellie Gordon to seek out another location. She discovered a vacant but dilapidated building near the Royal Palm Hotel and then outfitted the location and shifted operations.[33]

Miami resembled a frontier community. Both Brig. Gen. Gordon and his wife saw the makeshift unit as a necessity.[34] With tacit permission as a result of her spouse's military position, Mrs. Gordon personally nursed soldiers. She wrote to the Red Cross and Women's Christian Temperance Union (WCTU) for additional civilian nurses. Overall, Nellie Gordon undertook this momentous task without much military support (other than her husband's backing). "No time for journaling—my time has all been taken up with the Convalescent Ward—men keep coming in, & more, & more, & more cots & [mosquito] nets & camp stools and fans, & dishes & knives & forks had to be bought."[35] Conditions remained poor at Camp Miami.

Eventually, the convalescent ward moved to Jacksonville, Florida, and Nellie followed her husband when he was transferred to Puerto Rico.[36] Despite inadequate numbers at the camp, the nursing corps still discriminated against the use of women and African Americans. The civilian volunteer nurses, commonly military spouses and children, consequently endured a Herculean task in caring for the infected. They strove for minimizing mortality while simultaneously urging medical officers and line officers to accept their assistance and expertise against typhoid and other diseases resulting from poor sanitary conditions of the national encampments.

Camp Miami was not atypical. Camp Thomas, situated in the Chickamauga National Military Park near Chattanooga, Tennessee, declined into a "mass of putrefaction which no effort towards sanitation on our part, using quicklime and disinfectants, could prevent," according to a line officer with the 9th Pennsylvania Infantry.[37] The majority of the 425 deaths resulted from disease at Camp Thomas.[38] Located near Falls Church, Virginia, Camp Alger briefly served as the departure point for the 2nd Corps, but typhoid and other diseases forced the formal transfer of the corps to Camp George Gordon Meade near Middletown, Pennsylvania, by September 1898.[39] Typhoid fever affected all 92 regiments in the "First, Second, Third, Fourth, Fifth and Seventy Corps" in which "20,738 recruits contracted the disease (82 percent of all sick soldiers), and 1,590 died."[40] In short, typhoid represented the main source of contagion that killed both volunteers and regular army personnel before they could even leave the United States. Unrealistic expectations for hastily constructed encampments and a lack of preparedness proved deadly.[41]

Once recruits were deployed, disease played a significant role in the Cuban campaign. From July to November 1898, a typhoid fever epidemic was a defining feature of the war. Cirillo and other scholars acknowledged many of the issues discussed by contemporaries and surviving historical accounts:

> Disease (yellow fever, malaria, typhoid, and dysentery), woolen uniforms, relentless heat, dense foliage, daily rainstorms, scanty rations, no camp kettles or cooking utensils, insufficient tentage, a shortage of medical supplies, lack of indigenous food or fodder, roads and streams impassable for all but infantry and pack mules carrying half loads, and the lack of heavy siege cannon—all made the Santiago campaign the longest and hardest of the war.[42]

Following the major land engagements in Cuba, U.S. ground and naval forces saw success in Puerto Rico and the Philippines, with few casualties due to combat or disease. These later successes revealed that the army and the Medical Department, and not the other branches, required the most postwar reform. The Santiago ground campaign is illustrative of the broken nature of the army in the fight against nonhuman combatants in Cuba.[43]

As part of the ground invasion force instrumental to the Santiago campaign, journalist George Kennan observed that the supply of food and ammunition were sufficient, but he acknowledged that significant deficiencies "in the shape of cloth-ing and tentage, was not adapted to a tropical climate in the rainy season; it carried no reserve medical stores."[44] These shortages became clear with the later outbreak of typhoid, yellow fever, and malaria epidemics during the war. As in Camp Miami and other national encampments, Kennan reported the lack of hospitals and med-ical services found at Siboney, once the area was secured by American troops. Red Cross staff members found two makeshift hospitals—one for Cuban and the other for American sick and wounded. Both hospitals were in complete disarray:

> No attempt had been made to clean or disinfect either of the buildings, both were extremely dirty, and in both the patients were lying, without blankets or pillows, on the floor. . . . The army surgeons and attendants were doing, apparently, all that they could do to make the sick and wounded comfortable; but the high surf, the absence of landing facilities, the neglect or unwillingness of the quartermaster's department to furnish boats, and the confusion and disorder which everywhere prevailed, made it almost impossible to get hospital supplies ashore.[45]

From its inception, poor sanitary conditions, improper medical facilities, depen-dence on the Quartermaster's Department for medical supplies, and a limited civil-ian population to draw upon contributed to the impending public health crisis. In addition to the military hospital at Siboney, several hospital steamships operated in the harbor. Medical personnel and civilian Red Cross employees reluctantly brought into Cuba worked to the point of exhaustion caring for the wounded as well as individuals afflicted with typhoid. Several medical personnel and volun-teers even contracted yellow fever and became patients in a nearby camp set up for individuals stricken by that illness. Overwhelmed by the health crisis, Kennan placed blame on military leadership and not the medical personnel, Red Cross staff, and civilian volunteers.[46]

Even after preparations were made at the Siboney hospital for the arrival of additional wounded from the Santiago campaign, Kennan still complained about the lack of medical supplies, blankets, tents, and operating facilities.[47] He even devoted an entire chapter of his war memoir to the nature and work of the 1st Division field hospital of the Fifth Army Corps. This facility was established prior to the army's arrival, in preparation for any casualties from the attack on Santi-ago.[48] Nonetheless, the overflowing medical tents meant that wounded soldiers were forced to convalesce, often without food, water, or change of dressings, in an open field.[49] Lt. Col. Pope, the chief surgeon of the field hospital, drafted an order for additional supplies. Additional supplies were obtained, but it was not a sufficient amount to ensure proper care. Moreover, the tropical conditions severely complicated the recovery of the most seriously ill patients.[50]

Fears of contracting deadly diseases further complicated matters. Medical offi-cials and infantrymen, reassigned to work in the hospitals, refused to take care of infected individuals with either typhoid or yellow fever. These fears and the sheer "incompetence of corpsmen translated into human tragedy."[51] Yet, after a valiant display of heroism in the assault of San Juan Hill, the black 24th Infantry volunteered to care for typhoid and yellow fever patients in the quarantine hospital established near Siboney when 8 white regiments refused.[52] As a result, 167 men from the 24th Infantry contracted the disease, 24 died, and 40 received medical discharges from the regiment.[53] Fears of contracting disease, incompetence, and inadequate manpower prompted Surgeon General Sternberg to request authorization to employ women as nurses from the War Department. With official sanction, Sternberg worked with Dr. Anita McGee in the establishment of the Army Nurse Corps. These sanctioned nurses served primarily in the hospitals established in Florida and Puerto Rico, a decision resulting from the Medical Department's continued opposition to female nurses. Hence, the Cuban hospitals did not receive the necessary relief intended by Sternberg's request.[54]

Combating Typhoid with Emerging Science and Emerging Structural Support

While some U.S. Medical Department personnel displayed cowardice and criminal neglect, others rose to the occasion, as previously noted. William Crawford Gorgas played a significant role in the fight against typhoid and yellow fever in Cuba. Born on October 3, 1854, to Josiah and Amelia Gayle Gorgas, his father served as the chief of ordinance for the Confederate States of America. Upon his father's debilitating stroke and death, his mother raised the family while working as the university librarian, postmistress, and nurse at the University of Alabama. Gorgas graduated from the University of the South, Sewanee, Tennessee, in 1875, and received his medical degree from Bellevue Hospital Medical College four years later.[55] His passion for the eradication of the major diseases plaguing the military began when he joined the military. He was commissioned first lieutenant and appointed assistant surgeon of the U.S. Army on June 16, 1880, and then he was promoted to captain and assistant surgeon on June 16, 1885. His repeated promotions resulted from his service through two major yellow fever epidemics in Fort Brown, Texas, and Fort Barrancas, Florida. This prewar experience, and even his brief stint as a yellow fever patient at Fort Brown, not only gave him an immunity to yellow fever but enabled him to initially lead the reserve divisional hospital at Siboney and then the yellow fever hospital near Santiago, until he was stricken with typhoid fever.[56] Once recovered, Gorgas remained steadfast in the campaign of eradicating typhoid and other diseases affecting soldiers. Consequently, he was promoted to major and brigade surgeon of the U.S. Volunteers on June 6, 1898, and then major and surgeon of the U.S. Army following the conclusion of a typhoid fever epidemic in Santiago, Cuba, on July 16, 1898. Gorgas's experience was not atypical among the team composed by Maj. Walter Reed to eradicate the two major bacterial combatants and one protozoan parasitical disease. Gorgas and others took personal risks to ensure the readiness of the military and to curtail additional casualties.[57]

Military officials responded to repeated epidemics and calls for action with the creation of the U.S. Army Typhoid Board in August 1898. Maj. Walter Reed, Maj. Victor C. Vaughan, and Maj. Edward O. Shakespeare led the newly formed board tasked with the inspection of all primary and secondary encampments, systematically analyzing their findings.[58] Over a period of 21 months, the board characterized the root cause of the typhoid fever and many other diseases in the camps as the result of unsanitary conditions. "Camp pollution was the greatest sin committed by the troops in 1898," the board concluded.[59] They did place some blame on inexperienced volunteer officers and troops and the low number of regular army veterans "to teach the mass of volunteers self-reliance."[60]

Ultimately, the board concluded that "the line officers, by virtue of their command authority, must accept blame for the unsanitary conditions of the camps. 'Camp commanders should regard proper attention to the sanitation of the site occupied by their troops as one of their highest duties and its neglect as a crime.'"[61] The board recommended procedures and practices for prevention and treatment of typhoid and other diseases. Solutions included routine disinfection with a carbolic acid solution, proper diagnosis of typhoid from other diseases with diarrhea symptoms, and eradication of flies and other insects from the camps.[62]

In addition, the reality of the heavy toll on soldiers, physicians, nurses, and commands dictated the board's second charge: the systematic study of yellow fever, typhoid fever, and malaria diseases plaguing the military. Maj. Walter Reed led a team that included Gorgas, James Carroll, Jesse W. Lazear, and Aristides Agramonte. The team greatly benefited from the availability of new scientific research on the spread of diseases, specifically yellow fever in households; a new mosquito theory on the spread of infections; and the discovery that the various species of *Anopheles* mosquitoes were responsible for the spread of malaria.[63] After months of research, success occurred. Reed and his team proved that the *Aedes aegypti* mosquito was responsible for yellow fever. Success, however, came with a cost. In an effort to demonstrate the *Stegomyia* subgenus of the *A. aegypti* mosquito as the cause of yellow fever, Lazear tested his theory on himself and sacrificed his own life in the process.[64]

Building on the team's discoveries, Walter Reed outlined the necessary sanitary measures military commanders should follow to protect troops from further contagions. The board toured training camps and implemented Reed's reforms. Following the war, Reed continued his teaching duties, returning to Washington, D.C., in 1901. Unfortunately, he died of complications from an operation for appendicitis in November 1902. Gorgas remained in Cuba as the chief sanitation officer. There he undertook the daunting three-month task of trying to eradicate mosquito-breeding areas in Havana. According to a commendation made by an Alabama state legislator, Gorgas "cleaned up the pest holes, the hidden waste, the unclean places, the foul dens of the city, and by the use of kerosene and petroleum rendered inhabitable to the *Stegomya* its breeding places."[65] Gorgas received a promotion from surgeon to assistant surgeon-general with the rank of colonel in March 1903 as a result of his tireless service.[66] Within a year of the team's discoveries, yellow fever had been eradicated from Cuba. The end of American occupation in Cuba witnessed significantly fewer casualties from the three major diseases of typhoid, yellow fever, and malaria. Epidemic casualties were also reduced during the Insular Government of the Philippines, the American-led transitional government that operated from 1901 until independence in 1935.[67]

Following the medical disaster of the Spanish-American War, the War Department Investigating Commission began an investigation on the nature and conduct of military operations. Better known as the Dodge Commission, Chairman Maj. Gen. (Ret.) Greenville M. Dodge presented the commission's findings in February 1899. The commission concluded that the Medical Department had been ill prepared for the war, failed at investigating sanitary conditions in stateside military camps and abroad, suffered from an insufficient nursing force, and was hamstrung from a dependence on the Quartermaster Department for medical supplies.[68] Although successful in defeating Spain, the scathing nature of the findings revealed that the U.S. military, in particular the army, failed to meet the challenges of modern warfare, especially against disease in tropical and subtropical climes.

Combined Impact of Typhoid and War on Increasing Reforms

These findings ushered in several major reforms, initiated by Secretary of State Elihu Root. First, curriculum changes occurred at both the U.S. Infantry and Cavalry School (presently the Command and General Staff College) and the U.S. Military Academy at West Point. Future trainees had access to the latest scientific and medical knowledge for employment in the expanded U.S. Medical Department.[69] The enlarged department consisted of the Army Nurse Corps, Medical Corps, Hospital Corps, and Dental Corps. The restructure of the Medical Department also lifted restrictions on female nurses with the official establishment of the Army Nurse Corps (Female).[70] Second, the success of the Typhoid Board led to the creation of the Yellow Fever and Tropical Diseases Boards. Collectively, these boards contributed to a significant reduction of disease impacts on ground and naval forces operating in the Caribbean, Latin America, and the Philippines. They also contributed to the global advancement of scientific knowledge with their research on dysentery, cholera, yaws, and eventually dengue fever and beriberi.[71] It was the work of these boards that facilitated the development and mandatory administration of an antityphoid inoculation in the military.[72] Fourth, the army's reorganization resolved the supply problems experienced during the war, with the Medical Department receiving necessary medical supplies through the creation of a more efficient Quartermaster Corps. The new streamlined unit combined three departments (Quartermaster, Pay, and Subsistence).[73] In short, the Spanish-American War fundamentally changed how the U.S. Military Medical Department functioned, its organization, and its ability to treat both injuries and the ravages of diseases caused by nonhuman combatants.

The rapid movement from peacetime to war inevitably results in problems with the mobilization of forces and supplies. The lack of sufficient medical knowledge of diseases encountered in subtropical and tropical climes combined with the limited training of officers and medical staff made the movement into the Spanish-American War a costly one in terms of human life. Though not the only epidemic impacting American forces and volunteers during the conflict, typhoid was responsible for an astounding number of casualties due to the lack of understanding and insufficient training for officers on how the infection spread. In addition to impacting the conduct of the war, the outbreak of numerous typhoid epidemics at home and abroad resulted in positive military and medical advancements. These advancements did not eradicate typhoid, yellow fever, or malaria, but they better prepared the U.S. military to address the agelong dilemma of epidemics during wars, just in time for the buildup toward wars of the 20th century.

NOTES

1. Henry G. Beyer, MD, "The Dissemination of Disease by the Fly," *New York Medical Journal* 91, no. 14 (April 2, 1910): 682.
2. Kenneth E. Hendricks Jr., *The Spanish-American War* (Westport, CT: Greenwood Press, 2003), 73–82; James C. Bradford, ed., *Crucible of Empire, the Spanish-American War and Its Aftermath* (Annapolis, MD: Naval War College, 1993), xiii–xx; and Paul T. McCartney, *Power and Progress: American National Identity, the War of 1898, and the Rise of American Imperialism* (Baton Rouge: Louisiana State University Press, 2006), 258–273.
3. Vincent J. Cirillo, *Bullets and Bacilli: The Spanish-American War and Military Medicine* (New Brunswick, NJ: Rutgers University Press, 2004), 1.
4. Cirillo, *Bullets and Bacilli*, 2; For naval and marine operations during the war, see Jack Shulimson, "Marines in the Spanish-American War," in *Crucible of Empire* (Annapolis, MD: Naval Institute Press, 1993), 127–157; Hendricks, *The Spanish-American War*, 43–52, 58–61; and Brad K. Berner, ed., *The Spanish-American War: A Documentary History with Commentaries* (Madison, NJ: Fairleigh Dickinson University Press, 2014), 155, 183–184.
5. Cirillo, *Bullets and Bacilli*, 2.
6. Cirillo, *Bullets and Bacilli*, 1.
7. Anna E. Newton, Janell A. Routh, and Barbara E. Mahon, "Typhoid & Paratyphoid Fever," Centers for Disease and Prevention, accessed September 2, 2017, http://wwwnc.cdc.gov/travel/yellowbook/2016/infectious-diseases-related-to-travel/typhoid-paratyphoid-fever.
8. Newton, Routh, and Mahon, "Typhoid & Paratyphoid Fever."
9. Centers for Disease Control and Prevention, "Transmission of Yellow Fever Virus," accessed September 2, 2017, http://www.cdc.gov/yellowfever/transmission/index.html; and Centers for Disease and Prevention, "Anopheles Mosquitoes," accessed September 2, 2017, https://www.cdc.gov/malaria/about/biology/mosquitoes.
10. Centers for Disease Control and Prevention, "Transmission of Yellow Fever Virus."
11. Cirillo, *Bullets and Bacilli*, 20.
12. Cirillo, *Bullets and Bacilli*, 25.
13. Cirillo, *Bullets and Bacilli*, 26.
14. Cirillo, *Bullets and Bacilli*, 27.
15. Cirillo, *Bullets and Bacilli*, 28.
16. Cirillo, *Bullets and Bacilli*, 12; For overall strategy, see Joseph Smith, *The Spanish-American War: Conflict in the Caribbean and the Pacific, 1895–1902* (London: Longman, 1994), 56–63, 106–112.
17. Cirillo, *Bullets and Bacilli*, 59–60.
18. Cirillo, *Bullets and Bacilli*, 64–65.
19. Cirillo, *Bullets and Bacilli*, 57.

20. Cirillo, *Bullets and Bacilli*, 28.
21. Natalie J. Ring, "Mapping Regional and Imperial Geographies: Tropical Disease in the U.S. South," in *Colonial Crucible: Empire in the Making of the Modern American State*, ed. Alfred W. McCoy and Franscisco A. Scarano (Madison: University of Wisconsin Press, 2009), 306–308; Cirillo, *Bullets and Bacilli*, 3.
22. Berner, *The Spanish-American War*, 92.
23. Cirillo, *Bullets and Bacilli*, 21–22.
24. Cirillo, *Bullets and Bacilli*, 28.
25. Berner, *The Spanish-American War*, 98, 102–105.
26. Berner, *The Spanish-American War*, 68; Smith, *The Spanish-American War*, 101.
27. Cirillo, *Bullets and Bacilli*, 69.
28. Jacqueline Clancy, "Hell's Angel: Eleanor Kinzie Gordon's Wartime Summer of 1898," *Tequesta* 63 (2003): 41.
29. Clancy, "Hell's Angel," 40.
30. Clancy, "Hell's Angel," 43.
31. Clancy, "Hell's Angel," 43.
32. Clancy, "Hell's Angel," 44–45.
33. Clancy, "Hell's Angel," 45.
34. Clancy, "Hell's Angel," 47.
35. Clancy, "Hell's Angel," 51–52.
36. Clancy, "Hell's Angel," 55–57.
37. Clancy, "Hell's Angel," 69.
38. Berner, *The Spanish-American War*, 90.
39. Cirillo, *Bullets and Bacilli*, 70.
40. Cirillo, *Bullets and Bacilli*, 71.
41. Smith, *The Spanish-American War*, 105–106.
42. Cirillo, *Bullets and Bacilli*, 17; Berner, *The Spanish-American War*, 107–108; Smith, *The Spanish-American War*, 119–159.
43. Cirillo, *Bullets and Bacilli*, 18.
44. George Kennan, *Campaigning in Cuba* (1899; repr. Charleston: BiblioLife, 2009), 51.
45. Kennan, *Campaigning in Cuba*, 83.
46. Kennan, *Campaigning in Cuba*, 84–87.
47. Kennan, *Campaigning in Cuba*, 114.
48. Kennan, *Campaigning in Cuba*, 130, 132.
49. Kennan, *Campaigning in Cuba*, 135–137.
50. Kennan, *Campaigning in Cuba*, 145–147.
51. Cirillo, *Bullets and Bacilli*, 87.
52. Berner, *The Spanish-American War*, 134–135; Cirillo, *Bullets and Bacilli*, 92.
53. Cirillo, *Bullets and Bacilli*, 92.
54. Clancy, "Hell's Angel," 48.
55. "A Record of Brilliant and Gallant Service of More Than Twenty Years," in Articles, *Commoner*, Lincoln Nebraska, March 4–11, 1910, 13, in William Crawford Gorgas Papers, University of Alabama, Tuscaloosa, Alabama.
56. "A Record of Brilliant and Gallant Service of More Than Twenty Years," 14; Lister Hill, "William Crawford Gorgas—Speech of the Honorable Lister Hill of Alabama in the House of Representatives, March 28, 1928," 2, William Crawford Gorgas Papers, University of Alabama.

57. "A Record of Brilliant and Gallant Service of More Than Twenty Years," 14.

58. Cirillo, *Bullets and Bacilli*, 72–73.

59. Quoted in Cirillo, *Bullets and Bacilli*, 75.

60. Cirillo, *Bullets and Bacilli*, 77.

61. Cirillo, *Bullets and Bacilli*.

62. Cirillo, *Bullets and Bacilli*, 78–80.

63. "Yellow Fever: Cause for Concern?," *British Medical Journal (Clinical Research Edition)* 282, no. 6278 (May 1981): 1735; and Hill, "William Crawford Gorgas," 3.

64. William Crawford Gorgas, *The Scientific Monthly* 11, no. 2 (August 1920): 187; W. H. G. Armytage, "William Crawford Gorgas, 1854–1920," *British Medical Journal* 2, no. 4894 (October 1954): 985; and Mariola Espinosa, "A Fever for Empire: U.S. Disease Eradication in Cuba as Colonial Public Health," in *Colonial Crucible*, 294.

65. Hill, "William Crawford Gorgas," 4.

66. United States. Congress. Senate. Report on Senate Bill 2842, concerning Army promotion of Dr. W. C. Gorgas, February 6, 1903, in William Crawford Gorgas Papers, University of Alabama.

67. "Untitled," in Articles, *Commoner*, Lincoln Nebraska, March 4–11, 1910, 4–5, and Frank W. Boykin, Commemorative Exercises of the Thirtieth Anniversary of the Death of Major General William Gorgas at His Grave, Arlington National Cemetery, Speech of Honorable Frank W. Boykin of Alabama, House of Representatives, August 3, 1950, in William Crawford Gorgas Papers, University of Alabama.

68. Cirillo, *Bullets and Bacilli*, 103.

69. Cirillo, *Bullets and Bacilli*, 125–135.

70. Cirillo, *Bullets and Bacilli*, 111–112

71. Cirillo, *Bullets and Bacilli*, 120.

72. Cirillo, *Bullets and Bacilli*, 123–125.

73. James L. Yarrison, "The U.S. Army in the Root Reform Era, 1899–1917," US Army Center of Military History, 2001, accessed September 2, 2017, http://www.history .army.mil/documents/1901/Root-Ovr.htm; McCartney, *Power and Progress*, 145–146.

Chapter 8

Diphtheria in the Tajikistan War: Circumventing Post–World War II Medical Advances, 1992–1994

Rebecca M. Seaman

Diphtheria and other diseases rose and fell in direct relation to housing, nutritional improvement and wartime conditions, a factor taken into little account by those who consider vaccination to be the only relevant sacrament. The return of conditions of social dislocation and poverty will see an increase in all diseases which, under times of duress, have no respect for the vaccination status of anyone.[1]

—Hilary Butler

On September 9, 1991, Tajikistan reluctantly declared its independence from the Soviet Union, following the lead of its neighboring former Soviet Republics. With no experience in self-government over a diverse populace pieced together by the former Soviet Union, it is not surprising that the fledgling nation quickly devolved into a civil war that undermined its already weak economy and infrastructure. A diphtheria epidemic joined the new nation's many struggles amid this five-year-long civil war. Tajikistan witnessed the sharpest rise in reported diphtheria cases for all the Newly Independent States (NIS).

Diffusion of Diphtheria

Many have heard of diphtheria; yet, most people today cannot identify the disease or its symptoms. Ironically, more people are familiar with the Iditarod dogsled competition that annually commemorates the race to save a community suffering from diphtheria than they are with the disease itself. The cause of this bacterial infection is the bacterial organism *Corynebacterium diptheriae*. A highly contagious infection, diphtheria typically presents itself as a lesion on the membranes at the back of a patient's throat, tongue, nose, and airways. Today, the disease is rare in regions with high-quality medical care and vaccine protocols. In those nations where vaccinations are not regularly administered, diphtheria is more common. In particular, the disease thrives in societies where poverty, dislocation, and overcrowding are commonplace and medical care and hygiene are in short supply. Tajikistan's Civil War, from 1992 to 1997, provided conditions that spurred unprecedented growth of a diphtheria epidemic, especially during the first three years.

The method of diphtheria transmission is key to its rapid increase in periods of dislocation and duress. The disease is often found in respiratory mucosa and located in nasal passages and airways. The spray from coughing spreads the infection, as does contact.[2] The overcrowded conditions in Tajikistan, in particular in the region of Qurghonteppa (Kurgan-Tyube) that borders Afghanistan, facilitated the rapid spread of diphtheria. The disease also presents itself in extra-respiratory mucosa and cutaneous, or skin, lesions and can be spread by indirect contact through the sharing of utensils for eating as well as sharing clothing and bedding that are contaminated by droplets or discharges from the lesions.[3] Not surprisingly, the disease is more commonly acquired during the colder months of the year when common colds and coughs are the norm.

There are three main types of transmission of diphtheria from human carriers: through healthy carriers who transmit the bacillus to others but remain asymptomatic; through contact with people suffering from a mild case of the disease; and through contact with those recovering from the disease. The disease, occurring naturally, appears to be limited to humans, though scientists have infected animals with the strain and even produced fatal results.[4] Early diagnosis through bacteriological scrutiny is crucial to preventing the spread of diphtheria, but it is made difficult by virtue of the symptom presenting as a mild sore throat that is often perceived as not necessitating the services of a physician.[5]

The Identity and Symptoms of the Bacteria Responsible for Diphtheria

Not clearly diagnosed until the end of the 19th century, the disease historically ran its course through an infected population, with a wide range of fatality and survival rates. Left untreated, patients can experience further impediments that result in the hallmark pseudomembrane cover spreading into the larynx and trachea. The growth of this membrane causes disruptions in breathing and swallowing. The infection can result in complications by spreading throughout the patient's systems. The examination of victims from fatal cases of diphtheria reveals "sterile, hemorrhagic, and necrotic damage in many organs of the body."[6] Untreated patients display symptoms for approximately two weeks, but they often suffer complications that incapacitate them for months. This longevity not only results in the loss of human productivity—especially in a period of war—but also extends the period of possible transmission to others in close contact.

Named after the Greek word for leather, diphtheria was so designated in 1826 by Pierre Bretonneau, a French physician from Tours, long before the bacteria responsible for the disease was identified. For years, this dreaded disease was commonly associated with various respiratory diseases that involved throat infections. Tracing the impact of diphtheria upon societies and militaries is therefore inexact and problematic, typical of most retroactive diagnoses. Possible historical outbreaks include the second-century outbreak in Egypt and Syria designated "*malum Egyptiacum.*" A later outbreak on the Iberian Peninsula was labeled "*morbus suffocans*" or "*garrotillo*" for resemblance to the Spanish execution by suffocation.[7] Not recognized at the time as a bacterial infection, diphtheria outbreaks were identified by the observation of membrane lesions at the back of the throat and in nasal passages. In addition to the thick gray coating at the back of one's throat, common symptoms associated with diphtheria included chills and fever, a croupy cough, a sore throat, and swollen glands. Long associated with the strangling death of hundreds of thousands of children each year, diphtheria was endemic in many regions prior to the vaccine era.

In 1855, Bretonneau and fellow physician Armand Trousseau delineated the characteristic symptoms of diphtheria. It was not until 1883, when Swiss pathologist Theodor Albrecht Edwin Klebs and German bacteriologist Friedrich Loeffler discovered the diphtheria bacillus, that the cause of diphtheria was understood by the medical community. Over the course of the next decade, antitoxins were developed to counter the toxins produced by diphtheria. The development of these serums resulted in antitoxin administrations to patients that substantially lowered the incidence of diphtheria mortalities to 8 percent by 1905. By 1913, pediatrician Béla Schick had produced a diagnostic skin test that helped to identify those exposed to the disease, known as the Schick test.[8] By 1915, New York physician William Park had developed a vaccine that mixed toxin and antitoxin into an effective preventative measure.[9] During World War I (1914–1918), Maj. H. J. Bensted of the British Royal Army documented an epidemic of faucal (throat) and cutaneous (skin) diphtheria in the Middle East. This was the first historical documentation of diphtheria presenting as a skin infection. The use of Schick testing and immunization enabled the British to control the epidemic.[10]

By 1933, three strains of diphtheria had been identified. Gravis, the most severe, had many complications, including death and paralysis. The mitis strain is a mild form of the disease that resulted in no fatalities in the same 1933 report. The intermedius strain is not as severe as gravis but still resulted in complications. The gravis and intermedius strains both contain virulent bacteria.[11] Further investigations revealed that the bacilli gained entrance through a variety of locations, with the most common being the fauces, larynx, and nose, followed by genital areas, open wounds, and the eyes.[12] Unattended, faucal diphtheria in the throat or nasal passages can lead to strangulation as well as degenerate into other tissues and organs, including the heart, kidney, liver, and even the brain.

Following the identification of cutaneous diphtheria during World War I, further studies were conducted to understand the connection between the two diphtheria forms. Cutaneous diphtheria served to complicate existing wounds or breaks in the skin and may have resulted in part from patients with faucal diphtheria infecting their own skin. According to a study published in the *British Medical Journal* during World War II, lesions were often covered in crusts that disguised the greyish ulcers beneath. The use of saline baths "with glycerin magnesium sulphate or hydrogen peroxide" helped to remove the crusts for treatment. As with faucal diphtheria, antitoxins were applied, and patients were usually isolated from others. The isolation was crucial, as the infection quickly spread from patients to staff and then to other patients.[13]

Left untreated, cutaneous diphtheria can result in paralysis. Endemic in certain populations in the Pacific region, this form of the disease usually presented as mild sores or ulcers on the skin.[14] However, soldiers during World War I in Africa and the Middle East, and later during World War II in the Mediterranean, Africa, Pacific, and Indo-Burma theaters, encountered severe complications from cutaneous diphtheria, such as myocarditis (cardiac)[15] and debilitating skin ulcers resulting in the extensive loss of manpower hours despite the nonepidemic proportion of diagnosed patients.[16] The cutaneous form was also known as desert sores, tropical ulcers, ecthyma, and jungle rot, and it presented as lesions on the bodies and extremities of soldiers. The location of the ulcers, often on the feet of soldiers, accounted for the substantial levels of disabilities, hospitalizations, and even evacuations. Those returning to service often experienced recurring outbreaks, as the resumption of field activities disrupted the healing process, breaking through the thin scars and opening them to further contagion. The cutaneous form of diphtheria was also reported to be prevalent among prisoners in overcrowded prisoner of war camps in the Pacific and elsewhere.[17]

Diphtheria in Wars of the 20th Century

Diphtheria in its various forms was reported in army medical records during World War II, during the years 1942–1945. In sheer numbers, the most reported cases by the U.S. military occurred in the European theater (2,557 at a rate of 0.58 per 1,000). Though with fewer reported cases, the incident rate for the Mediterranean was higher, at 0.73 per 1,000 (with 1,087 reported cases). Taken cumulatively, the number of cases reported in the Pacific theater (southwest, central, and south) accounted for 1,134 reported cases. If China, Burma, and India are included, that number climbs to 1,342. Cutaneous diphtheria was the more common form of the disease for the U.S. Army in the Mediterranean, Middle East, China, Burma, and India and in the Pacific region. The British reported rates for diphtheria, especially in the African desert, that were far higher than those for the U.S. forces, with 1,350 reported cases in just the span of three months.[18]

All these reported cases come from records kept by military facilities during the war. However, not included in the numbers are those who suffered, and died, during such incidents as the Bataan Death March and the ensuing imprisonment at such places as the POW camp at Cabanatuan in the Philippines. Approximately 1,500 died at that one camp from a wide variety of diseases, including diphtheria.[19] Those included in the official records that survived the disease nonetheless added to the overall loss of service hours—or ineffective forces—due to the discomfort and the inconvenient locations of lesions (often on the feet, joints, and even eyes).

Diphtheria has historically been a dangerous disease, resulting in hundreds of thousands of people experiencing it annually and thousands dying. The rise of urban industrial societies shifted the disease from largely epidemic to endemic status, resulting in susceptible population clusters, especially young children and the elderly. Undiagnosed and unattended, tens of thousands of people continued to die annually when the disease emerged in the fall and winter.

Origin and Conditions of Tajik Civil War

The advancements in diagnosis, treatment, and prevention from the 1890s to the 1990s should have seen eradication or at least only rare occurrences of diphtheria in the world. Yet, the continuance of outbreaks in regions where social, political, economic, and military upheaval occurred demonstrated that knowledge and ability alone were not enough to exterminate the contagion. Thus, the dissolution of the Soviet Union, which left its former republics to fend for themselves, created the necessary turmoil and duress that proved a fertile ground for both civil war and epidemics.

A year before the fall of the Soviet Union, the landlocked country of Tajikistan was already experiencing internal upheaval. The nation has mountains covering 93 percent of its territory (8 percent of which are covered in glaciers) and possesses a largely agricultural economy, though only 6 percent of its land is utilized as croplands. Cut throughout by rivers and dotted with lakes (most lying in the eastern region), the nation is one of the highest producers of water per year; yet, during the civil war, this water became a source of disease—from hepatitis to typhoid and diphtheria. Of the water generated for use, most is directed toward agriculture, leaving only 8.5 percent for domestic use throughout the nation. Drinking water originates from a variety of sources, with a full 29 percent coming directly from rivers, streams, gorges, canals, irrigation ditches, and pools. The potential for contamination is great even in periods of internal peace.

Tajikistan's ensuing civil war meant that precautionary measures regarding water purity were sorely lacking in the early 1990s, especially after the water-quality laboratories were destroyed during the war. This same turmoil upset the internal controls that ensured the maintenance of irrigation systems for the cotton fields and drainage systems, which are necessary to maintain agricultural and public health. With 80 percent of the nation's productivity coming from its limited arable lands and the economy collapsing, the population resorted to subsistence farming that depended largely on the increasingly contaminated water sources. The disruption of water flow to irrigation ditches and fields affected at least 48 percent of the country, with as much as one-sixth of the nation's irrigated lands no longer receiving any water and far more of the nation receiving severely restricted water flow.[20] With a rugged geography and fragile economy, the country was susceptible to any internal or external trauma. That trauma came in the form of the Soviet Union's decline.

Dependent on the Soviet Union for trade, factions within Tajikistan were encouraged by rumors of the imminent demise of the communist dictatorship in 1991. The process of Sovietization conducted over the previous decades had met with resistance in the more rural and isolated regions that held strong clan, ethnic, and religious loyalties. A study conducted by Kirill Nourzhanov, a scholar of Central Asian politics and international relations, and his colleague Christian Bleuer revealed specific areas of concern affected by the civil war. The study asserted that the social elements of family, religious community, and subethnic regionalism successfully challenged "the monopoly of state agencies in making and enforcing rule in Soviet Tajikistan.[21]

Following the disastrous riots of August 1991, the Tajik Supreme Soviet opted for an independent republic the next month. According to a report by Global Security, the decision for independence was "a response to increasingly vociferous opposition demands and to similar declarations by Uzbekistan and Kyrgyzstan."[22] What followed was a series of weak attempts at coalition, democratic, and antireformist forms of government, some lasting only a few brief months and all preceded and followed by violent attempts to wrest power by opposition forces. The source of most of these struggles for authority came from long-held conflicts and factions already in existence within the diverse populace of Tajikistan.

While some blending of Soviet collectivization with the Tajik collective form had occurred in the decades of domination by the Soviet Union, the individualistic form of a modern Soviet society had never displaced the local self-consciousness of the Tajiks. Kinship and communal structures dominated, revealing a surprisingly more authoritative system than that used in the USSR. As Nourzhanov and Bleuer indicated, the newly independent government under recently elected Rahmon Nabiyev presumed to inherit an "absolute subordination to the will of 'the First,' which had existed before."[23] Meanwhile, the regional identities, already historically in place and politicized by the Soviets who had failed to consolidate them under a centralized system, became increasingly sensitive in the post-Soviet years.[24] Nowhere were these regional identities more sensitive than in Qurghonteppa, which also experienced the highest incidence of diphtheria during the ensuing civil war.

Located in the southwest of the country and bordered by Uzbekistan and Afghanistan, Qurghonteppa boasted the most diverse population in the country. Tajikistan possessed approximately 6 million people; the local Tajik, Arab, Turkmen, and Baluchi populations were augmented with Uzbeks, Russians, Germans, and others. The Russians emigrated out of the country in large numbers with the advent of the civil war, creating a vacuum and giving added emphasis to the factions remaining. The internal factions formed along the lines of kinship and religious orientation, localized regional subgroupings that perpetuated the age-old village-centric structure and asserted varying levels of reformist or conservative ideals. Even the religious factions were divided internally. Some secular groups targeted Islam as responsible for the slowing of progress. Others focused on using economic, nationalism, regional subgroupings, and desires for power to divide various religious communities. Islam, the largest religious population, was largely divided by factors that affected the other factions in Qurghonteppa and Tajikistan as a whole, namely, the dilemma of retaining their religious, cultural, economic, and political heritage versus using the opportunities of Soviet collapse and internal civil war to push through reforms and increase their influence over the region.

One interesting form of nationalism that emerged was in the Rastokhez populist movement that often targeted foreign elements in the society as responsible for all internal woes. Young Rastokhez activists called for a form of jihad to rid the country of foreigners, such as the Uzbeks, and even to secure and extend the border to incorporate Tajik populations that lived in neighboring Uzbekistan and Afghanistan.[25] Simultaneously, this somewhat democratic movement sought to model its new reformist government after foreign models, such as the Turkish and Pakistani Islamic models and liberal Western democratic structures. The attempt lacked sufficient support and was short-lived.

Adding to the overall negative atmosphere at the start of the civil war was the local economy. Even preindependence Tajikistan witnessed periods of economic weakness. Qurghonteppa in particular had a dismal annual GDP of negative 7.8 percent prior to the Soviet dissolution. The arrival of the civil war crippled the economy even further. It became the poorest of the former Soviet Republics, the second-poorest Central Asian republic (only Afghanistan fared worse), and one of the poorest nations in the world. The economy was dependent on two aspects: the local cotton production, which was nonmechanized and saw a sharp decline in output of over 80 percent during the civil war, and the typical Soviet-situated large industry that was not dependent on local labor, resources, or other small, localized industries. The severance of the Soviet Union and emigration of Russians by the start of the civil war undermined these industrial giants and left them ineffectual. Unemployment and inflation were consequently out of control, and the consumer price index rose 416 percent.[26]

The conditions of poverty, unemployment, and contaminated water as well as social and political unrest were ideal circumstances for the emergence of disease. But diphtheria was a disease presumably under check by immunization protocols. The start of the Tajik Civil War in 1992 disrupted the political structure and reallocated funding away from civilian needs. This reallocation precipitated the collapse of internal systems and facilitated the emergence of a diphtheria epidemic to further traumatize the already fractured population.

The void created by the former Soviet Union and the breakdown of civilian authority was replaced by emerging military leaders. Gaining their power through their ability to recruit people from among their own clan relations and economic and social ties, the leaders were often only recognized locally. These commanders initially targeted control of economic resources that could support their hold on power.[27] The lines of the war, like the lines throughout society, were drawn from a mixture of kinship, ideology, regionalism, and religious beliefs.

Ideologies typically formed around the desire to either resist reforms begun under Gorbachev's perestroika, to embrace Gorbachev's reforms, or to further revise his reforms. Revelations of such ideologies, and the accompanying support for anything Soviet or anti-Soviet, were construed in terms of one's level of nationalism and loyalty. With this localized mind-set and origin to the civil war, it is not surprising that the citizenry filled the ranks of the militias that were recruited throughout the country. Control of resources allowed military commanders to steer elements of the population and recruit them into military units, but not all of these commanders were from the best elements of society. According to Svetlana Lolaeva, in an article published through George Washington University's Institute for European, Russian and Eurasian Studies, "Tajikistan, stratified and suppressed for seventy years, was full of latent as well as active animosities and contradictions between sub-ethnicities, between the European-like cities and the backward countryside," as well as criminal elements that were made up of local gangs and mafias.[28]

The increased sensitivity displayed regarding affiliations and loyalties in the region around Qurghonteppa deepened the hostilities and thereby worsened conditions for the region's militia and the general population. Not surprisingly, Qurghonteppa suffered the heaviest losses from attacks by irregular forces against the coalition government and armed forces, other opposing forces, and citizenry associated with the various sides. Following the brief initial post-Soviet rule under President Rahmon Nabiyev, an attempt was made to form a pseudo-democratic structure under a coalition government, with Nabiyev still nominally in power. This brief coalition included members of the Rastokhez movement, the Islamic Renaissance Party, and the Democratic Party of Tajikistan. With such conflicting coalition members and ideologies, opposition to the new and somewhat unstable government quickly solidified throughout the nation, specifically originating in Qurghonteppa. The antireformist units sought to undermine the movement toward democratic reforms and to ensure that the initial short-lived coalition government could not incorporate underrepresented groups into the leadership structure as a means of building up continued support for its policies.

Led by a formerly convicted criminal, Sangak Safarov, the Popular Front opposition to the Islamic-Democratic coalition government forced the abdication of President Nabiyev. In his place, Akbarsho Iskandarov of the Pamiri clan was appointed as the acting president. Nonetheless, this new interim government was dominated by Islamists, giving rise to an assault upon the government by the anti-Muslim Popular Front. By December of 1992, the Supreme Soviet of Tajikistan had abolished the presidency, formed a parliament, and held elections that placed Emomali Rakhmonov as the leader.

Hopes for a return to peace were soon dashed. By July 1993, three military groups had clashed: former Russian Ministry of Security troops, Democratic-Islamists, and members of the local pro-Islamic mujahedin. Complicating matters were the influences and support given by forces from without, such as Afghanistan, Uzbekistan, and even the new Russian Federation. Each foreign group had its reasons (secular, political, economic, or territorial) that aligned with the individual Tajikistan groups they supported. The result was the escalation of hostilities and the further instability of the economy and society. Half of the remaining Slavic population fled as the war escalated in 1993, taking with them much of the skilled personnel that helped maintain communications, transportation, and infrastructure. Tens of thousands of locals also fled the southwestern region of Qurghonteppa, escaping across the border for safety. These expatriates returned occasionally, with radical ideologies and diseases in tow.[29]

Typical for periods of conflict, the Tajik Civil War saw looting and violence in the streets of cities and villages. People fled their homes to escape the depredations. Productivity plummeted in remaining local industries. The continued hostilities and constant political upheaval contributed to the rapidly declining economy; it also disrupted the maintenance of the general infrastructure. Silt remained in the canals and irrigation ditches, which hindered pumps and hampered the transference of water to fields. The record rainfalls and floods exacerbated this problem, helped create landslides, and further disrupted the functioning of irrigation pumps. The region was also beset with dust storms common to the cold desert and semiarid environment of Tajikistan.

Conditions of War That Facilitate the Spread of Diphtheria and Other Diseases

It was into the physical, political, cultural, and economic climate that the militaries, militia, and irregular forces encountered another foe—diphtheria. It is quite likely that the upheaval in neighboring Afghanistan, with its refugees fleeing to Tajikistan, carried the epidemic into the former Soviet Republic. Not the only disease that plagued the region, diphtheria was thought to be under control through vaccinations. This assumption resulted in the misdiagnosis of coughs and fevers by individuals and medical staff. Unfortunately, the disruption of governmental services in the wake of the Soviet withdrawal also reduced the number of children vaccinated and the lack of routine immunization and booster shots for adults.[30] Consequently, approximately half of the people who contracted diphtheria during the height of the Tajikistan war were over the age of 15.

Some of the common threads between the causes of diphtheria and the conditions in Tajikistan, especially in Qurghonteppa, include the following: The cold climate was especially conducive to the spread of the disease. However, climate alone does not account for the contagion in the early years of the civil war. Poor hygiene and insufficient dietary practices helped the disease to spread and facilitated the bacteria in infecting human hosts whose health was compromised by inadequate nutrition. Poor shelter furthered hygiene insufficiency and was a common condition for tens of thousands of Tajik citizens who fled their homes between 1992 and 1994. Exposure to the cold climate in the fall and winter seasons caused civil war refugees to gather in camps and close confines to share crude shelters and warmth, where they also shared the bacteria that spread diphtheria. The extreme rise in inflation, especially for food necessities, which saw a 416 percent increase, ensured that the majority of citizens and foreigners had inadequate diets, making it harder to fight off infections. Of the common food products produced in Tajikistan, only wheat retained a stable production; all other food crops saw a marked decrease in productivity between 1992 and 1994.[31]

Stress further undermined people's immune systems, brought on by fighting and the struggle to find the basic needs for survival. The standing water from floods, the failure of pumps, and inadequate filtration processes, also occasioned by the upheaval of war, provided another vector for the spread of the disease—contaminated water supplies. The high, mountainous terrain made movement from one region to the next difficult to impossible in the winter months.[32] This meant that once an epidemic began, the lack of proper medical facilities and care could not be supplemented from outside the region around Qurghonteppa, where the worst outbreaks occurred. The emigration of Russian personnel out of the region, with their aviation expertise and equipment, further complicated medical provisioning during the epidemic.

Evidence indicates that the rapid spread of diphtheria was directly related to the extent of immunization for children in the years leading up to the civil war. While the Soviet Sanitary-Epidemiological Service (SES) instituted widespread immunization, the number of follow-up boosters was inconsistent. Additionally, the recommended usage of the designated primary series for children (DTP or DT) was often replaced in rural areas with the administration of the adult (Td) primary series instead.[33] The SES was affected by the collapse of the Soviet Union. While SES subunits continued to operate in much the same fashion at the local, or *raion* level, the necessary supplies were restricted. In 1991, the dissolution of the USSR caused a disruption in vaccine supplies to all the republics except Russia. The disruption experienced in Tajikistan was extreme, with the closure of facilities, a dearth of vaccines, and the inability to test for infection or toxins due to a lack of electricity. Consequently, only the most severe cases were detected and reported by the limited medical facilities. This is a common problem with diphtheria in the best of situations, as its symptoms are often mistaken for a common sore throat. For those who were successfully diagnosed during the civil war, the normally administered protocols were challenging to implement because of the constant movement of the displaced populace.[34]

The Combined Impact of Diphtheria and War in Circumventing Disease Eradication

The diphtheria outbreak in Tajikistan occurred in 1993 and peaked in 1994. There was a 180 percent increase of reported cases in 1994, up to 1,907 identified cases from 680 the previous year. The majority of cases reported occurred in Qurghonteppa. The CDC report on diphtheria in Tajikistan indicated that the reasons for the epidemic in the NIS were not clear. However, careful examination of the combination of factors attributed to the spread reveals they were directly associated with the increased hostilities, human displacement, and the decline in health services and food production caused by the Tajik Civil War. This interpretation of the cause for the diphtheria epidemic helps explain why the epidemic was widespread in all the former Soviet Republics in 1993–1994, and yet the small country of Tajikistan had the highest incidence rates of all 15 republics.

Although recent historical outbreaks of diphtheria reveal that the bacterial infection is typically a childhood disease or one that affects children and the elderly, 50 percent of the cases reported during the Tajik Civil War came from people 15 years of age and older, with the highest numbers in the 15–17 and 40–49 age ranges.[35] Due to the lack of clear statistics designating which specific elements of the population contracted diphtheria, it is unknown whether the military forces or civilian populations were more affected by the epidemic. What is known is the extreme human impact in Qurghonteppa, Tajikistan. Evidence also reveals the corresponding conditions that enabled the spread of diphtheria and establishes that those conditions were caused by the outbreak of hostilities known as the Tajik Civil War of 1992–1997.

Periods of warfare throughout the ages have created conditions that facilitated the spread of contagious diseases. Despite the advances in identifying and combating diphtheria over the past century, the repeated occurrence of this bacterial infection during World War I, World War II, the Tajik Civil War, and other recent conflicts provides clear evidence that the conditions of war also undermine modern attempts to eradicate contagious diseases.

NOTES

1. Hilary Butler, "Diphtheria," accessed September 2, 2017, http://www.whale.to/m/butler .html.
2. James Grant, MD, DPH, "The Problems of Diphtheria," *British Medical Journal* 1, no. 4443 (March 2, 1946): 309, accessed May 13, 2017, http://www.jstor.org/stable /20365647; Tejpratap S. P. Tiwari, MD, "Diptheria," *VDP Surveillance Manual*, 5th ed. (2011): 1, CDC, accessed September 2, 2017, https://www.cdc.gov/vaccines/pubs/surv -manual/chpt01-dip.pdf.
3. Tiwari, "Diptheria."
4. A. M. Pappenheimer Jr. and D. Michael Gill, "Diphtheria," *Science, New Series* 182, no. 4110 (October 26, 1973): 357, published by American Association for the Advancement of Science, accessed September 2, 2017, http://www.jstor.org/stable/1737276.
5. "The Control of Diphtheria," *British Medical Journal* 2, no. 2276 (Aug. 13, 1904): 341, accessed September 2, 2017, http://www.jstor.org/stable/20281717.
6. Pappenheimer and Gill, "Diphtheria," 353.
7. "Diphtheria: Medical Research Council's Report," *British Medical Journal* 1, no. 3297 (March 8, 1924): 439, accessed September 2, 2017, http://www.jstor.org/stable/20435984.
8. Grant, "The Problems of Diphtheria," 309.
9. P. P. Mortimer, "Historical Review: The Diphtheria Vaccine Debacle of 1940 That Ushered in Comprehensive Childhood Immunization in the United Kingdom," *Epidemiology and Infection* 139, no. 4 (April 2011): 488, accessed September 2, 2017, www.jstor.org /stable/27975617.
10. "Cutaneous Diphtheria," *British Medical Journal* 1, no. 4345 (April 15, 1944): 534, accessed September 2, 2017, http://www.jstor.org/stable/20345103.
11. Grant, "The Problems of Diphtheria," 309.
12. Grant, "The Problems of Diphtheria."
13. "Cutaneous Diphtheria," 535.
14. Tiwari, "Diptheria."
15. Edward F. Bland, MD, "Heart Disease," *Infectious Diseases and General Medicine*, in Internal Medicine in World War II Series (Washington, D.C.: Office of Medical History, U.S. Army Medical Department): 431–432, accessed September 2, 2017, http:// history.amedd.army.mil/booksdocs/wwii/internalmedicinevolIII/chapter16.htm.

16. Aims C. McGuinness, MD, "Diseases Caused by Bacteria: Diphtheria," *Preventive Medicine in WWII,* Vol. 4, *Communicable Diseases, Transmitted Chiefly through Respiratory and Alimentary Tracts*, ed. John Boyd Coates Jr., MC, Ebbe Curtis Hoff, PhD, MD, and Phebe M. Hoff, MA (Washington, D.C.: Office of the Surgeon General, Department of the Army, 1958): 167, accessed September 2, 2017, http://history.amedd.army.mil/booksdocs/wwii/PM4/CH10.Diphtheria.htm.

17. Averill A. Liebow, MD, and John H. Bumstead, MD, "Cutaneous and Other Aspects of Diphtheria," in *Internal Medicine in World War II*, Vol. 2, *Infectious Diseases*, ed. John Boyd Coates Jr., MC, and W. Paul Havens Jr., MD (Washington, D.C.: Office of the Surgeon General, Department of the Army, 1963): 275, 307, accessed September 16, 2017, http://history.amedd.army.mil/booksdocs/wwii/infectiousdisvolii/chapter10.htm.

18. Liebow and Bumstead, "Cutaneous and Other Aspects of Diphtheria," 276–277.

19. Sherrilyn Coffman, "Margaret Utinsky: A Nurse Undertook Heroic Underground Activities in Support of American Prisoners in the Philippines during WWII," *American Journal of Nursing* 109, no. 5 (May 2009): 74, accessed September 2, 2017, http://www.jstor.org/stable/40384988.

20. Kristina Toderich, Munimjon Abbdusamatov, and Tsuneo Tsukatani, "Water Resources Assessment, Irrigation and Agricultural Developments in Tajikistan," *Kier Discussion Paper Series*, Kyoto Institute of Economic Research, no. 585 (March 2004): 3–8, accessed September 2, 2017, https://repository.kulib.kyoto-u.ac.jp/dspace/bitstream/2433/129519/1/DP585.pdf.

21. Kirill Nourzhanov and Christian Bleuer, *Tajikistan: A Political and Social History* (Canberra: Australian National University Press, 2013), 76.

22. Global Security.Org, "Tajikistan Civil War," accessed September 2, 2017, http://www.globalsecurity.org/military/world/war/tajikistan.htm.

23. Nourzhanov and Bleuer, *Tajikistan*, 291.

24. Nourzhanov and Bleuer, *Tajikistan*, 83, 90; and Svetlana Lolaeva, "Tajikistan in Ruins: The Descent into Chaos of a Central Asian Republic," George Washington University, 33, accessed September 2, 2017, https://www2.gwu.edu/~ieresgwu/assets/docs/demokratizatsiya%20archive/01-4_Lolaeva.PDF.

25. Nourzhanov and Bleuer, *Tajikistan*, 200–201.

26. Nourzhanov and Bleuer, *Tajikistan*, 103; Toderich, Abbdusamatov, and Tsukatani, "Water Resources Assessment," 10; and Jeffrey Hays, "Economy of Tajikistan," *Facts and Details* (April 2016), accessed September 2, 2017, http://factsanddetails.com/central-asia/Tajikistan/sub8_6d/entry-4896.html. The consumer price index helps to identify the extreme rise in the cost of food necessities during this time and is indicative of the substandard living conditions for the people in Tajikistan in general and specifically in Qurghonteppa.

27. Nourzhanov and Bleuer, *Tajikistan*, 333.

28. Lolaeva, "Tajikistan in Ruins," 34.

29. Lolaeva, "Tajikistan in Ruins," 40–43.

30. Mark R. Wallace et al., "Endemic Infectious Disease of Afghanistan," *Clinical Infectious Diseases* 34, Supplement 5, "Afghanistan: Health Challenges Facing Deployed Troops, Peacekeepers, and Refugees" (June 15, 2002): S197, accessed on September 2, 2017, http://www.jstor.org/stable/4461994.

31. Toderich, Abbdusamatov, and Tsukatani, "Water Resources Assessment," 10.

32. Shirin Akiner and Catherine Barnes, "The Tajik Civil War: Causes and Dynamics," from "Tajikistan: Disintegration or Reconciliation?," *Royal Institute of International Affairs*,

London (Spring 2001): 18, Conciliation Resources, accessed September 2, 2017, http://www.c-r.org/accord-article/tajik-civil-war-causes-and-dynamics.

33. "Diphtheria Epidemic: New Independent States of the Former Soviet Union, 1990–1994," *Morbidity and Mortality Weekly Report*, CDC 44, no. 10 (Mar 17, 1995): 178.

34. Charles R. Vitek, Erika Y. Bogatyreva, and Melinda Wharton, "Diphtheria Surveillance and Control in the Former Soviet Union and the Newly Independent States," *Journal of Infectious Diseases* 181 (Supplement 1): S25-6, accessed September 16, 2017, https://academic.oup.com/jid/article/181/Supplement_1/S23/842014/Diphtheria-Surveillance-and-Control-in-the-Former.

35. "Diphtheria Epidemic," 178, 179.

Part III

Viral Epidemics in the Context of Wars: Introduction

Rebecca M. Seaman

It was then (in December, 1914), that there began to appear and to multiply in the army, among the civilian population, in the hospitals, and above all among the prisoners of war, cases of illness which puzzled the doctors, who were overwhelmed with work owing to the number of sick and wounded. . . . Some doctors, having found the spirilla, asserted that is was relapsing fever. Others said that it was typhus. They were both right.[1]

—Voyislav Soubbotitch

The movement of people to form militaries, to fight wars, and to flee conflict creates interactions that facilitate exposure to and the transference of viruses. As a result, viruses have existed in conjunction with warfare throughout history. However, scientific understanding and identification of viruses occurred relatively recently. Consequently, the historical study of viral epidemics in wars of the distant past is imprecise at best. Part I, on unknown epidemics, postulates the possibility of viruses as the cause or source of those epidemics. Unfortunately, retroactive diagnosis of viruses is problematic, as the remnant viral physical evidence is often unstable and easily contaminated by contact with adjacent matter.

Viruses are not exactly living as living creatures are typically defined. They lack a "true viral metabolism" and have an "inability to reproduce on their own." Instead they must replicate inside the living cells of hosts. A recent study argues that the true identify of a virus is its "intracellular virus factory of infected cells" that survive via "an atypical reproduction method that requires infecting host cells."[2] How viruses replicate is based on the type of virus studied. Some viruses enter a host cell and immediately begin the process of replication. Others remain latent until appropriate stimuli induce them to begin replicating, at which point they produce disease symptoms in the host. One example of a long-term latent virus is chickenpox. In certain cases, like chickenpox, the resumption of replication may produce symptoms of a different but related disease (shingles). Additionally, some viruses cause cell lysis, or the destruction of the host cell in the process of replication.[3]

The chapters within this section introduce ancient and new viruses in the context of wars. Smallpox, one of the oldest known contagious diseases, has been associated with wars for over 2,000 years. Two wars were selected to highlight smallpox, examining the disease interactions on the invaded populations and the invading forces. In the case of Central America and South America, the Spanish were ill-equipped to defeat the warrior cultures that boasted far superior numbers. Even the Spanish weaponry proved inaccurate and cumbersome. It was not Spanish arms that defeated the numerous indigenous populations. Smallpox, in conjunction with other diseases and alliances, created poorly timed disruptions within the Aztec and Inca societies. The loss of indigenous leaders from smallpox prompted internal struggles for authority and opened opportunities for the smallpox-resistant Spanish to secure alliances and defeat otherwise powerful nations.

The American Revolution experienced smallpox in a different context. The colonial and indigenous populations in North America were more susceptible to smallpox than their British cousins and allies (respectively), though previous outbreaks had created some pockets of immunity. Prior to the conflict, inoculation against smallpox was introduced, providing a resource, albeit a risky one, to combat the epidemic spread of smallpox. The chapter traces George Washington's decision process to eventually inoculate the entire Continental Army and demonstrates how this potential colonial calamity ultimately proved an effective tool in ensuring the survival of the revolutionary armies.

The Haitian Revolt of 1802–1803 introduces yellow fever, another historic virus. This disease had emerged in epidemic proportions during previous wars. The timing of the Haitian epidemic, the immunity or resistance of the local Haitian population, and the typical lack of immunity on the part of the invading French created a reversal in the roles of colonial invaders versus indigenous populations. The superiority of arms, leadership, military structure, and training should have resulted in a French victory. Yet, the impact of yellow fever on the French military's health and unity of command assisted the local population in securing its independence.

Two chapters examine World War I and associated epidemics. The war created an opportunity for localized epidemics to spread into worldwide pandemics. Interestingly, measles emerged in numerous mobilization camps and transport ships, but it did not create a pandemic as a result. The medical and hygiene improvements, in conjunction with the push for medical research, helped to develop methods of containing the measles epidemics. The inability to identify the virus source allowed the virus to spread in the cramped conditions troops experienced in camps, trains, and ships. Yet, widespread contamination was averted.

The same cannot be said for the great influenza pandemic of 1918. Influenza also broke out in American mobilization camps and rapidly spread throughout society and abroad with the transfer of troops to the European theater of war. The chapter discusses the possible origins of the influenza, medical perceptions, and attempts to control and treat the virus. It also examines the impact of the sheer numbers of affected civilians and military personnel. The vast spread of this pandemic prompted the postwar movement to collaborate internationally in identifying and preventing future epidemics. Consequently, research that began with measles epidemics during World War I and expanded with the outbreak of the misnamed "Spanish flu" at the war's end eventually set the stage for rapidly improving medical research to eradicate epidemics globally in the future.

Despite international collaboration and improved medical research, epidemics continued to erupt, often in the context of wars. The last two chapters highlight the emergence of new and old viruses (HIV/AIDS and mumps, respectively). HIV emerged amid the disruption of social structures and refugees fleeing the African wars of the late 20th century. However, this retrovirus was misidentified and then identified incorrectly with only certain population sectors. The combination of disruptions from civil war, the breakdown of social structures and restrictions, and the flight of refugees within Africa and abroad, along with the misdiagnoses and presumption of disease association with restricted population groups, allowed HIV/AIDS to spread unchecked for decades, facilitating its spread into a global pandemic.

Medical personnel not only recognized mumps but also developed vaccinations that were disseminated to eradicate the disease. Unfortunately, the ethnic and religious conflicts of the Bosnian Wars during the 1990s disrupted the internal structures of the former Yugoslavia. Fragmented into numerous independent states with undetermined borders, the fluctuating governments and alliances diverted resources from social structures and medical protocols to military priorities. One can debate the efficacy of such resource reallocations in the short term, but the long-term impact from the Bosnian Wars of the 1990s emerged when unvaccinated children from the wars contracted mumps as young adults in 2010–2012.

Whether ancient in origin or newly encountered, viruses have the potential to produce disastrous results among peoples and nations at war. The existence of viral immunity or resistance by one side over the other typically aids those with immunity in defeating their foes. The discovery and use of inoculations or vaccinations can prevent the spread of viruses among military ranks and civilian populations. But war also causes societal disruptions that can impede effective medical protocols and health conditions that should avert the emergence of viral epidemics. Usually such interferences are observed during wars, but the impacts of military disruptions are occasionally felt long after the resumption of peace. Whether viral epidemics cause disruptions that facilitate the eruption of wars, emerge amid the commotion caused by war, or arise years later from the consequences of war, they are fundamentally connected to war.

NOTES

1. Voyislav Soubbotitch, "A Pandemic of Typhus in Serbia in 1914 and 1915," *Proceedings of the Royal Society of Medicine* 11 (1918): 32–33.
2. Arshan Nasir and Gustavo Caetano-Anollés, *Science Advances* 1, no. 8 (September 25, 2015): 18, accessed on September 2, 2017, http://advances.sciencemag.org/content/1/8/e1500527/tab-pdf.
3. Sheila C. Grossman and Carol Mattson Porth, *Porth's Pathophysiology: Concepts of Altered Health States*, 9th ed. (Philadelphia: Wolters Kluwer Health, Lippincott Williams and Wilkins, 2014), 254–256.

Chapter 9

Smallpox: Ensuring the Destruction of Armies in Colonial New Spain and Peru, 1518–1625

Angela Thompson

The pestilence of measles and smallpox was so severe and cruel that more than one-fourth of the Indian people in all the land died—and this loss had the effect of hastening the end of the fighting because there died a great quantity of men and warriors and many lords and captains and valiant men against whom we would have had to fight and deal with as enemies, and miraculously Our Lord killed them and removed them from before us.[1]

—Bernard Vazquez de Tapia

The Spanish introduced a host of European diseases into the New World in the 16th century that certainly facilitated Spain's conquest of the Americas. Old World diseases, such as smallpox, typhus, mumps, measles, plague, and influenza, among others, weakened native resistance in the fight against the conquerors and likely created significant psychological despair. More critically, these diseases helped spur a rapid decline of native populations. When European diseases first afflicted New World populations, they caused "virgin-soil" epidemics. This meant that the native peoples had no prior exposure to the microorganisms that caused those diseases and had thus not developed any natural immunity; consequently, they suffered very high mortality rates.

Both the extent of and reasons for native mortality are still under debate by demographers, medical historians, ethnohistorians, anthropologists, and others. Those debates usually focus on the extent of the demographic disasters these diseases caused and when, and what epidemics actually caused the disasters. But little doubt exists that disease played a major role in facilitating the conquest of Native Americans and in the subsequent serious decline in their populations, if not also in the complete disappearance of many native societies. Surely a convergence of many factors contributed to the devastation of native populations, but the combination of new virulent diseases spread during a period of warfare contributed to the lethal consequences.[2]

America Not "New" to Disease: Fertile Ground for Old World Viruses

The most terrifying and deadly Old World disease introduced to the New World was smallpox. Beginning in the early 16th century, it marched as a "conqueror" along with the Spanish conquistadors from the Caribbean to Mexico and Guatemala and from Panama into Peru. Smallpox was likely one of the "advance-guard" conquerors, reaching native communities ahead of the conquerors themselves, sometimes even decades before the Spanish and other Europeans arrived on the local scene.[3] The hardy variola virus is capable of spreading through the sharing of bedding, clothing, and utensils and even from contact with animals. This reality made the disease one that was easily communicated through trade and among soldiers, and it traveled wherever militaries moved in the era of exploration.

Because of their isolation from the Old World for thousands of years, Native Americans had suffered fewer virulent epidemic diseases than the people of the Old World. The North Asian steppes from whence ancient Native Americans migrated and the northwest of North America to which they migrated in small nomadic groups served as a "cold-filter" barrier to many diseases. In addition to the cold and ice of the Arctic region, the vastness of the Atlantic and Pacific Oceans protected America's First People. Furthermore, these Native Americans domesticated only a few animals prior to the period of sustained contact. Many Old World human epidemic diseases, such as smallpox, were shared with domesticated animals or related to diseases those animals carried.[4]

The New World, however, was not a disease-free environment. Human skeletal and mummified remains, as well as codices, sculptures, wall paintings, and other artistic representations, show the state of health and some of the ailments that people of New World suffered from, including cleft palate; clubfoot; leishmaniasis (an insect-born fungus that destroys facial tissue); Chagas disease (also caused by a tropical insect called the assassin or kissing bug that introduces a protozoa, *trypanosomiasis cruzi*, into the body); other parasites; respiratory and dysenteric diseases; skin diseases; blindness; dental problems; wounds and fractures; heart problems; tuberculosis; pneumonia; yaws; and syphilis.

Codices (or native books both pre- and postconquest), such as the *Badianus Manuscript*,[5] the *Florentine Codex*, and contemporary accounts and histories such as *The Royal Commentaries of the Inca*, provide information about medical treatments that existed among Middle and South American native peoples before the arrival of the Spanish in 1492.[6] Some of these treatments included tea made from chinchona bark for fevers, poultices from matico for skin ailments, tobacco for insect and snake bites, tea and leaves of the coca plant for altitude sickness. Stimulants included ground roots and herbs mixed with honey for sore throats and coughs, the root of the "divine cactus" *teonochtli* for toothaches, and resin, or the gum, from the guaiacum tree to treat syphilis. These and many other remedies are still used today (one can find them in local markets) in their traditional form or as derivatives in modern medicine. The chinchona tree contains quinine and similar chemicals that are effective for treating fevers and other ailments. Matico, a member of the black pepper plant family, was shown to be effective for skin diseases in the 19th century. A derivative of guiaicum is guaifenesin, a common expectorant in cough syrups sold today. Andean peoples still use coca for altitude sickness, and derivatives from the plant provide painkillers and stimulants as well as the recreational drug cocaine.

Before the arrival of the Spanish, healers among the Andean peoples effectively practiced trephination, which entailed removing a portion of the skull to relieve pressure on the brain in cases of skull fractures or other serious blows to the skull. Evidence indicates they had a 50–60 percent success rate in precolonial times. Meanwhile, when this procedure was used in the Old World, only 10 percent of patients survived.[7]

Native informants and codices indicated that disease and ill health had numerous causes: the gods and the supernatural, sorcery and magic, and imbalances in body and the natural order. These perceptions of disease and health were not unlike those of the Europeans. But while Europeans strove to balance the four humors (blood, phlegm, yellow bile, and black bile) and to avoid miasmas, or bad air, Aztecs strove to balance hot and cold, wet and dry. These efforts led to moderation in certain behaviors, such as in drinking alcoholic beverages, like the native pulque, or in sexual activity.[8] Perceptions that the gods and sorcerers had visited their wrath upon them were probably in the minds of Native Americans when confronted with a new pestilence as devastating as smallpox. Though not a direct impact on the population's health, such perceptions had a demoralizing effect.

Origin and Symptoms of Smallpox Virus

Smallpox, or variola pox, although unique to humans, belongs to a family of Old World viruses, the Poxviridae genus *Orthopoxvirus*, which affects numerous mammals. In addition to smallpox, the genus includes cowpox, vaccinia, monkeypox, camelpox, rabbitpox, and buffalopox, many of these perhaps a variation of vaccinia pox. Infection with one member of the genus confers special immunity against other members of the genus.[9] Although its exact origin is unknown, smallpox may have originated in Africa, perhaps among protohuman primates or other monkey species. It has probably afflicted humans for at least 3,000 years.

A highly contagious disease, smallpox may have spread from Africa to India and then on to China along trade routes. Mummies from ancient Egypt, such as that of Ramses V, who died in 1157 BCE, have scarring from pustules on the skin that indicate possible smallpox. Chinese sources from the first century BCE describe a serious disease with smallpox symptoms that arrived from the West. Since that time, and into the 18th century, accounts of presumed smallpox outbreaks describe similar symptoms to those used in modern medical literature. Typical descriptions include the sudden onset of fever and malaise, with the fever rising quickly; severe headache, backache, and vomiting; and a rash erupting as papules after two or three days on the face and upper extremities and then spreading to the rest of the body. The papules become pustular by the 5th day of the rash, reaching maximum size by the 9th day. Scabs form by the 13th day, and by the 20th day, most scabs have fallen off, leaving whitened and scarred areas on the skin.[10] Sources also describe much pain, suffering, and death. If death occurs, it usually does so during the second week.[11]

As a virus, smallpox has developed into different strains, some more lethal than others. Evidence suggests that the more deadly strain, *Variola major*, caused most of the recorded smallpox epidemics, at least since the 15th century and perhaps much earlier. *V. major* continued to cause epidemics with rates of 15–45 percent mortality into the 20th century. By the 19th century, mortality records indicate that a less lethal strain, *Variola minor*, had appeared, which caused fewer fatalities, perhaps as low as 1 percent. *V. minor* may have existed in Europe prior to the 16th century and survived along with *V. major*, causing minor cases with minimal rash and scarring but few deaths.[12]

Diffusion of Smallpox and the Impact on Societies: Endemic and Virgin Soil

As smallpox only infects humans, sustained transmission requires a certain level of human population and intimate contact as well as favorable environmental conditions to create an epidemic. The usual method of transmission is through airborne droplets passed over short distances that enter the body through the mouth or nose. Therefore, for infection to spread effectively, humans must live in close contact. Modern observations of susceptible populations show that 26–59 percent of those who live in the same household, compound, or dense neighborhood will contract the disease during an outbreak.[13] To sustain an epidemic of smallpox requires a population of around 250,000 susceptible individuals. Because the smallpox molecule is comparatively large, a certain level of humidity is required to carry the molecule from host to host in absence of direct or very close human contact. On the other hand, high humidity, particularly in warmer temperatures, may limit the spread over larger distances. Although smallpox can occur in any climate, it thrives better in a cool climate; thus, in some areas of the world, it occurred seasonally. Smallpox can also be spread through the pustule matter by direct human-to-human contact, entering through the mouth or nose or directly into the body and bloodstream through a cut. Rarely can infected bedclothes, linen, or clothing transmit smallpox, but in ideal conditions, the live virus can survive in dried scabs for a time, even outside the body. Although no clear evidence exists for transmission by food or water, it may be that contaminated water sources could transmit the virus within a very short time after contamination.[14] The incubation period before symptoms appear after becoming infected ranges from 7 to 14 days. An infected person is contagious from the onset of the rash until all the pustules dry up and scabs fall off, about three weeks.[15]

Smallpox is not only a terrifying disease due to the extreme pain, discomfort, and distress that it causes in its victims, but it has also historically caused high mortality. Numerous studies of unvaccinated populations in the 20th century record fatalities as high as 50 percent or more. Smallpox epidemics in previous centuries, even when it became primarily a childhood disease but before vaccination was readily available, also caused high mortality, 18–30 percent of those infected.[16] Such high infection and mortality rates over time and space in many different populations, including isolated peoples, indicate that smallpox was a lethal microbe. Only prior exposure, or some kind of inoculation or vaccination, prevented or reduced the severity of the symptoms and mortality. No other treatments have been very effective in reducing mortality.

Among Europeans in the 15th and 16th centuries, smallpox seemed to be an endemic childhood disease, meaning that it remained present in the population and affected mostly children and youths. It emerged in epidemic proportions only when a significant number of children had been born in an area in which population density was high enough to sustain an epidemic among the susceptible children. Those who survived epidemic and occasional outbreaks had immunity, which was probably lifelong. Additionally, many Europeans, adults and children alike, often lived in close contact with domestic animals, perhaps even some wild rodents. Exposure to animals that carried related orthopoxviruses also may have conveyed some immunity to smallpox, if not preventing it, perhaps reducing its lethality.[17] Prior exposure and domesticated animals may explain why Europeans remained virtually unaffected when smallpox struck native populations in the New World.

The first serious epidemic outbreaks of Old World disease occurred in the Caribbean within a short time after Columbus's 1492 encounter with the local native peoples. Records indicate that as early as Columbus's second voyage in 1493, both Spaniards and Indians had fallen ill. Although not conclusively identified, described symptoms indicate that influenza may have been the culprit for that and subsequent outbreaks, perhaps spread by the pigs that had accompanied the second voyage. Regardless of the causes of these epidemic episodes, the consequences were clear: the downward spiral and the eventual devastation of Caribbean native populations and their cultures. There is wide disagreement over the level of population at the point of contact, with estimates for the island of Hispaniola alone ranging from 50,000 to several million. In 1510, Diego Columbus reported 33,523 Taino on the island. By 1542, scarcely 2,000 were left.[18] Amid this decline, the timing of the arrival of smallpox unwittingly added a new weapon to the Spanish arsenal.

Tracking the Spread of Smallpox through New World Conflicts

Although some argue that smallpox arrived in the Caribbean as early as 1507, no contemporary evidence exists to confirm that date. Abundant eyewitness accounts and witness testimony, from or provided to Peter Martyr, Bartolome de Las Casas, Francisco Oviedo, and Hieronymite friars, indicated that an outbreak began in 1518 in the West Indian islands, including Hispaniola, Puerto Rico, and Cuba. These accounts indicate 30 percent or more of the natives died from the disease.[19] Oviedo, who always attempted to portray Spain's interactions with the native populations in positive terms, said smallpox left the islands desolated of Indians, "with so few that it seemed a great judgement from heaven."[20] Smallpox probably arrived directly from Spain, or perhaps from Africa, by ship. Thus, when Hernán Cortés began his adventure to conquer the land now called Mexico in February 1519, smallpox was already in the vicinity.

Cortés and the Advance of Smallpox across Mexico

Cortés organized his expedition from the Caribbean and then sailed to the mainland with over 400 men. Through a combination of diplomacy and fighting, the conquistador made his way to the interior. He enjoyed significant fortune, the arrival of smallpox during the conquest being just one example of a providential coincidence. For example, in a stop along the northeastern Yucatan coast before landing where he would march inland at present-day Veracruz, Cortés picked up a fellow countryman, Jeronimo Aguilar. Having been shipwrecked there for several years, Aguilar had learned the local Mayan language.

Shortly thereafter, Cortés landed on the western side of the Yucatan Peninsula, where a Mayan leader gifted Cortés several Indian maidens, no doubt to encourage the Spanish to go elsewhere. Among these young women was Malinalli (Doña Marina), who spoke both a Nahuatl language (the language family of most of the Aztec Empire) and a Mayan language. Through a three-way translation system that included Aguilar and Doña Marina, Cortés had the ability to communicate with virtually any peoples he encountered on his journey through the mainland to the Aztec capital, a consequence of another coincidence.[21]

After founding the port town of Veracruz in June 1519, which became his center of communication and supply, Cortés led about 300 of his men on a march inland. This expedition reached the center of the Aztec Empire and its capital, Tenochtitlan, by November of the same year. Cortés picked up native allies along the way, especially from the Tlaxcalans, who were traditional enemies of Moctezuma and the Aztec confederation. Stopping at the native city of Churultecal, now the town of Cholula, Cortés fortunately learned through his female translator, Malinalli, that local native warriors planned to ambush Cortés and his men. Cortés reacted swiftly by calling the local chieftains to come to him and then slaughtering them and many residents of the city. Having shown that he could be utterly ruthless, Cortés faced much less opposition on the remaining route to the central valley and Aztec capital.

The first encounter between the Spanish and the Aztec emperor Moctezuma occurred in the autumn of 1519 and was peaceful and full of ceremony. Moctezuma and his very large retinue of nobles and warriors met the Spanish outside the capital and accompanied them to the city. Once inside the city, relations soured quickly. As protection, Cortés took the emperor hostage.

In May 1520, Cortés received news that interrupted his efforts to solidify control of the Aztec capital and its environs. The Cuban governor, Diego Velazquez, was angry that Cortés had begun his adventure even though Velazquez had withdrawn his official permission and sanction of the expedition. Velazquez sent a force of 800–900 men or more against Cortés (the exact number is unclear). Led by Panfilo de Narvaez, this contingent was met and defeated by Cortés, who then recruited the survivors of the Narvaez expedition, compelling them to join his forces. Apparently, among this group was someone, a native or natives from Cuba or a young man, perhaps just a teenager, just recovering from smallpox contracted during the outbreak on the islands. He or they were obviously still contagious. Since this encounter occurred in the spring and summer of 1520, during the rainy season when it was generally cool and wet, creating the perfect environment for the spread of smallpox, the disease spread rapidly among a completely vulnerable native population. Cortés and his Spanish soldiers were not affected, a fact not lost on native observers, both ally and enemy alike.

Having neutralized the threat sent by Diego Velazquez, Cortés returned to Tenochtitlan with smallpox accompanying his newly expanded forces. Along the way, he learned that the contingent of Spanish he had left in the capital to guard Moctezuma was under threat and that natives in the countryside were up in arms. Cortés quickly returned to the capital. Finding the palace area under siege, where the Spanish soldiers were headquartered with the treasure they had collected and where they held Moctezuma as their prisoner, Cortés forced his way in to rescue his men. He then prepared his troops to flee the capital under cover of darkness, which they did the first of July. This episode is called *la Noche Triste* ("the Sad Night" or "the Night of Sorrows") because of the loss of many hundreds of Spanish soldiers as they fled. During the melee, Moctezuma was killed.

In the meantime, smallpox moved through the native population from coast to interior, dampening the revolts against the Spanish. While the Spanish soldiers seemed to be impervious to the infection, the disease dismayed Cortés. He wrote about his concern in his third letter to King Charles I, indicating that his native allies had suffered as did those natives he had sought to subdue and conquer:

> I remained with them two or three days and then left for the city of Tascalteca [Tlaxcala], which is six leagues from there; when I arrived all the Spaniards and the inhabitants of the city were very pleased to see me. On the following day all the chiefs of that city and province came to speak to me and told me how Magiscacin, who was their overlord, had died of the smallpox; they knew well how much this would grieve me, as he was a great friend of mine.[22]

Magiscacin was the overlord of Cortés's allies, the Tlaxcalans. Following the flight from Tenochtitlan in July, Magiscacin had provided refuge for Cortés and his wounded soldiers, after which they left to put down rebellions in neighboring communities. Upon their return to Tlaxcala, they found that smallpox had reached the city. The epidemic weakened the native forces Cortés had based his invasion hopes on. During that summer and autumn, the disease spread to many of the cities and provinces of the empire, including the capital and those in rebellion against the Spanish. Smallpox reached the Aztec capital after the flight of the Spanish and death of the emperor Moctezuma. Moctezuma's successor and brother, Cuitlahuac, who had instigated the rebellion against Cortés, rose to power in his brother's wake. His reign proved short-lived as he, too, died of the disease. A descendant of Aztec royal families, Fernando de Alva Ixtlilxochitl, wrote in the latter part of the century in his *Horribles crueldades* that Cuitlahuac had ruled no more than 40 days when he died during this terrible outbreak of smallpox. His death probably occurred sometime in August or September 1520, although most sources say he ruled 80 days, thus placing his death in November.[23]

An even more compelling account of the epidemic is in the Aztec version of the conquest in the work compiled by the priest Bernardino de Sahagun, *The General History of Things of New Spain*, also called *The Florentine Codex*. A sense of despair emerges in the description of the horror suffered:

> Twenty-ninth Chapter, in which it is told how there came a plague, of which the natives died. Its name was smallpox. It was at the time that the Spaniards set forth from Mexico.
>
> But before the Spaniards had risen against us, first there came to be prevalent a great sickness, a plague. It was in Tepeilhuitl that it originated, that there spread over the people a great destruction of men. Some it indeed covered [with pustules]; they were spread everywhere, on one's face, on one's head, on one's breast, etc. There was indeed perishing; many indeed died of it. No longer could they walk; they only lay in their abodes, in their beds. No longer could they move, no longer could they bestir themselves, no longer could they raise themselves, no longer could they stretch themselves out on their sides, no longer could they stretch themselves out face down, no longer could they stretch themselves out on their backs. And when they bestirred themselves, much did they cry out. There was much perishing. Like a covering, covering-like, were the pustules. Indeed many people died of them, and many just died of hunger. There was death from hunger; there was no one to take care of another; there was no one to attend to another.[24]

Records indicate the epidemic devastated the society and its leadership, military, and economy. In his analysis of various historical and primary accounts of the outbreak, historian Robert McCaa concluded, "The epidemic of 1520 enveloped other towns in Central Mexico and ravaged the ruling clans, weakening their diplomatic and military cadres."[25] Smallpox sickened and killed so many that there were no adults to provide food or care for the sick. Those who survived suffered scarring and blindness: "And many people were harmed by them on their faces; their faces were roughened. Of some, the eyes were injured; they were blinded. . . . At this time this plague prevailed indeed sixty day—sixty day-signs—when it ended, when it diminished"[26] (see Figure 9.1). When Cortés regrouped and returned to Tenochtitlan in late 1520, he encountered fierce fighting for months, but from a much weaker enemy than he had encountered only months before. The empire's capital fell to the Spanish and its native allies in August 1521 after a siege. Smallpox, too, was an invading ally, if an unwitting one.

In addition to the epidemic that had afflicted the Aztecs, a report submitted in the late 1560s indicated a plague had raged among the Yucatec Maya about 50 years previously. This outbreak coincided with the first documented outbreak of smallpox (1518–1519) on the Caribbean islands not far from the Yucatec

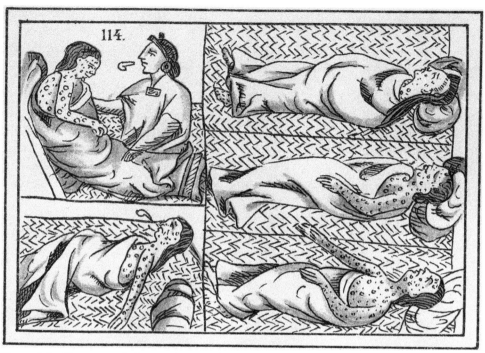

Figure 9.1   Florentine Codex, Book 12, Fol. 54. This image accompanied the description given above of the epidemic. (Courtesy of the Peabody Museum of Archaeology and Ethnology, Harvard University, PM# 2004.24.29636)

mainland. The Yucatec site was near where the Spanish were making coastal explorations at the time, although the Spanish did not attempt to conquer the Yucatec Maya until the 1540s. Diego de Landa wrote about the outbreak in his *Relacion de las cosas de Yucatan*: "After that there came again a pestilence, with great pustules that rotted the body, fetid in odor, and so that the members fell in pieces within four or five days."[27] Both the timing and the description strongly suggest that smallpox may have been the culprit in this case.

Not as conclusive, the *Annals of the Cakchiquels*, a codex of the Maya of highland Guatemala compiled later in the 16th century, date the beginning of a similar epidemic to 1519 and said that it had spread widely in 1520–1521. Although the description of this epidemic in the *Annals* is comparatively vague, leading to debate about whether the epidemic in this account was smallpox or measles or another rash-causing disease, the timing implicated smallpox. Likewise, when Cortés sent his captain, Pedro de Alvarado, to conquer the area in 1524–1525, evidence indicates Alvarado's task was doubtlessly made easier than that experienced by Cortés only three years prior.[28]

The smallpox epidemic that began in the Caribbean in 1518 spread farther than the mainland of Middle America; it perhaps even spread deep into South America, lasting well into the 1520s, perhaps until 1525–1528, and is thus referred to as a pandemic.[29] Beginning in the 1510s, expeditions from the Caribbean islands sailed to the Isthmus of Panama and went overland to the Pacific. From there, they explored down the Pacific coast of South America. A scourge accompanied them, invaded the area, and spread to parts of the Inca Empire that lay to the south.

Connecting Spanish Trade and Pizarro to Smallpox among the Inca

The epidemic that spread to the Inca was perhaps five to seven years before an expedition led by Francisco Pizarro, who marched inland and conquered the empire. Timing and descriptions by locals indicate that this scourge might have been smallpox. Whatever it was, it killed the reigning Inca emperor, Huayna Capac, and within hours his second son and designated heir, Ninan Cuyochi, sometime between 1525 and 1527.

From the *History of the Inca Empire* by Father Bernabe Cobo, written in the late 16th and early 17th centuries, comes a description of this epidemic based on evidence that Cobo collected while in Peru soon after the Spanish conquest: "Shortly after the first arrival of the Spaniards in this land, while the Inca was in the province of Quito, smallpox broke out among his subjects, and many of them died. . . . And later he got smallpox." Cobo went on to say that a healer told the Inca's aides to take him out into the sun (since the Inca ruler represented the sun, who was said to be his father), but he died nonetheless. The Inca historian Garcilaso de la Vega, in his *Royal Commentaries*, also refers to a fever as the cause of Huayna Capac's death. Whatever the cause of the fever, the deaths of Huayna Capac and his son threw the empire into a dynastic war between two half-brothers, Huascar and Atahualpa.[30]

In 1530–1531, another wave of rash-causing disease, perhaps measles, smallpox, or both, afflicted upper South America.[31] In 1532, Pizarro entered the scene during this civil conflict and epidemic crisis and took advantage of it. He captured the younger of the contentious bothers, Atahualpa. Pizarro held him hostage, enriched himself of the Inca's treasure, and conquered the Inca Empire. Pizarro was not only able to take advantage of an internal civil war among the Inca to assist his conquest, but he also was able to leverage the impact of disease to ensure his victory over the Inca.

Historical Accounts of the Combined Influence of Disease and Wars on Early America

Although evidence is less conclusive, smallpox and a host of other European diseases, especially measles, typhus, plague, and malaria, affected native peoples in the frontiers of the new Spanish viceroyalties of New Spain (Spanish North America) and Peru (Spanish South America). These diseases likely accompanied various exploratory expeditions even before these areas were conquered and settled in the 16th and 17th centuries. Expeditions into northern New Spain (northwest Mexico and Florida) were organized somewhere between 1530 and 1565 and included those led by Nuno Beltran de Guzman (1530–1531), Diego de Guzman

(1533), Cabeza de Vaca (1535), Fray Marcos de Niza (1539), Hernando de Soto (1539–1542), and Francisco de Ibarra (1563–1565). Reports from these expeditions described populated towns and "kingdoms," but without reference to specific population figures.[32] During some of these expeditions, reports indicate that both Spanish and natives suffered from various ailments, but natives more often died of them.

Furthermore, when the Jesuits accompanying the Spanish later moved in to establish missions in the same areas in the late 16th century and 17th century, many of the peoples described in earlier accounts seemed to have disappeared, and other communities were greatly diminished in population. The Jesuits also witnessed the consequences of simultaneous epidemics of measles and smallpox on native communities in northwestern New Spain in 1593–1594. The Jesuits were known for keeping better records than many Spanish conquistadors, explorers, and missionaries. They reported that most of the native population suffered and many died. In a letter, one Jesuit said that two-thirds of the children he had baptized had died during the epidemic.[33] Because the Jesuits themselves were not affected during this epidemic, and because they had tried to help and treat the natives who were, they more easily attracted natives to their missions. Disease thus likely facilitated the "spiritual conquest" of native populations.[34]

By the last quarter of the 16th century, epidemics and conquest had added to the devastation of native populations in upper South America, present-day Colombia, and Venezuela. These peoples likely suffered from the early epidemics of the 1520s and 1530s, although written evidence is lacking. Official reports, however, indicate high mortality, around 35 percent of the population in some areas, from a smallpox epidemic that affected the region from 1558 to 1560. Likewise, in the period 1558–1569, smallpox reached southern South America along the Rio de la Plata river system.[35]

Mortality and morbidity figures for specific epidemic episodes in the 16th century are imprecise, sketchy, and impressionistic at best. More accurate counts of native populations in some areas, from the 1540s to the 1620s, indicate that native populations declined precipitously wherever the Spanish traveled or settled. For example, four to five epidemic crises occurred in Mexico from 1520 to 1625 involving smallpox, measles, typhus, mumps, and other diseases. Some called the epidemics *huey zahuatl* or *matlazahuatl*, Nahuatl words that referred to diseases with a rash (see Table 9.1). These epidemics caused a 80–95 percent reduction in the native population in Central Mexico in just a century.

Scholars continue debating the level of the preconquest Mexican population, estimating that it was anywhere from 5 million to 25 million, with the majority of sources concluding that about 16 million people inhabited the region on the eve of the Spanish conquest.[36] Regardless of what the actual preconquest figure might have been, the population was large. Figures for 1548 to 1625 are fairly accurate and based on the Spanish tribute (native tax) records. Even with the least-case scenario, the population declined by 80 percent, from 5 million to 991,000 in just over a century, a catastrophic decline.

Table 9.1.   Indian Population Decline and Epidemics in Mexico, 1519–1625

Year	Indian Population	% Decline	Epidemic Years	Possible Diseases
1519	5,000,000 to 25,200,000 (range of estimates)			
			1520	Smallpox, "huey zahuatl"
			1529–1532	Measles, probably "zahuatl" but "small rash"
1532	16,800,000?			
			1545–1548	Matla(l) zahuatl, disease(s) with rash, possible typhus, smallpox, measles Indian deaths est. 800,000
1548	6,300,000			
			1550	Mumps (possibly)
			1559–1564	Various hard to identify diseases
1568	2,650,000	57.93		
			1576–1581	Matlazahuatl, various diseases Indian deaths est. 2,000,000
1580	1,900,000	69.84		
1595	1,375,000	78.17	1595	Measles, typhus, mumps, possibly
			1604	Smallpox, measles, mumps
1605	1,075,000	82.93		
			1613–1615	Smallpox, measles
1625	991,000	84.26		

Sources: Compiled from Sherburne Cook and Woodrow Borah, *Indian Population of Central Mexico* (Berkeley: University of California Press, 1960); and Hanns Prem, "Disease Outbreaks in Central Mexico during the Sixteenth Century," in N. D. Cook and George Lovell, *Secret Judgments of God*, (Norman: University of Oklahoma Press, 1992), 20–48.

The 17th century in New Spain (Mexico and Central America) experienced fewer widespread epidemics, although regional outbreaks occurred. Precisely because the native population had declined to just under a million, and the white and mixed population was comparatively small, under 200,000, the population was too small to sustain widespread epidemics until the end of the century. Smallpox needs a vulnerable population concentration of around 250,000 to sustain an epidemic, and few areas had such population density of unexposed people.

South America, conquered much later than most of New Spain, likewise experienced widespread epidemics in the 16th century and periodic regional epidemics in the 17th century. The diseases involved were the same as those that had afflicted New Spain, but they also included diphtheria, scarlet fever, and the plague (see Table 9.2). The plague affected people living in the Andes, where their domesticated llamas and alpacas harbored the fleas that caused plague in both humans and animals. Smallpox was involved in continent-wide epidemics at least three times between the 1520s and 1590s and many more regional outbreaks. The effect on the population was probably similar to the experience in Mexico, but comparable figures do not exist for all of Peru. The situation in Arequipa in 1589 is probably representative. There, smallpox caused over 25 percent mortality in an outbreak of the disease.

Smallpox and other European diseases helped Spain conquer an empire in the Americas. Disease alone did not result in the collapse of the Aztec and Inca empires. The combined impacts of native leaders succumbing to smallpox, large numbers of ailing and dying warriors, and fears of the disease combined with perceptions of the Spanish as impervious to the same all took their toll on both indigenous empires. Certainly, native sources indicated that a multitude of diseases were lethal, but smallpox may well have been the most frightening because of the dire symptoms the virus caused and the high mortality its victims suffered. It was viewed as one of the "horrible cruelties" perpetrated by the Spanish against its native subjects. Ironically, the Spanish Empire was also the most aggressive of the early modern European empires in trying to contain and prevent the spread of smallpox, most notably in the 18th century, when the disease returned in regular epidemic proportions and mainly affected children. By the 1780s, the Spanish

Table 9.2.   Major Epidemics in 16th-Century Peru

Years	Diseases
1524–1527	Smallpox, possibly; at least fevers
1531–1533	Measles, plague, fevers
1546–1548	Plague, possibly pneumonic form, perhaps typhus*
1558–1562	Smallpox, possibly measles, and possibly with influenza
1585–1591	Smallpox, measles, mumps, perhaps mixed with influenza and a vector-borne disease**
1597–1618	Outbreaks of measles, diphtheria, typhus, scarlet fever

*The concurrent illness of llamas and sheep—both susceptible to plague—strengthens the argument for plague; whereas, one form of typhus caused by rickettsia prowazekii is carried by lice, which live on the Andean guinea pig.

**In 1589, for example, Arequipa, Peru, reported infection rates for smallpox of 80% with 30% mortality, meaning 26.7% overall mortality.

Source: N. D. Cook and Lovell, *Secret Judgments of God.*

government had urged the voluntary use of inoculation or variolation (the injection of live smallpox matter, which was used as a folk preventative in the Middle East). This method was employed systematically in a 1797 outbreak with great benefit.[37]

After Edward Jenner's introduction of the smallpox vaccine, which injected related but less lethal cowpox or horsepox matter to provoke an immune reaction, it was the Spanish government that embarked on an ambitious effort to control smallpox in its colonies. It organized and funded an empire-wide expedition in 1803–1804, led by Spanish physician Dr. Francisco Balmis, to introduce Jenner's vaccine to its vast empire, from the Canaries to the Americas and on to the Philippines.[38] This proactive policy came too late for millions of Native American people in Central and South America who had died as a result of Spain's acquisition of its empire, in part through an unwitting "alliance" with an effective conqueror, smallpox.

NOTES

1. Bernard Vazquez de Tapia, quoted in Robert McCaa "Spanish and Nahuatl Views on Smallpox and Demographic Catastrophe in the Conquest of Mexico," accessed September 2, 2017, http://users.pop.umn.edu/~rmccaa/vircatas/vir6.htm.

2. Historians of the conquest such as William Prescott, writing in the 19th century, mention the presence of disease based on their reading of chronicles, published reports, archival material from Spain, and native codices. See William Prescott, *History of the Conquest of Mexico* (New York: Bantam Books, 1964), 482–486, first published in 1843. His *History of the Conquest of Peru*, published in 1847 by Harper and Brothers, scarcely mentions disease. Twentieth-century historians, however, using the tools of historical demography, evaluated the extent to which disease contributed to conquest and the subsequent fate of native populations. For example, see Eric Wolf, *Sons of the Shaking Earth: The People of Mexico and Guatemala—Their Land, History, and Culture* (Chicago: University of Chicago Press, 1959), 194–197. Eric Wolf, anthropologist and ethnohistorian, was among the first to highlight how significant disease, especially smallpox, was in the conquest of the Indians of Central America. Wolf relied on the historical demographic work of Sherburne F. Cook and Lesley Byrd Simpson, *The Population of Central Mexico in the Sixteenth Century* (Berkeley and Los Angeles: University of California Press, 1948) and Horacio Figueroa Marroquin, *Enfermedades de los Conquistadores* (San Salvador, Guatemala: Ministerio de Cultura, 1957). For an early general study of the consequences of disease during the conquest of all of the Americas, see P. M. Ashburn, *The Ranks of Death: A Medical History of the Conquest of America* (New York: Coward-McCann, 1947). Also see Alfred Crosby, *The Columbian Exchange: Biological and Cultural Consequences of 1492* (Westport, CT: Greenwood Press, 1972); and William H. McNeill, *Plagues and Peoples* (Garden City, NY: Doubleday Anchor, 1976).

3. Both the Bishop de Landa in 1566 and the Inca Garcilaso de la Vega, writing in the early 17th century, suggest the possibility that smallpox arrived among the Maya of the Yucatan and the Inca of Peru before the Spanish arrived to conquer those areas: Friar Diego de Landa, *Yucatan before and after Conquest*, trans. with notes William Gates (New York: Dover Publications, Inc., 1978), 18–19; and Garcilaso de la Vega, El Inca, *Royal*

Commentaries of the Inca and General History of Peru, trans. H. V. Livermore (Austin: University of Texas Press, 1966), part 1, book 9, chapters 14–15: 572–579. Other studies argue that disease traveled through many Native American communities before they had any direct contact with Europeans. See, for example, James West Davidson and Mark H. Lytle, "Contact," in *After the Fact: The Art of Historical Detection*, 6th ed. (New York: McGraw Hill, 2010), and F. J. Paul Hackett, *"A Very Remarkable Sickness": Epidemics in the Petit Nord, 1670–1846* (Winnipeg: University of Manitoba Press, 2002).

4. Native Americans domesticated dogs, turkeys, ducks, guinea pigs, and two camelos, the alpaca and llama.

5. Also known as the Codice de la Cruz-Badiano, the Codex Barberini, or the Aztec Herbal, produced by Martin de la Cruz, a medical student from the Colegio de Santa Cruz de Tlatelolco, a special college established by Spanish priests for sons of the Aztec nobility to facilitate native conversion to Christianity. It was the first known herbal and medical work written in the New World. The original, now lost, was in the Nahuatl language of the Aztecs. It was translated to Latin by Juan Badiano, an Aztec nobleman and collaborator of Martin de la Cruz, in 1552, as a gift to Francisco Mendoza, son of Viceroy of New Spain, Antonio de Mendoza, and titled, "Libellus de Medicinalibus Indorum Herbis." It made its way into the Spanish royal library and then to the family of Cardinal Francesco Barberini, from whence it moved to the Vatican Library. Pope John Paul returned the manuscript to Mexico, and it is now located in the library of the Instituto Nacional de Antropologia y Historia (INAH).

6. Bernardino de Sahagun, comp., *Florentine Codex: General History of Things of New Spain*, trans. Arthur J. O. Anderson and Charles E. Dibble, 2nd ed. (Santa Fe, New Mexico: School of American Research and University of Utah, 1975); and Garcilaso de la Vega, *Royal Commentaries of the Inca*.

7. John W. Verano and Douglas H. Ubelaker, "Health and Disease in the Pre-Columbian World," in *Seeds of Change: A Quincentennial Commemoration*, ed. Herman J. Viola and Carolyn Margolis (Washington, D.C.: Smithsonian Institution Press, 1991), 209–224.

8. Bernard R. Ortiz de Montellano, *Aztec Medicine, Health, and Nutrition* (New Brunswick, NJ: Rutgers University Press, 1990); and Gonzalo Aguirre Beltran, *Medicina y magia: El proceso de aculturacion en la estructura colonial* (Mexico: Instituto Nacional Indigenista, 1963).

9. Derrick Baxby, *Jenner's Smallpox Vaccine: The Riddle of Vaccinia Virus and Its Origin* (London: Heinemann Educational Books Ltd, 1981), 1–2; Frank Fenner, Donald A. Henderson, Isao Arita, Zdenek Jezek, and Ivan Ladnye, *Smallpox and Its Eradication* (Geneva, Switzerland: World Health Organization, 1988), 70–119; and Donald A. Henderson, "Smallpox: Clinical and Epidemiologic Features," *Emerging Infectious Diseases* 5, no. 4 (July–August 1999): 537–539.

10. Fenner et al., *Smallpox and Its Eradication*, 6–12, 210–216; and Centers for Disease Control and Prevention (CDC) and the World Health Organization (WHO), "History and Epidemiology of Global Smallpox Eradication" (Atlanta: Stephen B. Thacker CDC Library Collection, Centers for Disease Control and Prevention, U.S. Department of Health and Human Services, 2014), 33.

11. Henderson, "Smallpox," 537–538.

12. Peter J. Bianchine, MD, and Thomas A. Russo, MD, "The Role of Epidemic Infectious Disease in the Discovery of America," in Guy A. Settipane, MD, ed., *Columbus and the New World: Medical Implications* (Providence, RI: OceanSide Publications, Inc., 1995), 13–15; Fenner, *Smallpox and Its Eradication*, 96–97.

13. CDC, "History and Epidemiology of Global Smallpox Eradication," 23–25.

14. CDC, "History and Epidemiology of Global Smallpox Eradication," 19; Fenner, 70–119.

15. Henderson, 537–538.

16. Angela Thompson, "To Save the Children: Smallpox Inoculation, Vaccination, and Public Health in Guanajuato, Mexico, 1797–1840," *The Americas* 49, no 4 (April 1993): 440.

17. Fenner et al., *Smallpox and Its Eradication*, 117–118. Chapter 2 in Fenner provides a thorough discussion about related orthopoxviruses and the endemic and epidemic characteristics of the variola virus. For an explanation of endemic and epidemic smallpox, see Donald Hopkins, *Princes and Peasants: Smallpox in History* (Chicago: University of Chicago Press, 1983), 8.

18. For a discussion of population levels, disease outbreaks, and the debates surrounding them, see David Noble Cook, *Born to Die: Disease and New World Conquest, 1492–1650* (Cambridge: Cambridge University Press, 1998), 19–35.

19. Cook, *Born to Die*, 25–26, 60–63. Cook also provides an excellent map showing where smallpox spread from 1518 to 1528, 74–75.

20. Quoted in Cook, *Born to Die*, 63.

21. Cortés and the councilmen of the new Spanish town of Veracruz describe these events in the first, second, and third letters to the Spanish monarch Carlos I and his mother, Queen Juana, in Hernan Cortés, *Letters from Mexico*, trans. and ed. Anthony Pagden, with an intro. J. H. Elliott (New Haven, CT: Yale University Press, 1986). Also see the account written later by one of the Cortés's foot soldiers, Bernal Diaz del Castillo, *The Conquest of New Spain*, trans. and intro. John M. Cohen (London: Penguin Books, 1963), which Diaz del Castillo finished writing in 1568. Prescott used these and other documents in his very detailed narrative, *The Conquest of Mexico*.

22. From Fernando Cortés to Don Carlos, Emperor and King of Spain, May 15, 1522, in Cortés, *Letters from Mexico*, 165.

23. Fernando de Alva Ixtlilxochitl, *Horribles crueldades de los conquistadores de Mexico, y de los indios que los auxiliaron para subyugarlo a la corona de Castilla,* Suplemento a la historia del Padre Sahagun, redactado por Carlos Maria Bustamante (Mexico: Imprenta de Alejandro Valdes, 1829), 8.

24. Sahagun, *The Florentine Codex*, book 12: 83.

25. Robert McCaa, "Spanish and Nahuatl Views on Smallpox and Demographic Catastrophe in the Conquest of Mexico," from the *Journal of Interdisciplinary History* 25, no. 3 (Winter 1995): 397–431, accessed September 2, 2017, http://users.pop.umn.edu/~rmccaa/vircatas/vir6.htm.

26. McCaa, "Spanish and Nahuatl Views."

27. Landa, *Yucatan before and after Conquest*, 18–19.

28. Cook, *Born to Die*, 70–71.

29. See the map of the spread of this pandemic in Cook, *Born to Die*, 74–75.

30. Father Bernabe Cobo, *History of the Inca Empire*, trans. and ed. Roland Hamilton (Austin: University of Texas Press, 1979), book 2, chapter 17, 160–161; Garcilaso de la Vega, *Royal Commentaries of the Inca*, part 1, book 9, chapter 15, 576–578.

31. Cook, *Born to Die*, 92.

32. Daniel T. Reff, *Disease, Depopulation, and Culture Change in Northwestern New Spain, 1518–1764* (Salt Lake City: University of Utah Press, 1991).

33. Reff, *Disease, Depopulation, and Culture Change*, 132–140.
34. From the title of Robert Ricard, *Spiritual Conquest of Mexico*, trans. Lesley Byrd Simpson (Berkeley: University of California Press, 1966).
35. Cook, *Born to Die*, 112–114.
36. Thomas Whitmore, using a combination of studies of census data, studies of carrying capacity of the land, and backward projection, concluded that 16 million is a reasonable estimate for pre-Conquest Mexico in *Disease and Death in Early Colonial Mexico: Simulating Amerindian Depopulation* (Boulder, CO: Westview Press, 1992).
37. Thompson, "To Save the Children," 435–442.
38. Thompson, "To Save the Children," 442–446.

Chapter 10

Smallpox: Ensuring the Survival of an Army in Revolutionary America, 1775–1783

Arthur Boylston

That the Army may be kept as clean as possible of this terrible disorder [small pox], I have recommended it to every State, which is to send Troops to the Army in this department, immediately to begin upon the innoculation [sic] of their Recruits, and to continue till they have gone thro' the whole. . . . We intend for the present to keep the Matter as much a Secret as possible, and I would Advise you to do the same.[1]

—George Washington

Smallpox, caused by the variola virus, is characterised by the formation of white pus-filled domes on the skin, commonly known in the colonial era as "the pocks." In 18th-century America, the *Variola major* strain of the disease was the most deadly and had high mortality rates. The ability of the disease to survive and spread through clothing, bedding, and animals ensured that this fatal disease often traveled with militaries of the era. Those who survived experienced disfiguration, blindness, and other lifelong impacts. Knowledge of the death toll and lasting physical effects bred widespread fear of smallpox in the American colonies.

The 18th-Century Status of Smallpox

There were two ways to contract the infection in the 18th century: through close contact with a smallpox patient or their contaminated possessions or through a surgical procedure known as inoculation or variolation. For inoculation, a tiny amount of pus from a pock taken from a suffering smallpox patient was rubbed into a small cut or scratch on the upper arm of a healthy individual. A very mild case of smallpox usually resulted from inoculation, and the individual was immune to infection thereafter. These two forms of contracting smallpox played central roles in the American Revolutionary War and shaped the actions and responses of both the colonists and the British army to news of the disease's presence.

Though no longer "virgin soil" for smallpox epidemics, the American colonies still experienced devastating effects when outbreaks occurred. About 12 days after exposure to the virus, individuals developed a fever, followed by a headache and severe backache. Three or four days later, a rash appeared on the skin, causing such marked swelling of the face and eyelids that the patient was temporarily blinded. The rash gradually matured into pustules, small white, fluid-filled pocks, and in a typical case, the pustules turned into scabs and fell off about three weeks after the disease had commenced. Many experienced extremely sore throats that prevented them from eating or even swallowing water.[2] For most patients, the effects of small-pox lingered for weeks after the disease had passed. Extreme fatigue, muscle wasting due to inactivity, loss of appetite, and dehydration robbed recovering soldiers from full physical fitness and reduced the effective strength of colonial military units.

Survival hinged upon the patient's age and general health and nutrition. In healthy young male soldiers, the mortality rate was between one in three and one in five. The chances of dying increased if there was little or no supportive care or if the patient lay in filthy vermin-infested conditions, which encouraged secondary bacterial infections of the raw skin lesions. Survivors remained too weak to fight for weeks afterward. However, once recovered from smallpox, victims remained immune for life.

As soon as the rash appeared, the patient became infectious and remained so as the rash spread and finally dried up. Contagious individuals spread the infection through coughing and sneezing. Virus particles also helped spread the disease, as they settled on anyone in close face-to-face contact as well as clothes, bedding, and nearby furniture. Within military camps, the proximity and movement of soldiers between one tent and another encouraged the spread of disease.

Smallpox as a Weapon in Early 18th-Century Conflicts

In North America, people feared smallpox much like Europeans feared the plague. Described as a "sudden and terrifying scourge" by medical historian Patricia Watson, the disease attacked native and newcomer alike.[3] Rumors of outbreaks during warfare affected the recruitment of forces and increased desertion rates.[4] In 1690, during King William's War between New England and New France (Canada), colonists developed a plan to capture Quebec and all of French Canada using a two-pronged approach—attacking from both land and sea. The land army, intended to include 3,500 continental troops, 2,000 colonists, and 1,500 Native Americans, failed to produce the numbers necessary. Iroquois participants noticed that some of their intended native allies, the Hurons, had smallpox among them. Fearful of contracting the disease, the Iroquois refused to join, resulting in the cancellation of the ground force invasion. The naval party reached Quebec so damaged by diseases, especially smallpox, that the French easily defeated it. Thus, smallpox impacted armies in two different ways: fear of the disease led to individual and unit practices and policies aimed at avoiding contagion, and the disease could so incapacitate military forces that they were unable to fight effectively.[5]

Smallpox also found use as a weapon. In 1763, the British fought a confederation of Native Americans led by the Ottawa chief Pontiac. Sir Jeffery Amherst, the commander of all British forces in North America, wrote to Col. Henry Bouquet, inquiring, "Could it not be contrived to send the smallpox among these disaffected tribes of Indians?"[6] Bouquet replied, "I will try to inoculate . . . with some blankets that may fall into their hands, and take care not to get the disease myself." Amherst's successor approved an invoice for "Sundries got to Replace in kind those which were taken from people in the Hospital to Convey the smallpox to the Indians."[7] Whether this ploy succeeded in causing an epidemic among the Native Americans is unknown. However, historical documents account for the presence of smallpox epidemics in nearby forts where contaminated blankets were readily available.

The Devastation of Smallpox among Colonial Forces in Revolutionary America

The American Revolution began on April 18, 1775, with the Battles of Lexington and Concord. Following the Battle of Bunker Hill, on June 17 that same year, the British retired to Boston, only to be surrounded by the numerically superior colonists who settled down to besiege their enemies. The British could not fight their way out of Boston, and the colonists lacked sufficient artillery necessary to fight their way into the city. Fearful of the threat to the colonies if the British used Canada as a base to attack from the north, the Continental Congress authorized a two-pronged attack in August. One army, under Gen. Richard Montgomery, marched due north toward Montreal, while the other, under Col. Benedict Arnold, marched through the Maine wilderness to Quebec. Arnold's forces arrived outside Quebec on November 9, 1775. Montgomery's troops captured Montreal and then advanced to Quebec, where he joined Arnold on December 2, 1775.

On December 6, several cases of smallpox were detected among Arnold's forces.[8] As smallpox takes at least 12 days to become symptomatic, the date suggests smallpox infected Arnold's men before Montgomery's men arrived. Diaries by Arnold's men reveal that there was considerable contact between the civilians of Quebec and the soldiers. A British officer in Quebec confirmed smallpox's presence for some time, providing a source for the infection.[9] As the disease spread, colonial soldiers suspected the cunning commandant of the British troops had deliberately infected the citizenry. An American captain wrote, "The smallpox was sent out of Quebeck by Carleton, inoculating poor people at government expense for the purpose of giving it to our army."[10] A private, speaking of the deadly presence of smallpox in the American camp, noted, "There are spies sent out of Quebec every day and some are taken almost every day, both men and women."[11]

Approximately 200 of the small American force (about 1,100 men) were sick with smallpox. Despite his low number of effective forces, Montgomery felt compelled to attack the town because many of his men were on short enlistments and due to go home on January 1, 1776. He appealed to his troops' patriotism and comradeship, but he could not persuade men to reenlist, largely because they were terrified of smallpox. Seeing no alternative, Montgomery launched an assault on Quebec the night of December 31. It was a disaster. Montgomery was killed, and his second in command, Benedict Arnold, was severely wounded. Additionally,

454 men were killed, wounded, or captured.[12] The remnants returned to the houses that they had commandeered and undertook a leaky blockade of the city. Smallpox had played a role in forcing Montgomery into undertaking a flawed and unsuccessful attack.

Arnold appealed to Congress for reinforcements, but they responded by only sending a few men north. Upon arrival, these men also came down with smallpox. Attempts to quarantine sick soldiers failed because some men refused to enter the makeshift hospitals. Desperate, some began to inoculate themselves. The mild smallpox they contracted through self-inoculation spread to others, caused severe forms of the disease, and ensured smallpox was always present in the army.[13] The epidemic spiraled out of control; more became sick naturally, and others felt that they must inoculate themselves to survive. It became a vicious circle.

Arnold banned inoculation, but his men ignored his orders. Attempts to punish those inoculating themselves resulted in ingenious ways to escape detection. A large, obvious pock appeared at the inoculation site when inoculation was performed on the arm, so soldiers inoculated themselves with pins or needles inserted a short distance under their fingernails.[14] Seth Warner, the commander of one regiment of Green Mountain Boys, advised his men to inoculate themselves on the thigh so that their trousers covered the inflamed pox mark.[15]

By May, the American army in Canada consisted of about 1,900 men, with only 1,000 fit for duty. The strain on the healthy personnel to care for so many smallpox victims made an American attack on Quebec improbable. On May 10, 1776, British reinforcements arrived, forcing an immediate American retreat. Ordering a rapid withdrawal, the new American commander, General Thomas, developed smallpox himself and died on June 2. The already disorganized retreat became a shambles. Sick men were left behind, along with valuable equipment, as the shattered colonials attempted to retreat downriver. Desperate, sick soldiers tramped alongside healthy men in an effort to avoid being left behind, but their actions spread the deadly virus further among the ranks.

The army regrouped in Sorel, a small trading village on the St. Lawrence River, but approaching redcoats drove the colonists to a swampy island on the New York–Canada border. The site became a hellhole. One observer commented, "The most shocking of all spectacles was to see a large barn crowded full of men with (smallpox) many of whom could not see, speak, or walk. . . . No mortal would believe what these men suffered unless they were eye witnesses."[16] Two large pits, dug beside the camp, held the bodies of smallpox victims, numbering 15–20 bodies daily, each layer covered by a thin deposit of soil. Men from New England and New York suffered the most; few of them survived. The soldiers' squalid accommodations provided prime conditions for lice and maggots, which added secondary bacterial infections to the existing severe smallpox lesions. Conditions were so bad that Gen. John Sullivan, the next commander, feared his army would dissolve completely. On July 20, he ordered troops to move down Lake Champlain to set up camp at Fort Ticonderoga. Again, smallpox moved south with the army.

George Washington sent Gen. Horatio Gates north to assume command of the shattered forces. On July 29, Gates informed Washington,

> Every thing about this Army is infected with the Pestilence; The Cloaths, The Blanketts, The Air, & the Ground they Walk upon; to put this Evil from us, a General Hospital is Established at Fort George, where there are now between Two, & Three Thousand Sick, & where every Infected Person is immediately sent; but this Care and Caution has not yet effectually destroyed the Disease here, it is notwithstanding Continually breaking Out.[17]

Gates divided the army into two camps several miles apart. Any soldier who displayed signs of sickness was immediately sent to the hospital after swearing that he had not been inoculated or, if he had, naming the inoculator.[18]

On August 7, Gates wrote again, "The very great desertion rate from this army has, I believe, been principally occasioned by the dread of the smallpox. I am apprehensive that it will be extremely difficult to retain (soldiers) for another campaign."[19] However, Gates's strong quarantine measures succeeded in halting the epidemic. On August 28, he optimistically reported to Washington, "The smallpox is now perfectly removed from the Army."[20]

John Adams, a later president of the emerging republic, summed up the debacle when he stated, "Our misfortunes in Canada are enough to melt a heart of stone. The smallpox is ten times more terrible than Britons, Canadians, and Indians together. This was the cause of our precipitate retreat from Quebeck."[21] Canada remained British, due in part to the impacts of smallpox among the American invasion forces.

The Devastation of Smallpox among Native Americans in Revolutionary America

The American patriots were not alone in experiencing devastation from smallpox in Canada. Two incidents at the "Cedars" camp along the St. Lawrence River provide examples of the Native American experience. Col. Timothy Bedel, dispatched to the site by Gen. Arnold, was one who had inoculated himself against smallpox. Ailing from a mild version of the disease, Bedel ordered the construction of a stockade while he sought to sway the Kahnawake Mohawks to break the standing neutrality of the Iroquois Confederacy. Meeting with the Kahnawake leadership at the Council of Coughnawaga, Bedel's participation in passing the traditional pipe of peace likely spread smallpox among potential Native American allies. The number of funerals in the Kahnawake camp surged over the next year.[22]

While Bedel was away negotiating, the Americans at the Cedars were surrounded by a British and Native American force. The ailing and outnumbered Americans soon surrendered. Unaware of the surrender, American reinforcements, with smallpox among the ranks, approached the Cedars, where they were ambushed by the native allies of the British. Seeking to punish the Americans for prior losses, these native forces stripped the American reinforcements and donned the smallpox-infested garments. This fateful decision, combined with the presence of smallpox among the Kahnawake, started a widespread epidemic among the tribes in the north, largely allies or trading partners of the British. Canada remained British and maintained alliances with most of the regional tribes, but the deadly impact of repeated epidemics among the tribes over the next six years took its toll.[23]

Rumors of Weaponized Smallpox in the Revolution

While the American invasion of Canada faltered in part due to the ravages of smallpox, another campaign was underway at Boston, Massachusetts. In July 1775, Gen. Washington arrived in Massachusetts following his appointment as commander-in-chief of the Continental Army. His first concern was to ensure the health of his soldiers. Documented cases of smallpox had appeared in and around Boston two years prior to the war.[24] Colonial officials attempted to manage these outbreaks by strict isolation and quarantine of infected individuals, confining them to defined houses and tended by nurses and doctors already immune to the disease. Despite the best efforts of British officers and town officials, smallpox spread. For British soldiers this was not a serious problem, as most of them had contracted the disease in childhood or underwent inoculation upon recruitment into the British army. Those few still at risk were either segregated from the rest of the town or, more commonly, were inoculated. By late November, smallpox was again epidemic among the people of Boston, either due to natural infection or from inoculation.

George Washington, aware of the smallpox threat to his army, ordered the isolation of any soldier showing signs of the disease to a secure hospital. Furthermore, he commanded his men to avoid contact with civilians to prevent infection. The presence and threat of smallpox was an important part of his decision on whether to attack the town and contributed to his willingness to settle for a siege of Boston instead of invasion.

Gen. Sir William Howe, who had been appointed to command the British troops in October, quickly became aware of the susceptibility of the surrounding colonials to smallpox. Howe relied on colonial fears of infection to prevent any attempt to storm the town. As the siege wore on and winter drew in, food and fuel ran low in Boston. Howe's solution to the problem was to expel any citizens who were not Loyalists. He took the opportunity to order select groups of citizens to leave the city. According to some historians, this was an attempt to spread smallpox to Washington's army.[25] Others admit the possibility but acknowledge Howe may have simply expelled residents in an attempt to ensure sufficient provisions for his forces.[26]

A group of sailors warned Washington that some civilians coming out of Boston underwent inoculation by the British, who hoped to spread the disease to Washington's army. Initially doubting the British would attempt such tactics, Washington finally wrote Congress on December 11: "The information I received that the enemy intended spreading the smallpox amongst us, I could not suppose them capable of; I must now give some credit to it, as it has made its appearance on several of those who came out of Boston."[27] Fortunately, the general had ordered the segregation of all civilians from his forces. His soldiers were warned to stay away from enemy lines and to avoid anyone, patriot or otherwise, with recent exposure to the town.

Early Attempts to Combat the Spread of Smallpox among American Forces

Washington's precautions succeeded in preventing smallpox from afflicting his troops during the siege. However, the sudden end of the standoff exposed the Americans to a new and greater risk of the disease. The arrival in winter of 1776 of a former bookseller, Gen. Knox, with cannon from Fort Ticonderoga made the British position untenable. The American guns could fire on British shipping and the town itself, but Howe's forces could not storm the heights. Howe offered to evacuate Boston on condition that the Americans not attack; if they did, he would burn it to the ground.

With the British forces evacuated, Washington was compelled to deal with the dilemma of reoccupying Boston while it was still full of smallpox victims and infected houses. He ordered Gen. Israel Putnam and "one thousand men who had had the smallpox" to enter the town.[28] Returning citizens complicated the process and the potential spread of smallpox. The only solution was for the town officials to consent to general inoculation. Over 2,000 ordinary Bostonians and a whole regiment of New England volunteers underwent the operation. Fortunately, only 1 of the 500 inoculated soldiers subsequently died.

After abandoning Boston, the British moved their headquarters to New York. The colonial army closely shadowed this withdrawal, setting up an encampment in New Jersey to provide a screen between the British and the Continental Congress. In late autumn 1776, both sides settled down for the winter when campaigning was difficult.

George Washington faced a difficult problem. His army slowly dwindled as disease, cold, and malnutrition took their toll. Troops, whose enlistment had expired, were reluctant to reenlist. Some of these soldiers went home, while others, not yet eligible to leave, simply deserted. Few volunteers were prepared to join the poorly provisioned army with only sporadic victories. Recruitment was further deterred by the ongoing presence of smallpox. News of the disaster that had destroyed the northern army spread throughout the colonies. Wives and mothers were reluctant to see their men volunteer for a patriotic but outlawed cause only to die of smallpox. Many men were prepared to face British bullets but not to endure smallpox. Fear of the disease eroded the strength of the army and threatened to leave it too weak to take on the British. The American Revolution appeared on the verge of failure.

The Dilemma of Inoculation during a Period of War

Inoculation provided a possible solution by producing lifelong immunity; yet, Washington hesitated. Part of the problem lay in the quilt-like nature of the 13

American colonies. Each had its own laws, from a complete prohibition of inoculation in Connecticut, New York, and Rhode Island to freely available inoculation in Pennsylvania. Virginia allowed inoculation only if a father intended to protect his own family, and then public notices announcing that smallpox was present were required. In Boston, inoculation was only lawful when the selectmen agreed to it, and they usually required at least 20 families to suffer from the disease before they approved the procedure. Ships approaching Boston Harbor underwent inspection, and if smallpox was present or the ship had come from an infected port, officials redirected the ship to an island in the harbor, where it remained quarantined until the threat of smallpox had passed. In contrast, Philadelphia merchants felt that quarantines inhibited trade, so they allowed infected sailors ashore. Inoculation was widely practiced to counter the threat presented by the presence of infected men. As a result, smallpox was endemic to Philadelphia.

A letter from Jonathon Trumbull, the governor of Connecticut, demonstrates one example of the problems Washington faced:

> The retreat of the Northern army and the present situation has spread great alarm. . . . The prevalence of smallpox among them is in every way unhappy; our people in general have not had that distemper. Fear of the infection operates strongly to prevent soldiers from engaging the service and the battalions ordered to be raised in the colony fill up slowly. Are there no measures to be taken to remove the impediment? May not the army soon be freed from that infection? Can the reinforcements be kept separate from the infected? Or may not a detachment be made from the troops under your command and the militia raised in the several colonies be ordered to New York, sending such men as have had the smallpox to the Northern department. Could any expedient be fallen upon that would afford probable hopes that this infection may be avoided? The smallpox in our Northern army carries with it greater dread than our enemies. Our men dare face them but are not willing to go into a hospital.[29]

The governor did everything but say, "inoculate the army"; he could not advocate the practice because it was a criminal offense in Connecticut.

There were important practical considerations as well as legal strictures. Men receiving inoculation required isolation from the rest of the army for about a month. Removing substantial numbers of soldiers from active duty at one time risked insufficient numbers to resist an enemy attack. Furthermore, immune soldiers were needed to guard the hospitals containing the inoculated men and to provide basic care. There was also the problem of "preparation." The standard method of inoculating involved a period of preparation on a meat-free diet, often bread and water only, for two weeks before the procedure. The practice sought to rid the body of the "fuel" that supported smallpox. Soldiers found that this diet was near starvation and complained of feeling weak while on it. Between preparation and the disease, soldiers were out of action for at least a month. Despite these concerns over widespread inoculation, the inoculation of only small groups of soldiers risked spreading smallpox through the army.

Adding to Washington's problems was the proximity to Philadelphia. Soldiers visited the town, expediting their exposure to the smallpox that frequented the city's streets. While strict isolation of any soldier showing symptoms of infection might have succeeded in preventing the infection from spreading, the risk that one or more men might escape detection raised the chances of a catastrophic outbreak.

In January 1777, Washington decided inoculation of the entire army was necessary. He wrote to William Shippen, the director of the Army Medical Department:

> Finding the smallpox to be spreading much, and fearing that no precaution can prevent it from running through the whole of our army, I have determined that the troops be inoculated. . . . Necessity not only authorizes but seems to require this measure, for should the disorder infest the army in this natural way and rage with its usual virulence, we should have more to dread from it than from the sword of the enemy.[30]

While awaiting approval of this drastic measure, the situation became more urgent. Smallpox was spreading, and it was impossible for Washington to contain the disease by mere isolation. He ordered Dr. Shippen to begin inoculating troops as soon as they arrived in Philadelphia.

Washington also undertook to overturn the prohibition on inoculation in Virginia, writing to Governor Patrick Henry, "I am induced to believe that the apprehensions of the smallpox and its calamitous consequences have greatly retarded enlistment. But may not those objections be easily done away with by introducing inoculation into the state?"[31]

Washington argued that soldiers from Virginia would inevitably be exposed to smallpox and would carry the infection home with them when they returned from duty. Inoculation of recruits would remove this threat to the health of the whole colony. His appeal succeeded. Volunteers were inoculated as they joined the army. They were treated as soon as they arrived so that little time was lost and were simultaneously fitted with boots, rifles, and uniforms.

Inoculation centers were set up as part of the recruitment process in several colonies. Brig. Gen. Samuel Holden Parsons wrote to Washington in March 1777 that he had established several hospitals in Connecticut alone. Between the number of recruits required to receive inoculation and those needed to maintain the hospitals and protection, Parsons indicated "Innoculating [sic] the Troops renders it impossible for me to make a Descent on Long Island with continental Soldiers."[32]

Men went from inoculation hospitals directly to the main army based in Morristown, New Jersey, but this presented a difficult problem. These newly inoculated troops needed new clothes or to have their original clothes carefully laundered; otherwise, they carried the smallpox virus into the main camp. It was clear that the whole army required inoculation before the summer campaigning season began. However, there was a grave risk that the British might attack if they learned the American army was incapacitated by the inoculation process. Washington gave orders that no news should escape the camp. He commandeered two churches to serve as hospitals where whole regiments underwent inoculation at the same time. Men already immune to the disease stood guard at these hospitals to prevent the virus from spreading into the still susceptible parts of the army.

The results in Morristown were spectacular. Whole regiments underwent the procedure without a single fatality. The soldiers recovered quickly and were available for duty within a few days. The Americans succeeded in inoculating a whole army in the face of the enemy for the first time. Sadly, although the soldiers did well, the virus escaped into the civilian population, and several citizens of Morristown died of the disease.[33]

Washington's audacious action did not completely eliminate the dangers of smallpox for the Continental Army. Groups of volunteers received inoculation at their enlistment centers before marching to join the main force. At some centers, the commanding officers chose to hang on to their inoculated soldiers to provide protection and nursing care for newly inoculated men. Other commanders simply ignored or countermanded Washington's orders, sending new recruits along to continental forces without inoculations. When men without inoculations arrived at headquarters, they were prime candidates for contracting smallpox. Such recruits became a drain on resources while recovering and necessitated isolation from the local civilians.

The winter of 1777–1778 saw the Continental Army encamped at Valley Forge, Pennsylvania, which became famous for the hardships suffered by the troops. Many had no shoes and left bloody footprints in the snow. Food was in short supply, and the men were crowded into small huts for protection from the cold. Such conditions were difficult enough, but the risk of smallpox in this inhospitable environment threatened to exacerbate the struggles. To Washington's dismay, he found that many of these men had somehow avoided inoculation, and the conditions in the winter camp provided a near-perfect setting for an epidemic of smallpox. Of his roughly 14,000 soldiers at Valley Forge, 3,000–4,000 required immediate inoculation to prevent the virus from spreading through the camp.

During this awful winter, the army dwindled through desertion and expiring enlistments. By March 1778, almost half the troops had disappeared, and Washington found himself with only about 7,000 men fit for duty, far too few to resist a British attack. The Continental Army was in desperate need of reinforcements, but recruits trickled in slowly, as the process of inoculation often delayed their arrival. Additionally, the continued trend of local commanders to delay sending men forward for a variety of reasons slowed the process of replenishing the ranks with much-needed reinforcements.

New Strategies for Inoculation during the Revolution

Eventually, Washington and his medical officers were forced to change their strategy for inoculation. Volunteers went directly to Washington's main camp, where they received inoculation upon arrival. While marching to the army, these men traveled circuitous routes to avoid any chance contact with smallpox patients in the countryside. Then the new recruits were encamped three days' march from Valley Forge so that camp doctors could prepare for their arrival.[34]

Inoculation at Valley Forge was successful. Army doctors were familiar with the new Dimsdale/Suttonian method of inoculation that did away with the strenuous restricted diet required by older methods. The operation itself now consisted of a simple, shallow, almost pinprick-sized jab with a small lancet. Using the best methods reduced the mortality of inoculation to about 1 in 500 or less. Many Continental Army regiments did not lose a single man to inoculation.

By the end of 1778, Washington had an army that was largely immune to smallpox. Occasional soldiers that had avoided inoculation came down with the disease, but the threat of a disastrous epidemic within the army was over, as was the concern that the effective strength of the Continental Army would be undermined by sizeable epidemics. But the threat still remained for the general civilian population, including slaves.

The Impact of Smallpox on the British and African Americans during the Revolution

When the Revolution broke out in 1775, the royalist governor of the colony of Virginia, the largest colony in North America, was John Murray, the 4th Earl of Dunmore. Months before the start of hostilities, Murray realized conflict was inevitable and that his handful of a few hundred British soldiers would be overwhelmed by the rebels. He created a new, and for the rich planters of Virginia, terrifying strategy. Lord Dunmore encouraged slaves to abandon their patriot owners and join the British. The response was immediate. Numerous slaves escaped their masters and headed for anywhere that the British were in control. On November 7, 1775, Dunmore issued his famous proclamation: "And I do hereby further declare all indentured Servants, Negroes, or others free . . . that are able and willing to bear Arms; they joining his Majesties Troops as soon as may be, for the more speedily reducing this Colony to a proper sense of their Duty, to His MAJESTY'S Crown and Dignity."[35]

The inclusion of indentured servants along with slaves was an important part of Dunmore's Proclamation. By the mid-18th century, indentured servants traveling to Virginia and its neighboring colonies increasingly migrated from the Scottish Highlands, fleeing economic ruin in the aftermath of the 1745 rebellion. The transportation to the colonies of the more destitute was paid for by a period of servitude for 7 or 14 years, a period that was sometimes extended. Those still serving their indenture saw the Revolution as an opportunity to regain their dignity. For them, as for the slaves, the promise of freedom proffered by Lord Dunmore was a powerful lure.[36]

Within a few weeks, over 800 able-bodied slaves and servants joined with Dunmore's 300 British soldiers and a few Virginia Loyalists. Through poor planning and naïve leadership, this force lost its first battle and retreated to several boats to form a sort of floating guerrilla army. They sailed up and down the coast of Chesapeake Bay, raiding small towns and destroying rebel property.

Dunmore's forces might have presented a considerable threat to Virginia by destroying and confiscating valuable property, damaging the plantations from which the slaves fled, and pinning down many Virginian rebels who might otherwise have marched north to join George Washington. Instead, Dunmore's force was struck by smallpox. The Scottish members, originally from the Highlands region in Scotland, had escaped exposure to epidemics more common to children in England and lower Scottish cities. Slaves, raised in rural Virginia, were as susceptible to the contagion as their white colonial masters. In January 1776, the virus first appeared among men aboard the floating army and spread rapidly through the crowded ships. Simultaneously they experienced a "putrid fever," probably typhus.

Dunmore tried to establish a land base, but the threat of approaching Virginian soldiers prevented these plans. His surgeons recommended inoculation, but the base was too insecure to take the risk. Dunmore moved his camp to Gwynn's Island, where his troops were so sickly they needed support from their Royal Marine colleagues to dig trenches and latrines. Despite the sickness raging in Dunmore's army, as many as eight escaped slaves managed to reach the camp daily. Sadly, they immediately fell prey to smallpox. Even when inoculated, the continuing effects of typhus sapped the strength of the little army. Dunmore eventually abandoned Gwynn's Island, leaving behind a horrifying scene. Unburied bodies were scattered everywhere over a two-mile stretch of land, and many survivors remained on the shore, unable to march with the retreating forces. Witnesses estimated that at least 500 men died there.

It became clear that the devastating losses due to infection made further attempts to form a powerful army of unexposed recruits without inoculations certain to fail. Dunmore abandoned his enterprise and sailed away. He lamented, "Had it not been for this horrid disorder I should have had two thousand blacks; with whom I should have had no doubt of penetrating into the heart of this Colony."[37]

In late 1777, British general John Burgoyne devised a plan to end the Revolution. He proposed to march an army south from Canada to split the New England Colonies from those south of New York, which were already in British hands. An American army, now smallpox-free, managed to muster equal numbers of men and surround Burgoyne's army. After a battle at Saratoga, Burgoyne surrendered his entire force. The victory was a crucial turning point for the Revolution because it convinced France that the American rebellion had a good chance of defeating the British. France entered an alliance with the colonists, promising advice and the provision of naval support and ammunition.

The Impact of Smallpox on Intended French Strategies for Supporting the Revolution

The Americans, British, and Native Americans were not the only ones impacted by smallpox during the Revolution. The French realized their old enemy, Britain, was overstretched, with most of its soldiers in North America and most of its ships patrolling the 700-mile American coastline and the Caribbean. They approached Spain with a plan to form a joint force composed of ships from both navies. The French planned to form an army of 50,000 battle-hardened soldiers who would be stationed along the French side of the English Channel. The plan was to use the combined French and Spanish naval force to attack and capture a vulnerable point on the south coast of England. Then, having secured a base and disposed of the outnumbered British fleet, the soldiers would be ferried across the Channel to mount an invasion of Britain.

On paper, the plan seemed likely to succeed. Britain, forced to defend holdings at home and abroad, felt compelled to hire 30,000 Germans troops (Hessians) to fight in North America. The British home fleet along the south coast of England numbered about 35 ships, while the combined Franco-Spanish armada had 66 first-class ships and 14 smaller and faster frigates. The armada headed for the Isle of Wight and the important naval base at Plymouth with the intention of capturing the forts and the huge stores of supplies kept there. Four hundred transports waited on the French coast to carry the army across the Channel once the armada cleared a landing site. The allies had a clear picture of Britain's weakness and vulnerable points, and the British had no idea what was heading in their direction.

When the French fleet set off in June 1779, it carried both smallpox and putrid fever (typhus).[38] Fighting ships were perfect incubators for the rapid spread of disease. With hundreds of men crammed into a small space so that their hammocks touched each other, it was impossible to prevent smallpox from spreading through the crews. The combined fleet reached the British coast and was clearly visible from the land, but no attack came. On several ships, only half the crew were fit for duty. There were too few to man the guns or maneuver the sails in battle. They were too weak to ride out a gale and were barely able to sail in fine weather. The invasion was abandoned and the army dispersed. The homeland of Britain was not threatened again during the American Revolution. The outbreak of smallpox and typhus on French vessels had forced a shift in strategy and thus delayed the hoped for assistance by the French in the American colonies.

The Combined Impact of Smallpox and Warfare during the American Revolution

Smallpox affected the American Revolution in several ways. When the disease broke out among a susceptible group of soldiers, it soon rendered the force too weak for battle. The catastrophes of the invasion of Canada, Dunmore's slave army, and the Franco-Spanish armada that had threatened Britain are examples of this. A more subtle influence was fear of the disease, which was widespread among the American colonists, who realized that they were at risk. Washington could not attack Boston for fear that his soldiers might become infected there. Meanwhile, the British within Boston tried to infect the colonial army by sending individuals who were infected with smallpox into the American camp. Washington was obliged to establish strict quarantine for these individuals and to do everything to prevent his own men from contracting contagion. Furthermore, fear of smallpox severely inhibited men from volunteering to join the Continental Army.

As his army shrank, Washington took the dangerous step of inoculating his entire force, the first and largest mass inoculation ever undertaken. With a history of immunity and inoculation, the British started with an advantage over the

American patriots. However, the British Native American allies experienced the same fears and susceptibility to smallpox contagion as the colonists. This reality, not effectively countered by the British, led to deadly epidemics among their native allies and inconsistent support during the war.

With the threat of smallpox behind them, the Continental Army was able to face and eventually defeat its British opponents. The French alliance's promise of aid was delayed, in part due to the impact of smallpox. However, with the success of mass inoculation, Washington was able to increase the number of recruits and conduct successful campaigns with balanced forces to oppose the large British forces until the French allies were able to recover and strategically assist the Americans. Instead of allowing the fears and devastation of smallpox to undermine his forces, Washington used inoculation against smallpox as part of his military strategy for success in the American Revolution.

NOTES

1. George Washington to the New York Convention, February 10, 1777, Founders Online, National Archives, accessed September 2, 2017, http://founders.archives.gov/documents/Washington/03-08-02-0320; in *The Papers of George Washington*, 8:299–300.
2. C. W. Dixon, *Smallpox* (London: J&A Churchill, 1962), 5–57.
3. Patricia A. Watson, *The Angelic Conjunction: Preacher-Physicians of Colonial New England* (Knoxville: University of Tennessee Press, 1991), 15.
4. Ann M. Becker, "Smallpox in Washington's Army: Strategic Implications of the Disease during the American Revolutionary War," *Journal of Military History* 68 (2004): 383.
5. Becker, 68: 408–411.
6. Francis Parkman, *The Conspiracy of Pontiac and the Indian War after the Conquest of Canada*, 6th ed., Vol. 2 (Boston: Little, Brown, 1886), 39.
7. Elizabeth A. Fenn, *Pox Americana: The Great Smallpox Epidemic of 1775–82* (New York: Hill and Wang New York, 2001), 88–89.
8. Becker, "Smallpox in Washington's Army," 68, 405–407.
9. Becker, "Smallpox in Washington's Army," 68, 407.
10. Becker, "Smallpox in Washington's Army," 68, 408.
11. Becker, "Smallpox in Washington's Army."
12. Kenneth Roberts, *March to Quebec: Journals of the Members of Arnold's Expedition* (New York: Doubleday, 1938), 40.
13. Roberts, *March to Quebec*, 238.
14. Roberts, *March to Quebec*.
15. Israel Warner, Letter to Henry Stephens, January 15, 1846, in "Papers of Seth Warner," *Proceedings of the Vermont Historical Society* 11 (June 1943): 111–112.
16. Douglas R. Cubbison, *The American Northern Theater Army in 1776: The Ruin and Reconstruction of the Continental Force* (Jefferson, NC: MacFarland and Co., 2010), 127.
17. "To George Washington from Major General Horatio Gates, 29 July 1776," Founders Online, National Archives, last modified December 28, 2016, accessed September 2, 2017, http://founders.archives.gov/documents/Washington/03-05-02-0369. [Original source: *The Papers of George Washington*, Revolutionary War Series, vol. 5, *16 June 1776–12 August 1776*, ed. Philander D. Chase. Charlottesville: University Press of Virginia, 1993, 498–501.]

18. Fenn, *Pox Americana*, 77.

19. "To George Washington from Major General Horatio Gates, 7 August 1776," *Founders Online,* National Archives, accessed September 2, 2017, http://founders.archives.gov /documents/Washington/03-05-02-0451. [Original source: *The Papers of George Washington*, vol. 5, 597–602.]

20. Fenn, *Pox Americana*, 78.

21. Hugh Thursfield, "Smallpox in the American War of Independence," *Annals of Medical History*, Series 3, 2 (1940): 312.

22. Colin Calloway, *The Indian History of an American Institution: Native Americans and Dartmouth* (Dartmouth, MA: Dartmouth College Press, 2010), 46; Fenn, *Pox Americana*, 72–73.

23. Calloway, *The Indian History of an American Institution*, 48.

24. Becker, "Smallpox in Washington's Army," 394.

25. James E. Gibson, *Dr. Bodo Otto and the Medical Background of the American Revolution* (Springfield, IL: Charles C. Thomas, 1937), 88.

26. Fenn, *Pox Americana*, 50; and Philip Cash, "1775: Smallpox Epidemic in the American Revolution," in *Disasters, Accidents, and Crises in American History: A Reference Guide to the Nation's Most Catastrophic Events*, ed. Ballard C. Campbell (New York: Facts On File, 2008), 39.

27. Cash, "1775," 89.

28. Cash, "1775," 90.

29. Cash, "1775," 99.

30. Cash, "1775," 131.

31. Jared Sparks, *The Writings of George Washington; being his Correspondence, Addresses, messages, and Other Papers, Official and Private, Selected and Published from the Original Manuscripts: with a Life of the Author, Notes and Illustrations* Vol. 10/11 (Boston: American Stationers' Company, 1838), 390.

32. "To George Washington from Brigadier General Samuel Holden Parsons, 6 March 1777," Founders Online, National Archives, accessed September 2, 2017, http://founders .archives.gov/documents/Washington/03-08-02-0553. [Original source: *The Papers of George Washington*, Revolutionary War Series, vol. 8, *6 January 1777–27 March 1777*, ed. Frank E. Grizzard Jr. Charlottesville: University Press of Virginia, 1998, 527–529.]

33. Richard B. Stark, "Immunization Saves Washington's Army." *Surgery, Gynecology and Obstetrics* 144 (1977): 425–431.

34. Becker, "Smallpox in Washington's Army," 427.

35. S. Mintz, "Lord Dunmore's Proclamation," *Digital History*, accessed September 2, 2017, http://www.umbc.edu/che/tahlessons/pdf/Fighting_for_Whose_Freedom_Black _Soldiers_in_the_American_Revolution_RS_4.pdf.

36. David Griffith, "Local Knowledge, Multiple Livelihoods, and the Use of Natural and Social Resources in North Carolina," in *Traditional Ecological Knowledge and Natural Resource Management* (Lincoln: University of Nebraska Press, 2006), 157–158. The Scottish immigration to the colonies following the '45 was most pronounced in North Carolina, which included highlanders that initially settled in Virginia and then fled to North Carolina to escape their indenture prior to the Dunmore's Proclamation.

37. Fenn, *Pox Americana*, 58.

38. George Otto Trevelyan, *George the Third and Charles Fox: The Concluding Part of the American Revolution* (New York: Longmans, Green& Co, 1912), 184–200.

Chapter 11

Yellow Fever: Unexpected Ally in the Haitian Revolution, 1802–1803

Christopher Davis

Take courage, I tell you, take courage. The French will not be able to remain long in San Domingo. They will do well at first, but soon they will fall ill and die like flies.[1]

— Jean-Jacques Dessalines

Since the arrival of Columbus's ships in 1492, the island of Hispaniola has experienced its fair share of uninvited guests from across the seas, many negatively affecting those already living there. The original inhabitants of the island, known as the Taino, were the first known victims of this transatlantic contact. Their encounter with the Spanish resulted in the swift extinction of their civilization. Ultimately, this was due to their lack of resistance to unfamiliar European diseases as well as their enslavement by the Spanish to support the establishment of Spain's first colony in the New World. The use of slavery in Hispaniola, along with the unwitting introduction of foreign pathogens into the ecosystem and the human population, proved to be recurring themes throughout the history of what eventually became the nations of Haiti and the Dominican Republic.

Origins of Yellow Fever among the Haitian Population

The high mortality rate of the Native American slaves, from both disease and the physical demands imposed by their Spanish masters, eventually made the Spanish realize that establishing an agriculturally profitable colony required an alternative source of labor. Thus, the dawn of the 16th century witnessed the beginning of the Atlantic Slave Trade. From the 16th and well into the 19th centuries, enslaved Africans were brought across the treacherous Middle Passage of the Atlantic to work on plantations throughout the Caribbean and elsewhere.

The entirety of the island remained in the hands of the Spanish until 1697, when the Treaty of Ryswick formally brought the western third of Hispaniola under French control, and it was renamed Saint Domingue. After the treaty was signed, ships under the flag of France began importing African slaves to the colony, which would be renamed once again in 1804 as Haiti. Shipping records preserved from the era indicate the first French slave ship to Hispaniola, the *Nicolas*, departed Saint-Malo in December 1677; arrived at the port of Cacheu in the Senegambia region of West Africa (modern-day Guinea-Bissau), where it took on 120 African slaves; and then arrived in Port-Paix on February 25, 1697, with the 92 Africans who had survived the crossing.[2] What no one at the time could have known is that those ships carried more than goods essential for the survival of the colony of Saint Domingue. The vessels also transported the two catalysts by which the French colony would ultimately be destroyed: the Africans whose descendants eventually rose up against the plantation masters and a far less conspicuous migrant that proved just as deadly to the French.

Aedes aegypti, a species of mosquito that made its way to the Americas aboard the same ships that brought millions of African slaves, undoubtedly seemed a nuisance to the Europeans as they adjusted to the tropical climate of the Caribbean. These mosquitos carried with them a devastating disease referred to as "yellow fever," due to its tendency to produce jaundice in victims during its final stages. A variation of *Flavivirus*,[3] this disease has previously been known as Yellow Jack, Bronze John, and Mal de Siam.

Historians have long accepted its introduction to the Americas via the slave ships traveling from Africa during the age of European expansion overseas. However, recent genetic research helped to scientifically confirm that assumption. A large geographically diverse data set of viral isolates, taken over the course of several decades from Africa and South America, confirmed observations made concerning the origin of the virus.[4] The data corresponds with the accepted diffusion pattern expected if the importation of African slaves to the Americas were the catalyst for the virus's transmission across the Atlantic. According to these observations, the migration of the virus first emerged somewhere in East Africa before being carried into West Africa. Slaves obtained along the western periphery and the interior of the continent were then forced onto ships bound for the Americas.

Understanding the Yellow Fever Virus, Its Symptoms, and Impact on Humans

The structure of the yellow fever virus is a single RNA strand surrounded by a protein capsid that is encased in a lipid membrane. These form the three structural proteins of the virus. There are an additional seven nonstructural proteins on the exterior of the lipid membrane (NS1, NS2A, NS2B, NS3, NS4A, NS4B, and NS5), which are used to attach the virus to the human host's cells. Once attached, the intruder inserts its RNA into the cell, and the genome begins to modify the host cell to begin replicating the virus, whose copies will eventually burst from the host cell to seek out and infect others. One aspect of the virus's genetic structure makes it especially efficient at quickly spreading from one cell to the next. The RNA strand possesses a positive-sense RNA genome that enters the host cell with the correct order for that cell to directly copy and replicate the viral proteins.[5] A more efficient weapon did not exist in 19th-century Haiti.

For the French troops who arrived in Saint Domingue in the spring of 1802, this weapon proved to be as deadly as it was efficient. Once the infection spread among the cells of the host, the host began exhibiting two stages of worsening symptoms. During the initial, acute stage of infection, the victim experienced symptoms of sudden fever, chills, fatigue, nausea, vomiting, and severe headaches, along with back pain and body aches.[6] If the victim was fortunate, these symptoms passed without escalating to the next phase. Recovery at this stage was difficult to determine, as those still suffering from the disease also entered a brief remission period before the final toxic phase. For those who resumed experiencing symptoms after the roughly 24-hour remission period, the next toxic phase included high fever, the characteristic jaundice from which the disease got its name, bleeding, and eventually death from multiple organ failure.[7] From the moment a mosquito transmitted the virus by biting its victim, it only took three to six days of incubation before the host became symptomatic.[8] The disease was able to incapacitate an enemy French soldier in less than a week.

The assistance provided to the Haitian rebels, by both the mosquito and the yellow fever virus it carried, was of course not based on any conscious favoritism toward the Haitians or animosity toward the French. Rather, a variety of conditions made the French more susceptible to infection than the native Haitians. The vast majority of the population of Saint Domingue was either of African import or descent; therefore, those who rebelled against the French benefited from an immune system already familiar with the disease, as both the virus and the mosquito species that carried it shared their African heritage. Additionally, the local population typically fled coastal cities for the countryside and mountains during the fever season. Consequently, most Haitians remained uninfected, were asymptomatic, or recovered from a milder form of the disease. Those who developed symptoms and recovered typically enjoyed a lasting immunity to the virus.[9] Having inherited a greater level of resistance to the virus, the Haitians therefore were not significantly incapacitated during new outbreaks of yellow fever.

For the French who came to Saint Domingue, the virus was completely alien to the list of pathogens their immune systems were prepared to combat. Though aware of the disease and European susceptibility to it, the disease had yet to pose a direct threat to the French military superiority before the Haitian Revolution. When Charles Victor Emmanuel Leclerc, a French army general and brother-in-law to Napoleon Bonaparte, landed the French expedition in Saint Domingue in 1802, multiple factors consolidated to diffuse the virus among his forces. The disease first struck in Cap Français, where the cramped conditions of a military occupation helped to accelerate its spread among the French population, as did the climate and poor nutritional health of the recent French arrivals. Because rebels controlled the countryside, the French forces and loyal population were forced to huddle within the towns, thereby giving the virus multiple victims in close proximity.[10] Local social customs also made the French more susceptible. Mosquitos are most common at dusk, which was the main social hour in Cap Français and the time to indulge in the local pastime of taking an evening stroll.[11]

Conditions Supporting the Prevalence of Yellow Fever among the French

Before their forces arrived in the colony, there were additional problems that were specific to the Leclerc expedition that aided the spread of the disease upon arrival. Leclerc himself described supply problems experienced by the French early on, each of which aided in the spread of any epidemic. He complained about the food supply: "the wine is bad, the biscuit no good."[12] Poor nutrition could easily account for a higher mortality rate, as malnourishment diminished the body's ability to fight off the disease. Poor nutrition was not the only factor that made the French more susceptible to contracting the disease.

Leclerc's letters revealed that his forces were in desperate need of "thirty thousand pairs of shoes" because supply problems left his troops "barefoot."[13] He complained further that he needed hats for his troops and more medical supplies to "preserve the soldiers from sunburns that send them to the hospital."[14] The lack of adequate covering for the French troops, in the form of shoes and hats, contributed to their vulnerability to the disease's vectors. With more skin being exposed, the French had less protection against mosquitos that spread the virus as they fed on the military forces. The combined impact of inadequate protection, poor nutrition, vulnerable immune systems, and the shortage of medical supplies placed the French at a tremendous disadvantage. Even the hospitals, where sunburnt soldiers sought assistance, proved fatal refuges.

Not only was the expedition short on medical supplies, it was also short on doctors. Before the expeditionary fleet left the port of Brest, Leclerc determined that the medicines requested were unfit. He fatefully decided to leave his entire pharmacy and many of his medical officers in France.[15] Once the expedition arrived at Saint Domingue, Leclerc vainly attempted to make up for these shortcomings. As the spring campaign of 1802 began, he ordered the immediate organization of hospitals, but the short supply of buildings, nurses, and food meant that the wounded received substandard care.[16] Presented with these challenges in the spring, the French suspected worsening conditions with the arrival of summer.

Perhaps the most significant and enabling factor that contributed to the diffusion of yellow fever was the lack of knowledge regarding how the disease was transmitted. In fact, the exact method for the spread of yellow fever continued to be a source of intense debate among medical scientists for another century. U.S. Army surgeon general George Miller Sternberg, Walter Reed, and his lab assistant, James Carroll, examined the bacterium theory espoused by Italian scientist Giuseppe Sanarelli in 1897. They concluded that *Bacillus icteroides* was merely a variety of the common hog cholera bacterium and not causally related to yellow fever.[17] The debate was not resolved until 1900, when Walter Reed determined the culprit was a virus and developed a vaccine to prevent its spread. It was a significant moment in medical history, but one that did nothing for the French troops in Saint Domingue in 1802. Left to guess how it spread, the French never suspected mosquito bites, nor understood the importance of protective clothing.

Occurrence of Yellow Fever before and after the Haitian Revolution

With the cause and prevention unknown, the virus continued unchecked and significantly impacted events in the history of the Americas before and after 1802. One such instance, though still highly debated, is the theory that yellow fever was the unidentified plague that struck the Native American population of New England between 1616 and 1619. Few records survived from that time to give a clear indication of what disease was responsible. Sources from the time implied it began with a French shipwreck in Massachusetts Bay in which the locals captured sailors.[18] This would certainly not be a unique occurrence for Europeans to introduce an unfamiliar pathogen to a Native American community that in turn decimated that community. Daniel Gookin, a colonist, was told by "old Indians who were then youths, who say that the bodies all over were exceedingly yellow, describing it by a yellow garment they showed me, both before they died and afterwards."[19]

Further evidence for yellow fever as the culprit includes a linguistic argument. The name by which Native Americans referred to this plague not only differed from their word for smallpox (the usual suspect in European to Native American transmitted illnesses), but it literally translated as "a bad yellowing."[20] Though the descriptions of the victims match well the symptoms of yellow fever, the absence of the necessary vectors, in the form of *Aedes aegypti* mosquitos, makes yellow fever an unlikely candidate. Many scholars additionally dismiss yellow fever as the cause because, despite the description of the victims, the epidemic was also described as occurring year-round between 1616 and 1619. Even if the necessary mosquitos were present, they could not have survived during the New England winters to transmit the virus.[21]

A more conclusive appearance by the disease prior to the Haitian Revolution was the Philadelphia epidemic of 1793. That summer, residents of the city exhibited symptoms consisting of chills, high fever, headaches, and extreme pain in the back and extremities, which briefly passed only to be followed by a returned fever, yellowing eyes and skin, and bleeding of the nose, gums, and intestines.[22] While it was initially unclear to local physicians what the disease was, Dr. Benjamin Rush, one of the Founding Fathers and a signer of the Declaration of Independence, eventually made the final determination. Based on an earlier epidemic in 1762, Rush declared that the disease in question was indeed yellow fever.[23] The disease persisted through the summer until winter temperatures rid the city of mosquitos and, consequently, also the yellow fever virus. The inability of doctors to treat or even determine the cause of the illness contributed to what remained one the worst epidemics in American history.

Yellow fever again left its mark on American history during the Civil War. Much like the French troops who had to adjust to the humid climate of the Caribbean at the turn of the century, Union troops invading the American South during the Civil War ran into the same issues. Mosquitos became as much a regular feature in the warmer months of the American South as they were in Saint Domingue.

Consequently, yellow fever was no stranger to the Southern states, and, much like the Haitians before them, the Confederates fled cities for the countryside during the fever season, if at all possible. Knowing that the armies of the North would occupy tidewater regions of the Southeast, the Gulf Coast, and the areas around the marshes of the Mississippi River, the Confederates hoped that the summertime diseases of malaria and yellow fever would disrupt Northern advances into Southern territory.[24] The Confederates even attempted to utilize a form of biological warfare, whereby Confederate agents sold what they conceived were yellow fever–infected clothing to the population in Washington, D.C. The attempt failed, as infected clothing did not provide an adequate vector, but fears of the "sickly season" did reduce the Union incursions in the deep South during much of the war.[25]

One likely benefit the Confederates gained over their Union enemies was due to the darker colors worn by the Union forces, colors that attracted mosquitoes more easily than the Confederate gray. It is also likely that Union soldiers removed or opened layers of their uniforms at night in an effort to escape the unbearable heat and humidity of the South—thereby exposing themselves to a more deadly enemy than their Confederate foes, much like the insufficiently clad French were previously exposed to disease-carrying mosquitoes. Confederate soldiers also fell ill to yellow fever when the virus was introduced to soldiers from isolated rural communities who had never encountered it before.[26] Compared to the earlier epidemic and circumstances in Saint Domingue, the South was too large and not interconnected enough to make yellow fever an effective weapon. In the Civil War, this yellow fever afflicted friend and foe alike.

Before the end of the 19th century, yellow fever had played a major role in one final conflict before the mystery behind its transmission was finally solved. When America engaged in war with the Spanish in 1898, the American military knew all too well the dangers of fighting a war in the Caribbean during the summer months. The casualties that their Spanish enemy had already suffered in Cuba while putting down the rebellion made the danger quite clear. According to statistics, between 1895 and 1898, an estimated 16,000 Spanish troops died from yellow fever.[27] In 1898 alone, a Spanish force of 230,000 was reduced by disease to only 55,000 fighting men, and a Spanish garrison of 18,000 at Manzanillo had 6,000 in fever wards.[28] The Cubans learned the lesson from Haiti that the summer months were their ally against a European army. The same could not be said for the Cuban American allies. The primary focus of army medical efforts was on the threat of yellow fever.[29] Without a clear understanding of how the disease was spread, the U.S. Army set up yellow fever hospitals and camps in preparation for the worst, and it even assigned personnel to these facilities from black regiments and any other soldiers who were believed to be immune to the disease.[30] The army was desperate to keep the knowledge of their forces' medical condition from the Spanish, fearing that their army would become demoralized and negotiations with the Spanish would collapse if knowledge of the number of ailing U.S. soldiers became public.[31] Acting on these fears, the United States engaged in subterfuge to hide its medical circumstances, and eventually the Americans managed to achieve a victory in Cuba.

Origins of the Haitian Revolution

One of numerous yellow fever outbreaks throughout modern military history, the 1802 epidemic in Saint Domingue, provided insight into the long-ranging impacts such an epidemic could have on local, regional, and even global events. Though the initial Haitian rebellion began in 1791, it was not until 1802 that France directed its massive military force directly against the population of Haiti. The slave uprising of 1791 against the plantation owners in Saint Domingue was only the beginning of a complex struggle in which multiple factions fought for various goals.

The initial uprising consisted of the combined slave population of the colony, under the leadership of mulattos, with the free people of color against the white planters. However, this alliance was not based on mutual goals between the two groups. The slaves were motivated by a desire for emancipation, and the mulattos and free people of color sought social and political footing equal to the white planter class. This did not necessarily mean that they were in favor of ending slavery in the colony; in fact, many either sought or already possessed slaves themselves to work their own plantations.

The Saint Domingue planters unsuccessfully sought assistance from the French government to put down the rebellion, as the mother country was experiencing its own revolutionary upheaval. Having begun in 1789, the French Revolution raised questions about the nature of political authority and the rights of citizens. These questions reverberated from Paris to the farthest corners of France's empire. In French-controlled Haiti, the conflicts between revolutionary and counterrevolutionary forces were felt in the socially and racially tiered society of Saint Domingue. French society had long been divided among social lines of the clergy, the nobility, and the rest of the population that fell into what was known as the *third estate*. In Saint Domingue, society was racially divided, with the white planter class at the top, the slave population at the bottom, and those of mixed African and European lineage and free people of color often somewhere in between.

In revolutionary France, the Declaration of the Rights of Man, as well as the growing influence of the abolitionist group Les Amis des Noirs, eventually brought about the abolition of slavery. However, because the end of slavery within the French empire at this time proved both gradual and impermanent, the Haitian Revolution continued to parallel France's revolution through its various phases for more than a decade. Republican values trickled into Saint Domingue, inspiring mulattos and free people of color to pursue a more equal standing with the white planters and for slaves to rebel against their masters. Meanwhile, the white planter class reacted with greater repression of nonwhites and fought for greater autonomy from France. France's official abolition of slavery in 1794 was based as much on practicality as it was ideology. Following the execution of Louis XVI, France experienced invasions by the other European powers, both on the continent as well as in France's overseas colonies. The British and Spanish forces that invaded Saint Domingue offered emancipation to slaves who joined them in their fight against the French. Forced to respond in kind or lose a colony already enduring its own revolution, France proclaimed the end of slavery.

The Role of Slavery and Abolition in the Haitian Revolution

For Haiti, the abolition of slavery resulted in leading figures of the Haitian Revolution, such as Toussaint Louverture and Jean-Jacques Dessalines, abandoning their original support for Spain in favor of France. The mulatto, free people of color, and former slave populations of Saint Domingue rallied against the remaining Spanish and British forces. For a brief period, it seemed as though Saint Domingue would enjoy both slave emancipation and a degree of political autonomy within the French empire. Napoleon Bonaparte's rise to power in 1799 changed that perception, after a brief period of ambiguity regarding the effect of Napoleon's rule on France's policy of abolition. Fears of the reestablishment of slavery triggered the final phase of the Haitian Revolution. Ultimately, Napoleon interpreted the revived revolution in Haiti as a direct challenge to his authority, and he decided to invade and resubjugate the colony and its leader, Toussaint Louverture, under direct French control.

Historians debate whether Napoleon always intended to reestablish slavery. Within weeks of seizing power in November 1799, he had removed colonies from the purview of the French Constitution.[32] While his motivations or intentions for this decision are unclear, the effect it had on the population of Saint Domingue was certain. Rumors circulated across the Atlantic, and the colony's vast population of former slaves feared their newfound freedom was about to be ripped away. Early hopes that the emperor would respect the loose autonomy of the colony resulted in the population repelling France's enemies. Consequently, Toussaint Louverture, as governor-general of Saint Domingue, was initially viewed by Napoleon as an asset whose army and location in the Caribbean might assist France's extension of its power in the region.[33]

By 1801, Napoleon clearly perceived Louverture as a rival who exerted his own authority within the colony without the emperor's consent. Louverture had made unilateral decisions the year before Napoleon came to power, such as the promotion of religion within the colony, the provision of amnesty to colonists previously in support of the British or Spanish, expulsion of his political rival General Hedouville from the colony, and even the negotiation of a treaty with Britain and the United States to expel French privateers from the colony.[34] But it was not until 1801, when Louverture issued his own constitution for the colony of Saint Domingue, that Napoleon decided the governor-general could no longer be trusted.

The initial fears concerning rumors of France reestablishing slavery were exponentially magnified once word of the impending arrival of the Leclerc expedition reached Saint Domingue. For many inhabitants, the imminent arrival of roughly 20,000 French troops could only mean one thing. For the French, the objective was to remove Toussaint Louverture and reestablish control, but the status of slavery was not certain. The population of Saint Domingue believed the reestablishment of slavery was the main objective, and, as such, Leclerc's forces landed on an island with a hostile population ready to fight to the death against a clear and present threat to its liberty.

The Impact of Yellow Fever on French Efforts to Reestablish Control over Haiti

The Leclerc expedition arrived on Saint Domingue in February 1802 and initially enjoyed significant military success. The spring campaign was marked with French forces quickly taking strategic locations throughout the colony and with the capture of Toussaint Louverture. The local population, convinced that the French were there to reenslave them, persisted in their resistance of the army's presence through guerilla attacks and scorched-earth tactics that denied the French needed resources to make up for their severe supply shortages. Resistance continued as the summer months approached, and with the heat came the outbreak of yellow fever.

The first attack by the yellow fever virus in 1802 was recorded during late April in Cap Français (Le Cap), where it was believed that the virus had come from British Jamaica.[35] This corresponds with the time frame of the HMS *Cerberus* arriving in port on April 20 after having sailed from Kingston, where yellow fever was present, and the epidemic beginning in Le Cap in the final week of April.[36]

The epidemic of 1802 appears to have been the result of a particularly virulent form of yellow fever. Despite having nearly 20,000 troops at his disposal, Leclerc soon had 200 men admitted to army hospitals daily, losing more men to yellow fever than field combat.[37] Though French doctors noted a lull in the illness by the third to fifth day in most cases, they also noted that many patients died before reaching that point. Furthermore, symptoms often returned to patients, and 80 percent of those died.[38] Details recorded by doctors described a truly horrific experience for the infected. The disease manifested itself with a violent bout of fever and a headache behind the victim's eyes, followed by a diminished headache but with acute kidney pain, vomiting, and thrashing about as patients experienced the sensation that their skin was burning.[39] For those who did not die during the acute phase, the worst was still to come. Their skin turned yellow once the toxic phase set in, followed by foul-smelling black blood that oozed from the mouth and nose, as well as black vomiting and diarrhea, before death occurred.[40] French medical records revealed an even greater and more horrifying element in this epidemic. Doctors reported that the fevers suffered by patients rarely included the delirium normally associated with such conditions, allowing most of the patients to remain lucid during the various phases of the disease.[41] Consequently, the victims of yellow fever from Leclerc's expedition were fully aware of their fatal experience, from beginning to graphic end.

From Le Cap, the virus continued to spread. Several ports experienced outbreaks as ships from Jamaica continued to arrive. The second-largest city in the colony, Port Républicain, reported patients shortly after the May 11 arrival of the frigate

La Franchise.[42] By June, Arcahaye had cases of infection, and by July, the southern region was also affected.[43] Only Mole Saint-Nicolas and the neighboring colony of Santo Domingo remained free from contagion, but complacency and a lack of understanding of the disease brought an end to these last pockets of resistance. By August, assumptions about the health of the region of Mole Saint-Nicolas led to the construction there of a large hospital to accommodate the sick from other areas, thereby introducing the virus to this last holdout.[44] Between the rebellion and the epidemic, Leclerc fought a war on every front.

The yellow fever epidemic impacted the events of the Haitian Revolution beyond simply reducing the numbers and fighting ability of the French forces. It also changed the character of the French campaign from one of reestablishing control to one of desperately trying to survive in hostile territory. While rebels remained largely impervious to the extreme ravages of this virulent outbreak of yellow fever, Leclerc's army lay in ruins. Though he desperately needed more support from the local population until reinforcements could arrive from France, rumors that his army intended to reenslave elements of the population spread as rapidly as the virus. To make matters worse, in May of 1802, Napoleon confirmed France's intentions regarding the end of abolition. On May 20, Napoleon announced that slavery would be maintained where it had been abolished and that the French slave trade would be reinstituted.[45] While this did not imply that slavery would resume in Saint Domingue, the events in Guadeloupe later that summer of returning blacks to slavery made French intentions clear.

Napoleon's overall intentions regarding the West also deserve scrutiny. Shortly after announcing the reinstitution of the French slave trade, the French ruler revealed another objective involving Santo Domingo in a letter to his minister of the navy and colonies, Denis Decrès, dated June 4, 1802:

> My intention, Citizen Minister, is that we take possession of Louisiana with the shortest possible delay, that this expedition be organized in the greatest secrecy, and that it have the appearance of being directed on St. Domingo. The troops that I intend for it being on the Scheldt, I should like them to depart from Antwerp or Flushing.[46]

The outbreak of yellow fever in Santo Domingo, which devastated the French forces sent to put down the Haitian rebellion, also undermined Napoleon's goal for a subsequent invasion of Louisiana.

Correspondence between Leclerc in Santo Domingo and his French superiors shows that the French knew how the news would affect the already struggling campaign in Haiti. In a letter dated July 14, 1802, to Leclerc from Decrès, Leclerc was advised how to handle the reinstitution of slavery in the colonies. "For a little while longer, it will be necessary that vigilance, order and a discipline both rural and military replace the positive and official slavery of people of color in your colony . . . [until] the moment has come to force them back into their original condition, whence it has been so fatal to have removed them."[47] With the removal of ambiguity over the status of slavery in Napoleon's empire, vital support for the

French by Jean-Jacques Dessalines and others slipped away from an already desperate Leclerc. He pleaded with his superiors to forestall such a policy for the sake of the campaign:

> I had asked you, citizen consul, to do nothing that might make [the blacks] fear for their freedom until I was ready, and I was making rapid progress toward that moment. All of a sudden there arrived the decree that legalizes the colonial slave trade along with letters from merchants in Nantes and Le Havre asking whether they can sell blacks here. . . . Now that your plans for the colonies are known to everyone, citizen consul, if you want to keep Saint Domingue, send a new army here, and especially send money. I am telling you that, if you abandon us to our own devices as you have done up to now, this colony is lost, and once lost, you will never get it back.[48]

Leclerc's plea became prophetic as word of France's resumption of slavery spread alongside yellow fever, with more and more soldiers falling ill.

With a dwindling army, increased desertion of blacks and mulattos among his forces, and shrinking public support, Leclerc changed his approach as summer turned to fall. Yellow fever had robbed him of the forces necessary to hold strategic positions across the island colony. To compensate, Leclerc took what was left of his forces and began a policy of genocide. Writing to Napoleon in October 1802, Leclerc recommended that, "We must destroy all the blacks of the mountains—men and women—and spare only children under twelve years of age."[49] The hope was to eradicate the revolutionary generation and ensure the younger population would be less resistant to renewed slavery.

Leclerc did not survive to see through the attempted extermination of the black adult population. On November 2, 1802, he succumbed to infection by the yellow fever virus. As the brother-in-law of the emperor, Leclerc was the virus's most high-profile victim, but only one of the estimated 22,000–24,000 troops killed out of the 34,000 sent to Saint Domingue between February and October 1802.[50]

The genocidal policy continued in its implementation by Leclerc's successor, General Donatien Rochambeau. Though the yellow fever season had waned, its impact on the French expedition set the course for how the French conducted the remainder of the war. Rochambeau began executing black troops out of fear of betrayal by tying weights around their necks and dumping them into the harbor as well as suffocating prisoners by locking them in ship holds with burning sulfur.[51] These acts sought to eradicate the population and to spread a campaign of terror. Ironically, it had the opposite effect; the colony was further galvanized against the remaining French forces. Haitian forces, then under Jean-Jacques Dessalines, vowed to destroy the French. The inhabitants of the colony ground down Rochambeau's army until it surrendered after the Battle of Vertières, on November 18, 1803. The French atrocities committed after the disease had left the French army so vulnerable drove the rising animosity of the Haitian people and carried them to a military victory. As Dessalines declared Haitian independence on January 1, 1804, part of his proclamation included the eradication of the remaining French civilians of what became the Republic of Haiti, impacting Haiti's foreign relations for years to come.

The Combined Impact of Yellow Fever and War Strategies on the Outcome of Revolution

The American, French, and Haitian revolutions were responsible for this period being called the Age of Revolutions. Each of these movements marked a significant turning point in the history of the Atlantic region. The Haitian Revolution has not traditionally received the same level of attention as its American and French counterparts. Nevertheless, the birth of the Haitian Republic not only created the second independent nation in the Western Hemisphere, but it also became the first and only country to be created through a successful slave rebellion. The emergence of a republic of freed slaves in 1804 added fuel to arguments both for and against abolitionism throughout the region as the 19th century pressed on. Therefore, despite the lesser attention it has traditionally been paid, the Haitian Revolution was a watershed moment for the history of slavery in the Americas as well as the beginning of a complex and intertwined history between Haiti and the United States.

Given the impact of the revolution on the history of the Atlantic region, understanding the role of the yellow fever outbreak in 1802 in determining the outcome of that event becomes all the more essential. Had it not been for an outbreak of a particularly virulent form of the disease that summer, the Haitian rebels would have contended with a large professional army that may have proven more effective in the conflict. Based on Napoleon's correspondence, it is also possible that the absence of yellow fever, or even a less virulent outbreak in Saint Domingue in 1802, might have resulted in the French launching their planned invasion into Louisiana. Such action would have reshaped French-American relations just prior to the resurgence of Napoleonic warfare in Europe during the first decade of the 19th century.

One cannot conclusively speculate that the Haitians would have lost had it not been for the disease. Rather, the resistance of the African-descended population to yellow fever and the practice of avoiding coastal cities and low-lying areas during the fever season, combined with the French susceptibility and poor provisions, tipped the balance of the conflict in the Haitians' favor. The rumored French intention to return slavery gave further momentum to events. This in no way diminishes the Haitian rebels' agency in their success against the French. The Haitians, like any clever military force, had seized upon an opportunity provided within their environment and used it to their advantage. However, acknowledging the environmental factors of disease and disease vectors that had enabled a Haitian victory reveals that our understanding of military history cannot remain limited by the assumption that humans are the only actors in these events. The Haitian Revolution, therefore, stands as an example of how a momentous event in the history of human rights was impacted, and perhaps decided, by a nonhuman participant.

NOTES

1. C. L. R. James, *The Black Jacobins: Toussaint L'Ouverture and the San Domingo Revolution* (1963; repr., New York: Vantage Books, Random House, 1989), 314.
2. The Trans-Atlantic Slave Trade Database, accessed September 2, 2017, www.slavevoy ages.org/voyage/33528/variables.

3. The overall Flaviviridae family of arthropod-borne viruses includes other noted diseases, such as West Nile, dengue fever, and even the recently emerged Zika virus. "Scientists illustrate how host cell responds to zika virus infection," in Biotechin.Asia, accessed September 2, 2017, https://biotechin.asia/2017/05/09/scientists-illustrate-how-host-cell-responds-to-zika-virus-infection.

4. J. E. Bryant, E. C. Holmes, and A. D. T. Barrett, "Out of Africa: A Molecular Perspective on the Introduction of Yellow Fever Virus into the Americas," *PLoS Pathogens* 3, no. 5, e75 (May 2007): 0669, accessed September 2, 2017, http://dx.doi.org/10.1371/journal.ppat.0030075.

5. Amanda Robb, "Yellow Fever Virus: Structure and Function," Study.com, accessed September 2, 2017, http://study.com/academy/lesson/yellow-fever-virus-structure-and-function.html.

6. Centers for Disease Control and Prevention, "Yellow Fever: Symptoms and Treatment," last modified August 13, 2015, accessed September 2, 2017, https://www.cdc.gov/yellowfever/symptoms/index.html.

7. Centers for Disease Control and Prevention, "Yellow Fever."

8. Centers for Disease Control and Prevention, "Yellow Fever."

9. Centers for Disease Control and Prevention, "Yellow Fever."

10. Philippe R. Girard, *The Slaves Who Defeated Napoleon: Toussaint Louverture and the Haitian War for Independence, 1801–1804* (Tuscaloosa: University of Alabama Press, 2011), 161.

11. Girard, *The Slaves Who Defeated Napoleon.*

12. Laurent Dubois, *Avengers in the New World: The Story of the Haitian Revolution* (Cambridge, MA: Belknap Press, 2004), 268.

13. Dubois, *Avengers in the New World.*

14. Dubois, *Avengers in the New World.*

15. Girard, *The Slaves Who Defeated Napoleon*, 160.

16. Girard, *The Slaves Who Defeated Napoleon.*

17. John R. Pierce and James V. Writer, *Yellow Jack: How Yellow Fever Ravaged America and Walter Reed Discovered Its Deadly Secrets* (Hoboken, NJ: John Wiley & Sons, Inc., 2005), 98.

18. Sherburne F. Cook, *An Expanding World*, Vol. 26, *Biological Consequences of the European Expansion, 1450–1800*, edited by Kenneth F. Kiple and Stephen V. Beck (Aldershot, UK: Variorum, Ashgate Publishing Limited, 1997), 253.

19. Cook, *An Expanding World.*

20. Cook, *An Expanding World.*

21. Cook, *An Expanding World*, 253–254.

22. Jim Murphy, *An American Plague: The True and Terrifying Story of the Yellow Fever Epidemic of 1793* (New York: Clarion Books, 2003), 13–14.

23. Murphy, *An American Plague*, 15.

24. Andrew McIlwaine Bell, *Mosquito Soldiers: Malaria, Yellow Fever, and the Course of the American Civil War* (Baton Rouge: Louisiana State University Press, 2010), 20.

25. Bell, *Mosquito Soldiers*, 103–110.

26. Bell, *Mosquito Soldiers*, 20.

27. Pierce and Writer, *Yellow Jack*, 103.

28. Pierce and Writer, *Yellow Jack.*

29. Pierce and Writer, *Yellow Jack*, 105.

30. Pierce and Writer, *Yellow Jack.*

31. Pierce and Writer, *Yellow Jack*, 106.

32. David Geggus, *The Haitian Revolution: A Documentary History* (Indianapolis: Hackett Publishing Company, 2014), 168.

33. Geggus, *The Haitian Revolution*.

34. Geggus, *The Haitian Revolution*, 139.

35. Girard, *The Slaves Who Defeated Napoleon*, 161.

36. Girard, *The Slaves Who Defeated Napoleon*.

37. Girard, *The Slaves Who Defeated Napoleon*.

38. Girard, *The Slaves Who Defeated Napoleon*.

39. Girard, *The Slaves Who Defeated Napoleon*.

40. Girard, *The Slaves Who Defeated Napoleon*.

41. Girard, *The Slaves Who Defeated Napoleon*.

42. Girard, *The Slaves Who Defeated Napoleon*.

43. Girard, *The Slaves Who Defeated Napoleon*.

44. Girard, *The Slaves Who Defeated Napoleon*.

45. Geggus, *The Haitian Revolution*, 172.

46. John S. Marr, MD, and John T. Cathey, MS, "The 1802 Saint-Domingue Yellow Fever Epidemic and the Louisiana Purchase," in *Journal of Public Health Management and Practice* 19, no. 1 (January 2013): 81, accessed September 2, 2017, https://www.researchgate.net/publication/233738388_The_1802_Saint-Domingue_Yellow_Fever_Epidemic_and_the_Louisiana_Purchase.

47. Geggus, *The Haitian Revolution*, 172.

48. Geggus, *The Haitian Revolution*, 172–173.

49. Laurent Dubois, *Haiti: The Aftershocks of History* (New York: Picador, 2012), 40.

50. Girard, *The Slaves Who Defeated Napoleon*, 179.

51. Dubois, *Haiti: The Aftershocks of History*, 40.

Chapter 12

Measles in World War I: Pestilence within Mobilization Camps and Transport Ships, 1915–1919

Sonia Valencia and Rebecca M. Seaman

I got the measles. . . . I don't know where I got them. . . . I didn't say anything until we got on the boat. . . . Because I knew if I did and it leaked
that I did have something, I might be out of the company or something,
and I didn't want that, so I didn't say nothing.[1]

—Pvt. William J. Lake

In 1914, failed diplomacy among European nations led to a war that ravaged
Europe. Known at the time as the Great War or the War to End All Wars, the conflict involved 30 nations and colonies from around the globe. Some nations joined
at the outset of the war, and others were gradually pulled in due to alliances or
the expansion of hostilities. Consequently, there was a constant process of mobilization and transport of military personnel from their homes and home bases to
the war zones. It was through the process of recruiting, training, and moving units
from civilian life to scattered military fronts that a new foe made its appearance in
World War I. This foe, the measles virus, indiscriminately undermined the effectiveness of armed forces.

Measles was found in military camps globally, but it managed to have a considerable influence on American and Australian military personnel during mobilization efforts for World War I. Though not typically fatal itself, measles undermined
the health of personnel, leaving them open to secondary infections that often did
prove fatal. This unseen enemy moved among raw recruits, especially those from
remote rural regions. It sent them to military hospitals and accounted for weeks
of noneffective-duty status. Not all contagious individuals were identified or quarantined prior to their deployment, resulting in the spread of the virus within the
cramped confines of trains and ships as troops were moved to distant battlefields.

The complications caused by measles and secondary infections also affected
the mobilization of military units and thereby impacted the timing and prosecution of the war. The sheer number of those impacted, the resulting loss of effective fighting capabilities, and delays in transportation to active combat disrupted

the strategies of political and military commanders, which indirectly extended the war.[2] The quarantine delays for measles were significant and did impact the war, albeit indirectly and in a manner difficult to measure. However, the same epidemics prompted extensive research efforts to reduce casualties from disease and ultimately helped the development of medical reforms, thereby reducing similar delays for future conflicts.

Understanding the Measles Virus, Its Symptoms, and Transmission

The measles virus is a member of the *Morbillivirus* genus in the Paramyxoviridae family. It shares characteristics with the rinderpest virus that once affected cattle.[3] One theory on the origin of the measles virus stated that the virus crossed over into the human population during the 11th and 12th centuries BCE, as a result of the shift from a nomadic lifestyle to a sedentary existence and the consequent presence of domesticated livestock. People living in close proximity to cattle had an increased risk of contracting disease.[4] Initially restricted to the Eurasian and African continents, the era of exploration inadvertently introduced the virus to the native populations of South America, North America, and Australia.

The virus presents itself as an acute febrile rash. The rash is usually generalized over the body and maculopapular in nature (red and flat). People who contract measles typically have temperatures over 101°F accompanied by a cough and even conjunctivitis. Fevers are known to rise as high as 105°F. Though typically mild, the resulting malaise ensures a lengthy recovery.[5] Those patients who experience more severe cases often also encounter such complications as pneumonia, encephalitis, otitis media, streptococcus, and even death.

The measles virus is a highly contagious acute respiratory disease. The pathogen is transmitted by physical contact or by way of respiratory droplets suspended in the air due to the coughing or sneezing of an infected person. Once exposed to the virus for the first time, the disease progresses in three stages. The first stage is the incubation period, which generally lasts 10–14 days. The infected person does not exhibit any symptoms but may be contagious. During this time, the virus replicates in the respiratory tract and later spreads to the lymphoid tissue and organs, such as skin and the intestinal tract.[6]

The second stage is the preeruptive stage, which begins with the first physical symptom: a fever ranging from 100 to 105 degrees. The fever is followed by conjunctivitis (red eyes) and inflammation of the upper respiratory tract; this leads to coughing, sneezing, and nasal discharge. In some cases, small white spots, known as Koplik spots, appear inside of the mouth. This stage lasts an average of four days and ends with the first sign of eruption.

The final stage is the eruptive stage, and it is indicated by a rash that forms on the face and spreads along the hairline, behind the ears, down the neck, over the torso, and to the extremities. Without complications, the patient will recover and gain permanent immunity.[7] Previously mentioned complications can occur in cases of cross-infection, whereby the compromised immune system of a measles victim is introduced to a pathogen that cannot be fought. Bronchopneumonia, otitis media, and lobular pneumonia are the most frequent secondary infections of measles. These complications increase the likelihood of death.

Historic Occurrence of Measles during Mobilization for Wars

Periods of war particularly felt the impact of measles epidemics. During the American Revolution (1775–1778), the Continental Army struggled with crippling diseases, such as measles and smallpox, that broke out among the troops. The occurrence of measles not only impacted the health of recruits and rippled through the army, it additionally discouraged potential recruits and encouraged desertion. George Washington employed a process of inoculation for smallpox to combat problems with health and troop mobilization.

Despite the advent of inoculation, measles continued to make its appearance over the centuries in mobilization camps as the fledgling American nation fought to ensure its independence and growth. In the War of 1812 (1812–1815), infectious diseases outpaced the deaths from combat. Diseases such as dysentery, typhus, and measles claimed the lives of approximately 17,000 soldiers out of a total mean strength of approximately 286,730.[8]

These same diseases wreaked havoc on Confederate and Union soldiers during the Civil War (1861–1865). Many Civil War deaths were attributed to camp diseases, such as chronic diarrhea, dysentery, and measles. Measles persisted as the most common ailment during early mobilization and induction of new troops, especially African American troops, and the accompanying secondary infections, such as pneumonia, were the third leading cause of death in the Civil War.[9] Measles often affected new recruits who lacked previous exposure and, therefore, had no immunity.

Climate also played a role in the outbreak of disease in periods of military conflict. During the Spanish-American War (1898–1902), approximately one-third of the 306,760 troops reported to a military hospital for disease, and 2,061 deaths were attributed to disease. Measles morbidity was very low, however, as the arena for the Spanish-American War was in warm tropical climates where measles outbreaks were less common. As a result, the incidence of measles cases dropped from the 2.0 percent during the Civil War to 0.32 percent per 1,000 troops for the Spanish-American War.[10]

Efforts during World War I (1917–1918) were also complicated by disease. Toward the end of the conflict, a worldwide influenza epidemic affected troops in just about every continent in 1918. Prior to the influenza epidemic, smaller and scattered, yet virulent, epidemics spread misery throughout the mobilization camps. From the outset, the process of mobilizing forces for the war also brought people together, those with diseases and those with limited resistance. By the middle of 1915, the Australian Imperial Force's escalation of recruitment following the Australian and New Zealand Army Corps' (ANZAC) landing at Gallipoli resulted in massive numbers of new troops placed in overcrowded camps that were ill prepared to deal with the sanitary and medical needs. Insufficient housing, dirt floors, and continuous rains contributed to conditions that allowed for the rapid spread of respiratory infections. By October of 1915, camps in Australia boasted well over 70,000 troops. Efforts to build new camps and shift growing numbers of recruits to additional camps were incapable of keeping up with the massive influx of volunteers. Disease kept pace with the growing number of recruits. By June 1916, a total of 61 percent of the cases reported to camp hospitals were from respiratory ailments, and at least 20 percent of those cases were due to measles.

The late involvement of the United States in the war delayed the need for mobilization until 1917. Unfortunately, despite efforts for "preparedness" by reform-advocate Elihu Root, the additional time was not used in preparing sufficient numbers and improving the quality of military camps and hospitals. The total breakdown of American military deaths during World War I accounts for 112,422, including those in the United States and in the American Expeditionary Force. Of those deaths, 51 percent were attributed to disease, and 30 percent of the 51 percent were deaths due to disease at military bases located in America.[11] From April 1, 1917, to December 31, 1919, measles cases were responsible for 98,255 admissions to military hospitals, 2,370 deaths, and 1,877,955 sick days, directly affecting the effective strength of the U.S. military during the war.[12] As the staging ground for mobilization and training of military forces for the war, the impact of measles and other illnesses affected the ability to prepare and deploy troops in a timely fashion.

The number of deaths may not seem that high when considering the total mean strength of the Australian and U.S. militaries. For the US Army, the total mean strength was 4,128,479, and the total number of deaths was 112,422, of which 56,991 were caused by disease.[13] Indeed, once the camps were developed and supported by hospitals, the decline in disease was a testament to the lessons learned by Australia in the first two years of World War I as well as lessons learned by the U.S. military in the Civil War, the Spanish-American War, and eventually World War I. Yet, despite the improvements, pneumonia, influenza, and measles spread throughout the ranks and in the medical wards.

The fact remained that the medical communities were ill prepared to handle respiratory epidemics due to their lack of knowledge and experience. The alarming rises in measles cases, both among troops and in nearby cities, stirred medical professionals into action. The measles epidemics of 1917–1918 in the United States especially provided opportunities for the medical community to investigate factors enabling its proliferation. Using this information, they developed methods of prevention. These tools were later used during the subsequent influenza epidemic of 1918.

Understanding the Complexities of Measles Diffusion during World War I

"Measles was one of the most prevalent and one of the most fatal of the infectious diseases that occurred" among U.S. military forces in the fall of 1917. The mortality of the disease was in large part due to the complications that accompanied the contagion.[14] To better understand the prominence of the measles epidemics during World War I, three aspects of disease contagion should be examined: the demographics and diffusion of contagion during mobilization, the impact of insufficient facilities and provisions for sheltering mobilized troops, and the circumstances encountered in military medical facilities that contributed to further diffusion and complications of measles. The timing of the outbreaks is also important and reflects the timing of the U.S. entry into World War I. Having been late to enter the war, the United States attempted a rapid deployment that experienced multiple measles epidemics and crippled its mobilization efforts, further delaying its movement of troops to the Western Front.

The United States managed to maintain neutrality for more than two years of the war. However, repetitive attacks on U.S. vessels by German U-boats crumbled diplomatic relations with Germany and threatened American security on its southern border with Mexico and with commercial interests. On April 16, 1917, President Wilson joined the Allied effort and declared war against the German alliance, despite the fact that the United States was not fully prepared for the demands of war.[15] Between April and May 1917, American field administration for the War Department was in the process of decentralizing its functions into territorial departments throughout the United States. The decentralized departments of the army consisted of the Northeastern, Eastern, Southeastern, Central, Southern, and Western divisions and were vital for carrying out mobilization functions. But the recent declaration of war and rapid mobilization found these departments in a state of transition from peacetime to wartime.[16]

The United States traditionally maintained a minimum of essential personnel in its permanent army, demobilizing its forces after each conflict. Grossly understaffed in April 1917, recruiting programs went into effect to build the ranks. Throughout 1917, recruiting programs successfully enlisted 155,455 new recruits and reenlisted 3,725 soldiers. These numbers, while a tremendous growth of the existing military, were insufficient. The United States needed to mobilize and transport over 2 million soldiers to Europe as soon as possible.[17] To compensate, President Wilson passed the Selective Service Act of May 1917, which authorized the conscription of men with desirable traits into military service. In June 1917, 10 million men were registered for the draft, but only 2,810,296 successfully entered into the armed forces during the next year and a half.[18]

Many brave and patriotic young men answered President Wilson's call to arms in April 1917, similar to the earlier Australian response of 1915. Volunteer recruitment jumped from 6,374 volunteers in March 1917 to 29,027 volunteers in April. The number of volunteer enlistments continued to rise in subsequent months and peaked at a total of 141,931 in December. For the months that followed, volunteer enlistments averaged 24,901 volunteers per month. This patriotic pattern came to an end in August 1918 after President Wilson discontinued the practice of admitting volunteers and news emerged of a virulent influenza epidemic.[19]

On July 20, 1917, the first draft was held to increase the number of men required, and approximately 180,000 men were conscripted into the armed forces, complementing the numbers who had already volunteered. The mobilization of conscripted men began in September, and the first examinations at the cantonment camps were scheduled for September 6, 1917. Not surprisingly, the number of measles cases sharply increased at mobilization camps starting in September. Conscripts and volunteers received physical examinations, which admitted 70 percent of those still eligible after occupational, citizenship, and dependency deferments and exemptions. Later, an officer of the Medical Department of the Army conducted a second and more thorough physical examination. This examination was performed shortly after arrival at the assigned camp, resulting in up to 8 percent additional rejections. However, the precautions, intended to ensure healthy volunteers and conscripts, were often bypassed, as the immediate demand for troops far exceeded the number enlisting voluntarily or through conscription in the summer months of 1917.[20] Without the requisite physical exams, no barriers protected susceptible rural recruits and conscripts from contagious individuals.

The health of recruits sometimes changed dramatically from the initial physical exam until troops boarded trains to assigned camps. Measles, contagious prior to infected individuals showing the onset of symptoms, was spread to nonimmune individuals during the mobilization process. Urban centers were more prone to measles epidemics because their dense populations experienced a continuous influx of susceptible populations, resulting in endemic conditions; consequently, urban populations boasted higher rates of immunity. Urban areas experienced epidemics that occurred on an annual or biannual cycle, depending on the number of previously unexposed people available and the climate. This endemic presence of measles helped ensure the probability of exposure to susceptible new military recruits arriving at military camps from rural areas with little or no history of measles exposure.

For troops in the middle of deployment from distant regions, such as Australia, exposure often occurred on crowded ships at ports where the ships stopped on their way to the Middle Eastern and European theaters of the war, especially during the winter and early spring, when the weather was cold and huddling for warmth in poorly ventilated quarters was more common.[21] In the United States, exposure usually occurred on crowded troop transports en route to mobilization camps or at the camps.

Using Medical Research as a Strategy to Combat Measles in World War I

Medical professionals A. G. Love and Charles B. Davenport conducted investigations of circumstances pertaining to the occurrence of measles in the mobilization camps in an effort to understand why these camps were vulnerable to measles epidemics. Their research, based on detailed military medical records and recruit demographics, supported the conclusion that the "highest morbidity and mortality rates have been from camps that drew from sparsely populated areas of the Southern Atlantic and Gulf States, and to a less striking extent from the sparsely settled states of the West."[22] Their findings were later supported by analysis conducted by

Dr. G. Dennis Shanks of the Australian Army Malarial Institute. By comparing the outbreak of measles and case fatalities at specific military mobilization camps with the homes of origin of measles patients, Shanks discerned that recruits from rural areas and climates typically warmer year-round had a greater incidence of measles in World War I mobilization camps of Australia and the United States, along with other camps included in his study.[23]

Military personnel and medical experts went to the camps most severely affected by measles epidemics to study what factors had contributed to the increase of cases and high rate of secondary infections. These camps were primarily located in the Southeastern and Southern Departments, with the Central Department following close behind. According to a population study conducted by Love and Davenport, these states were sparsely settled and had few urban centers.[24] The rate of measles admissions was lower in the Northeastern, Eastern, and Western Departments, in part because these departments had fewer camps, were located in more urban areas, drew recruits from urban areas where measles was often endemic, and drew recruits from states that were densely populated and, therefore, more likely to have increased immune populations in their camps.[25] The camps that had record numbers of measles admissions or deaths included Camp Wheeler, Georgia, and Camp Pike, Arkansas.

By the end of the war, Camp Pike had mobilized 116,236 men. Of these recruits, some had brought measles with them and spread it to others en route to the camp or shortly after arrival. By April 1919, there were 3,100 hospital admissions for measles. The rate of admissions continued to grow; by December 31, 1919, the camp had experienced a total of 6,730 measles cases, 209 deaths, a death ratio of 4.22 percent per 1,000 men, and a case fatality rate of 2.97 percent. The high morbidity rate at Camp Pike inspired medical professionals to develop and test a vaccine for measles and some of its complications. The vaccine was made using the Tunnicliff coccus. Unfortunately, the rapid mobilization process and consequential shifting of troops from one location to the next undermined the vaccine experiment. While testing the vaccine on 1,500 troops, all but 176 were transferred out of the camp before receiving all three doses. Frequent transfers interfered with experiments at Camp Pike and elsewhere and rendered the results inconclusive.[26] It was not until 1963 that an effective measles vaccine was finally developed.

Camp Bowie, in Fort Worth, Texas, was another camp with high rates of measles cases. In September 1917, troops from Arkansas and Louisiana were redirected from Camp Pike to Camp Bowie. New recruits from these states, as well as various parts of Texas, brought illness with them. When the camp and its hospital opened on September 24, 1917, measles and pneumonia patients filled the hospital beds. Up until January 1, 1918, medical personnel struggled with 3,624 measles cases.[27]

Likewise, Camp Sevier and Camp Jackson, in South Carolina, ranked in the top 10 total numbers of measles admissions reported from April 1, 1917, to December 31, 1919. Camp Jackson, an army camp located near Columbia, South Carolina, ranked eighth on the list of top measles admissions, with 3,022 admissions and 66 deaths. Camp Sevier ranked fourth on the list of highest measles admissions from September 1917 to December 1919, with 3,685 admissions and 110 deaths. The camp drew new recruits from the Southeastern Department states of Alabama, North Carolina, and South Carolina as well as Kentucky.[28] All these states were considered rural and sparsely populated and more likely to be unexposed to measles. Military medical officers Warren Vaughan and Truman Schnabel investigated pneumonia and empyema cases at Camp Sevier and noted that the health of the camp was surprisingly good until late October, when the arrival of 8,000 recruits triggered a measles epidemic. According to Vaughan, "Many of the new men coming from other camps had the measles rash on arrival, and others had only recently been in communities where the disease was endemic."[29]

Camp Wheeler, Georgia, provides another excellent example of measles being transported into the ranks. On October 14, 1917, Camp Wheeler welcomed 4,000 conscripts and another 10,000 more two weeks later. According to epidemiologist Victor C. Vaughan, "not a troop train reached Camp Wheeler in the fall of 1917 that did not have measles onboard from one to six cases of well-developed measles."[30] Measles cases soon appeared in the hospital. The seven cases present on October 19, 1917, multiplied into 44 cases four days later. Patients were typically nonimmune men who had traveled on the train with infected individuals. The epidemic swept through the camp. By November 22, 1917, measles cases had risen to 174 admissions.

The epidemic was severe enough for William Crawford Gorgas, the surgeon general of the U.S. Army, to make a personal appearance at the camp to inspect the situation himself. Gorgas speculated that the epidemic had been caused in part by "the fact the men came from surrounding southern states which are sparsely settled and therefore the inhabitants do not, as a rule, have measles in childhood."[31] Fortunately, the number of cases had subsided by December 7, after the virus had run its course through the camp.[32] Scenarios such as these occurred throughout all the cantonment camps as they received new recruits. The confined environment of trains occupied by a mix of immune, nonimmune, and infected was the catalyst that sparked epidemics, but the poor conditions at the camp ensured maximum virulence.

Camp Travis, Texas, which experienced a measles epidemic shortly after it opened its own hospital, provides an example of contagion through transporting troops as well as insufficient facilities for troops upon arrival.[33] Initially sparked by the arrival of new recruits from the rural states of Oklahoma and Texas, the camp's low rejection rate of 3.03 percent for those examined upon arrival and an insufficient number of accommodations led to overcrowding in barracks and mess halls and contributed to the exchange of pathogens that triggered measles outbreaks among susceptible troops. During this epidemic, there were 4,203 measles cases. The epidemic subsided in mid-January 1918, but the camp was soon hit with another measles epidemic in March of that year, only a little over a month later. This second epidemic was less virulent and lasted only two months. In all, from November 1917 to December 31, 1919, Camp Travis incurred a total of 4,821 measles cases and 57 deaths, which caused serious delays in the mobilization cycle of World War I troops.[34]

The housing of new recruits during the rapid mobilization for World War I proved problematic, especially in regard to the spread of measles. At the time war was declared, existing facilities at U.S. camps were only capable of housing 124,000. To accommodate the flow of recruits, the Office of the Quartermaster General created the Cantonment Division in July. This new division immediately began construction of 32 additional mobilization cantonments and camps capable of housing approximately 1 million men. Sixteen camps were allocated to the National Guard, and the other 16 were allocated for the National Army.[35]

In September 1917, 180,000 conscripts, hailing from all areas of the United States, were placed onto trains and sent to army camps for training. To their dismay, upon arrival, they discovered that the camps were still undergoing preparations. Even though the organization and construction of the mobilization camps began in July 1917, construction was still incomplete in September. The camps were ill-equipped with military supplies as well as uniforms, undergarments, shoes, coats, socks, canvas, and blankets.[36] Barracks were often overcrowded, and accommodations in tents were no better, as the men often had less than 50 square feet of space.[37] Both barracks and tents were not yet equipped with adequate heating as an extremely cold winter approached. Huddling to keep warm was inevitable, as was the spread of infectious respiratory illnesses.

The overall sanitary conditions at U.S. military facilities during World War I were far superior to those of the Spanish-American War 17 years earlier. The improvement in medical and scientific knowledge regarding bacteria, bacterial contaminations, and the ability to treat or prevent infection was partially responsible. Additionally, military medical reforms under the leadership of Surgeon General Gorgas and the preparedness reforms of Elihu Root resulted in modified training facilities and policies designed to assist in improved hygiene and environments. Unfortunately, these reforms were not consistently adhered to under the urgent pressures of war.

Placing cohorts of men with varying disease histories into poorly heated and overcrowded accommodations during a supply shortage and prior to an exceptionally cold winter ensured that the greatest mobilization effort in America would be teeming with the spread of disease. It did not take long before the close-knit camp communities became disease ridden. In the fall of 1917, as the mobilization effort began, measles cases appeared in great quantities among the various camps. The number of cases and duration of the epidemics varied for each camp, but, in summary, from October 1917 to January 1918, over 47,000 cases of measles were reported among the training camps.[38] The rate of measles cases fluctuated in tandem with mobilization and the introduction of new recruits, especially among those who were susceptible. It made no difference on the death rate whether the men were housed in National Guard tents or army barracks; both groups suffered equally.

Another camp with high incidents of measles due to overcrowding and insufficient provisions for the new recruits included the aforementioned Camp Wheeler, ranked fifth highest in the number of measles cases. The high measles admissions at Camp Wheeler had a direct correlation to the cohorts of immunes, nonimmunes, and infected troops. Enlisted and conscripted men from Florida, Georgia, Louisiana, Mississippi, and Alabama were sent to this camp as well as the active guard troops that operated on the Mexican border. Approximately 3 percent of the border guard troops were sick with both pneumonia and measles.

On October 14, 1917, the first wave of conscripted men arrived. There were approximately 4,000 men in all. Subsequent waves of new recruits poured into the camp so that by October 28, 1917, 10,000 new recruits had arrived. Approximately 30 percent of these men were nonimmune, and many showed signs of measles upon exiting the train. Measles cases filled the hospital, and by December 7, 1917, there were 3,000 measles patients, all of which were new recruits.[39] Gorgas visited the camp to inspect the situation and suggest improvements. He observed the overcrowded conditions at the camp and the lack of warm clothing for the men and blamed the epidemic in part on these factors as well as the immune status of the recruits. Gorgas recommended that woolen garments be supplied to the men and that at least 50 feet of floor space be given to each man, even if this meant building more shelters. He also recommended that the camp stop accepting new men until the epidemic subsided.[40] Unfortunately, the realities of rapid mobilization and budgetary restraints made implementing his recommendations nearly impossible, though modified reforms were employed. More tents were added to the camp so that instead of nine men per tent, the number was reduced to five. New recruits continued to be accepted, but they were segregated from the other troops into observation tents to deter the spread of measles.

Camp Gordon, Georgia, also experienced a measles epidemic in December 1917. Startled by the high rate of respiratory infections in the camps, F. T. Woodbury, MD, a U.S. Army colonel, visited Camp Gordon and published his findings in April 1919. He observed the overcrowded conditions in the barracks. When the new recruits arrived at the camp in September 1917, there were only enough accommodations for fewer than two-thirds of the men. Woodbury believed the spread of infection was due to "crowding in poorly ventilated dormitories or squad rooms, which reduces resistance and directly favors irritative laryngeal and nasal reflexes whereby coughing and sneezing are promoted, which in turn spread the infection."[41] Woodbury recommended reducing overcrowding, providing proper ventilation, and reducing cold drafts with the use of cloth screens in the windows. He also recommended providing proper heating of the barracks as a means of preventing the spread of respiratory diseases. He went on to sketch out and describe what he considered to be "a model barrack for a company," whereby he recommended sanitary features such as sleeping quarters that were separated from lounging rooms and the separation of beds by hanging sheets or wooden boards between them. Windows should be screened, and restrooms should be provided in the barracks to prevent recruits from exiting into the cold outdoors to use these facilities.[42] Woodbury's suggestions became the model for 20th-century barracks improvement in the United States.

Aside from exposure to measles on troop transports and in overcrowded camp barracks, the most important means of diffusing measles was related to the circumstances encountered in military medical facilities during and immediately after World War I. Circumstances differed from camp to camp, but certain factors repeatedly emerged as measles epidemics were investigated: overcrowding in hospitals, misdiagnosis of measles and other contagious diseases, insufficient isolation of measles patients from other contagious respiratory and other diseases, and resulting cross-infections that complicated measles and increased mortality rates.

The camp holding the record for the highest number of measles admissions and deaths was the army cantonment Camp Pike. On September 17, 1917, the base hospital at Camp Pike opened and was immediately flooded by recruits suffering from respiratory diseases. The hospital ran out of space for its patients; therefore, a barracks was used to house the rest. The camp epidemiologist observed that of the 538 measles patients treated in the hospital, 51 contracted secondary infections, which caused 11 deaths. Out of the 256 measles patients treated in the fairly isolated barracks, 4 contracted secondary infections, resulting in 1 death. It was concluded that crowded conditions in the hospital had increased the risk of cross-infections and complications, as the rate of secondary infection was much lower in the barracks.[43]

The close proximity of Camp Travis to a fully equipped base hospital provided the opportunity and resources for medical officials to study the epidemiological nature and reaction of pathogens. On January 3, 1918, medical officials from Fort Sam Houston and Camp Travis gathered to determine which pathogens were responsible for causing pneumonia in measles cases. The medical officers, James Cumming, Charles Spruit, and Charles Lynch, set out to study the prevalence of pneumococci and hemolytic streptococci in measles patients. At the same time, Gorgas sent a commission of contract surgeons and medical officers to Fort Sam Houston and Camp Travis to study the same subject. The research of Cumming, Spruit, and Lynch demonstrated that over one-third of measles patients had contracted hemolytic streptococci, and one-third of that subset of patients had developed streptococci pneumonia.[44] Cole and MacCallum also studied measles patients in the ward and found hemolytic streptococci in 56.6 percent of them. They went a step further and took throat samples from measles patients as they were admitted and continued to take throat samples for consecutive days. They discovered that 11.4 percent of measles patients were positive for hemolytic streptococci upon admission; the number increased to 56.8 percent after 8 to 16 days. These findings indicated measles patients contracted hemolytic streptococci while in the hospital wards.[45] The logical conclusion was that overcrowding of the hospital facilities had led to cross-contamination of already weakened measles patients with other respiratory infections.

Logan Clendening, MD, the chief of the medical services at Fort Sam Houston, felt that the scope of Cole and MacCallum's report was too narrow and did not take into account the incidence of bronchopneumonia in all the measles cases. He was perturbed that they also failed to offer up any methods of prevention. Conducting his own research regarding hemolytic streptococci infection in cases of lobar pneumonia, measles, and scarlet fever, hemolytic streptococci had appeared as a complication in all the aforementioned diseases, and, of the 716 measles cases, hemolytic streptococci had complicated 14.8 percent of these cases. Realizing that patients might be contracting hemolytic streptococci in the wards, Clendening created a system of isolation and study in the hospital. Patient wards were isolated according to diagnoses, sheets separated beds, and weekly cultures were taken from patients' throats to ensure reinfection did not occur. This practice resulted in a dramatic reduction in bronchopneumonia cases.[46]

James Greenway, Carl Boettiger, and Howard Colwell investigated measles and pneumonia cases at Camp Bowie. They admitted to the difficulties encountered in properly identifying and diagnosing measles cases as well as recognizing complications. The team observed that two weeks after the start of the measles epidemic, there was a peak in pneumonia cases, reaching a total of 973 in just over three months.[47] As the cases dwindled, 6,000 new recruits arrived and sparked another epidemic just as virulent as the first. They asserted hemolytic streptococci was the culprit to the complications among measles patients and increased the likelihood of death.

Warren Vaughan and Truman Schnabel's investigation of pneumonia and empyema cases at Camp Sevier revealed this illness was not a new disease but instead a secondary infection caused by the well-known streptococcic bacteria introduced to measles patients. To limit cross-infection in measles cases, patients were confined to beds surrounded by wooden frames draped with sheets. Persons entering the room wore protective gowns, and patients were given their own thermometers, towels, drinking cups, washbasins, and bedpans. All items used by patients were frequently washed and disinfected. These practices were put into effect on December 1, 1917, along with attempts at achieving an accurate diagnosis. Vaughan reported the death rate was lowered to 10 percent due to the new precautions avoiding cross-infection.[48]

As with the attempt by medical professionals at Camp Pike to create a measles vaccine, the doctors at Camp Gordon sought to create a vaccine against streptococcus infections. Fifty measles patients were given an experimental streptococcus vaccine, and another 50 were given a placebo. Of the patients who received the vaccine, two developed streptococcus bronchopneumonia or empyema, whereas 14 measles patients in the placebo group developed the same illness. Doctors at Camp Gordon continued to administer the vaccine, and an overall lower death rate and incidence of measles complications was recorded.[49] Unfortunately, the urgencies of war delayed the perfection of a consistently effective vaccine for five more decades.

Medical officers Robert L. Levy and H. L. Alexander realized the severity of measles cases occurring in the camps and that serious secondary infections not only increased the number of days spent in the hospital but increased fatalities due to bronchopneumonia and empyema complications. Levy and Alexander went to Camp Taylor, Kentucky, to study this phenomenon. They decided to establish a measles-receiving ward. In this ward, new admissions of measles patients had their throats swabbed and tested for hemolytic streptococcus. Those who tested positive were sent to a ward for hemolytic streptococcus–positive patients, and those who tested negative were sent to a ward with others who had tested negative.

Both groups were required to wear gauze facemasks that were changed daily. They hoped separating measles patients based on whether or not they had hemolytic streptococcus would reduce the cross-infection rate. The team tested 388 measles patients, of which 299 were positive for hemolytic streptococcus. Complications occurred in 36.8 percent of those cases. Of the cases where measles patients did not test positive, only 6.4 percent of them developed minor complications, such as tonsillitis, demonstrating the success of the process of testing and isolation.[50]

Communicating Successes in Medical Strategies for Treating Measles Outbreaks

As epidemics emerged, research and findings struggled to keep pace. Lessons learned at one hospital were shared with others, though the ability to implement the reforms was restricted to the circumstances at individual camps and hospitals. Hospital quarantines were quickly picked up and implemented where room allowed. It was the policy of hospitals with available space to quarantine a ward that became infected with another disease for the duration of a week. Unfortunately, frequent quarantines delayed the discharge of healthy patients and prevented the admission of new cases.[51] To prevent cross-infections and the stifling quarantines that ensued, a cubical system was employed in the base hospital at Camp Grant, Illinois, whereby bed sheets were hung from metal wires around the cubicle. This practice was believed to prevent the spread of infectious respiratory droplets, but it failed to take into consideration that patients rarely stayed in their cubicles; washrooms remained communal. As such, patients who were protected from cross-infection by the cubicle system forfeited this protection when they got up to use the restroom.

Military physician Joseph A. Capps devised a system of facemasks and protective gowns used by the staff to prevent introducing or contracting infections. In the case of staff members, this practice worked, and they experienced fewer illnesses. Unfortunately, patients still contracted secondary infections. Capps required that patients in wards with recent cross-infection episodes must wear the masks at all times when outside of their cubicles. He even ordered patients to wear masks while riding the ambulances to the hospital to prevent cross-infection between multiple patients in the ambulance.[52] His precautions bore fruit. Out of the 1,132 measles cases that occurred from early mobilization to December 31, 1919, only 10 cases led to fatalities. Consequently, the use of facemasks by patients and staff became a standard practice in base hospitals where contagious infections were detected.[53]

Another factor played a role in the numbers of cross-infections with measles patients during World War I. Misdiagnosis of measles, confusing it with scarlet fever or rubella, was a common occurrence. The milder, or three-day, version of measles was not considered serious, and patients thus diagnosed often remained in wards with other patients, exposing the other patients to measles. Some patients with rubella who were diagnosed as having the severe form of measles were isolated in wards with measles patients, subsequently contracting the more severe form of the disease following their episode with rubella. Likewise, misdiagnoses of measles and scarlet fever resulted in patients with these diseases being placed in the same wards.

While Victor Vaughn's research on misdiagnoses acknowledged that such actions also happened in civilian hospitals, these mistakes in the large, overcrowded military hospitals had serious consequences.[54] Misdiagnoses at Camp Cody, New Mexico, and Camp Lewis, Washington, demonstrated the impact of the problem. Those diagnosed with the milder rubella form were placed in wards that allowed continued exposure to other complicating illnesses. Additionally, the records kept on patient diagnoses reflected the erroneous data. The numbers recorded for measles cases and deaths from complications experienced at Camps Cody and Lewis reflect inaccurate data as a consequence.[55]

As recruits completed their training at mobilization camps, they were sent by railroad to an embarkation camp and then deployed abroad. To maximize the number of troops shipped, Maj. Gen. Peyton March devised a plan in conjunction with Adm. Albert Gleaves that increased the number of bunks per room. Hammocks were lined along hallways and hung in the mess hall. These changes in accommodations led to a 40 percent increase in the number of troops shipped overseas per vessel.[56] It also led to overcrowding, already identified as a main cause of disease contagion. Not surprisingly, when the United States began transporting troops overseas, measles reappeared among passengers of troopships. In June 1917, seven cases were reported, and by January 1918, the number of measles cases had risen to 507. Approximately 100–200 cases were reported per month during the spring, and 800–900 cases per month by the late summer.[57]

On August 6, 1918, General Order 72 mandated medical officers to conduct physical examinations of soldiers ordered to embarkation camps.[58] The order attempted to reduce the spread of diseases, especially respiratory illnesses, onboard ships en route to France. Those troops identified with symptoms were quarantined, as were nonimmune troops that had been exposed to troops with symptoms. The process slowed mobilization and troop movement abroad for 12 months following the U.S. declaration of war. While this improvement reduced the number of cases, the system was not consistently effective, as evidenced by Pvt. Lake's quote at the start of this chapter.

Measles cases among transported troops aboard troopships peaked in September 1918 and then gradually declined until the armistice. Out of approximately 2,036,103 American troops finally sent overseas to join the American Expeditionary Forces, 9,168 additional soldiers were admitted for measles while deployed, and 358 of these men died from complications.[59] The army reported that these cases were contracted in training camps and resulted in the infection of nonimmunes during transport in highly overcrowded and poorly ventilated transport ships.

Combined Impact of Measles, Medical Research, and Mobilization in World War I

In November 1918, an armistice brought an end to the war. By this time, over 2 million U.S. servicemen had been recruited, drafted, trained in camps, and shipped overseas to assist in the war. Almost 100,000 of this total had been admitted to hospitals for measles, and close to 2 million days of effective-duty status had been lost from illness. Additionally, of the over 421,809 Australians who had served in the Australian Imperial Forces, 28.7 percent had been admitted to hospitals for primary diseases, of which 61 percent were respiratory in nature (20 percent were clearly identified as measles, or almost 15,000 measles patients).[60] The impact of disease, particularly measles, was felt on these two nations, especially in the more rural military camps and populations. Negative impacts were felt most in the delays of mobilization and deployment, the loss effective-service days, and the illness and even death of troops.

In the brief period of U.S. involvement in World War I, measles epidemics appeared at almost every mobilization camp across the United States. Those camps with high numbers of rural recruits mixed with recruits from regions where measles was endemic saw epidemic outbreaks. Overcrowded camps, even those that maintained good hygiene protocols, typically suffered higher rates of contagion than smaller camps. Camps in the south and west, more rural in nature, tended to experience higher morbidity rates than those in the east and northeast. Hospitals with overcrowding, especially those that failed to segregate measles patients from the outset, saw increased complications and, consequently, high mortality rates among measles patients. The makings of disaster were present, but efforts to research and improve conditions increased with reports of new outbreaks, resulting in positive and lasting reforms from the measles epidemics.

The investigations by numerous medical staff helped improve protocols and research on measles in the United States and Australia. Improvements in housing, testing of recruits as they arrived at mobilization camps, and varying means of isolating those contagious with measles and postmeasles infections improved the odds of a quick recovery and survival. While some reform recommendations were not implemented immediately due to space, time, and budgetary constraints, most military camps instigated basic protocols designed to restrict the diffusion of measles among the population. Improved efforts to isolate and treat measles patients did cause further delays, as repeated quarantines were implemented to reduce further epidemic spikes.[61] Although cases of measles continued to appear in camps among the new recruits, especially those recruits from rural areas, the case numbers did eventually decline when the new protocols were carefully followed.[62]

The impact of measles epidemics causing delays in mobilizing and deploying World War I troops, while obvious from military records, will never be known in terms of specific quantifiable impacts on the war itself. The numbers of personnel that contracted the illness, especially considering the likelihood of underreporting due to misdiagnoses, were staggering. Military documents reveal that at least "one and a half million days were lost from duty." The Americans had the highest ratio of noneffective personnel in World War I due to illness. Indeed, the study produced on measles in the war indicated that "no disease was more closely allied to mobilization than was measles."[63]

Yet, of equal significance to the study of measles epidemics in World War I were the medical research and reforms implemented to stop the spread of measles, reduce the outbreaks, and lessen the number of days that would have otherwise been lost to recovery from the disease. More importantly, the medical discoveries and reforms implemented during the measles outbreaks helped contain to some degree the spread of the ensuing great influenza pandemic of 1918 that rippled around the globe at the tail end of World War I.

NOTES

1. Richard Rubin, *The Last of the Doughboys: The Forgotten Generation and Their Forgotten World War* (Boston: Houghton Mifflin Harcourt, 2013), 340.
2. Carol R. Byerly, "The Politics of Disease and War: Infectious Disease in the United States Army during World War I" (PhD diss., University of Colorado, 2001), 2.
3. William J. Moss and Diane E. Griffin, "Measles," *The Lancet* 379, no. 9811 (2012): 153, 155.
4. Jennifer Manley, "Measles and Ancient Plagues: A Note on New Scientific Evidence," *Classical World* 107, no. 3 (2014): 394, 396.
5. Preeta Kutty, MD, et al., "Measles," in *Manual for the Surveillance of Vaccine-Preventable Diseases*, Centers for Disease Control and Prevention, accessed September 2, 2017, https://www.cdc.gov/vaccines/pubs/surv-manual/chpt07-measles.html.
6. Moss and Griffin, 156.
7. Mayo Clinic Staff, "Symptoms," *Diseases and Conditions: Measles*, accessed September 2, 2017, http://www.mayoclinic.org/diseases-conditions/measles/basics/symptoms/CON -20019675.
8. Vincent J. Cirillo, "Two Faces of Death: Fatalities from Disease and Combat in America's Principal Wars, 1775 to Present," *Perspectives in Biology and Medicine* 51, no. 1 (2008): 123.
9. Friedrich Prinzing, *Epidemics Resulting from Wars*, ed. Harald Westergaard (Oxford: Clarendon Press, 1916), 177–179. African American troops continued to suffer higher rates of measles and complications during World War I.
10. David M. Morens and Jeffery K. Taubenberger, "A Forgotten Epidemic That Changed Medicine: Measles in the U.S. Army, 1917–18," *The Lancet: Infectious Diseases* 15, no. 7 (2015): 852.
11. Leonard P. Ayers, Col., "Health and Casualties," *The War with Germany, a Statistical Summary* (Washington, D.C.: Government Printing Office, 1919), chapter 9.
12. Henry C. Michie and George E. Lull, "Measles," *Communicable and Other Diseases*, Vol. 9, *The Medical Department of the United States Army in the World War* (Washington, D.C.: U.S. Government Printing Office, 1928), 413.
13. Ayers, "Health and Casualties."
14. "Influenza, Pneumonia, and Common Respiratory Diseases," *Annual Report of the Surgeon General for Fiscal Year 1919*, Vol. 1 (Washington, D.C.: GPO, 1919), 640.
15. Charles Robert Mowbray Fraser Cruttwell, *A History of the Great War: 1914–1918*, 2nd ed. (Chicago: Academy Chicago Publishers, 1991), 200–203, 380.
16. Marvin A. Kreidberg and Merton G. Henry, *History of Military Mobilization in the United States Army 1775–1945*, Department of the Army pamphlet, no. 20-212 (Washington, D.C.: Department of the Army, 1955), 218–219.
17. Kreidberg and Henry, *History of Military Mobilization*, 223–228.

18. Timothy J. Perri, "The Evolution of Military Conscription in the United States," *Independent Review* 17, no. 3 (2013): 432, 437; Kreidberg and Henry, *History of Military Mobilization*, 249–250; and Anthony W. Smiley, "The Homefront: World War One at Home" (Air Command and Staff College thesis, Air University, 2000), 11.

19. Kreidberg and Henry, *History of Military Mobilization*, 228, 250–251.

20. Kreidberg and Henry, *History of Military Mobilization*, 267–274.

21. Moss and Griffin, "Measles," 154.

22. A. G. Love and Charles B. Davenport, "Immunity of City-Bred Recruits," *Archives of Internal Medicine* 24, no. 2 (1919): 152.

23. G. Dennis Shanks, "Measles Epidemics of Variable Lethality in the Early 20th Century," *American Journal of Epidemiology* 179, no. 4 (February 15, 2014), accessed September 2, 2017, https://academic.oup.com/aje/article/179/4/413/128401/Measles-Epidemics -of-Variable-Lethality-in-the.

24. Love and Davenport, "Immunity of City-Bred Recruits," 131.

25. Kreidberg and Henry, *History of Military Mobilization*, 313–314.

26. Michie and Lull, "Measles," 419, 442.

27. James C. Greenway, Carl Boettiger, and Howard S. Colwell, "Pneumonia and Some of Its Complications at Camp Bowie," *Archives of Internal Medicine* 24, no. 1 (1919): 1.

28. Michie and Lull, "Measles," 417, 419.

29. Warren T. Vaughan and Truman G. Schnabel, "Pneumonia and Empyema at Camp Sevier," *Archives of Internal Medicine* 22, no. 4 (1918): 441.

30. Victor C. Vaughan, *Epidemiology and Public Health: A Text and Reference Book for Physicians, Medical Students and Health Workers*, Vol. 1 (St. Louis, MO: C. V. Mosby Company, 1922), 177, accessed September 2, 2017, https://books.google.com/books?id =J4saAAAAMAAJ.

31. American Association for the Advancement of Science, "Medical Inspection of Camp Wheeler," *Science* 46, no. 1197 (1917): 558, accessed September 2, 2017, http://science .sciencemag.org/content/46/1197/558.

32. Michie and Lull, "Measles," 421.

33. F. W. Kiel, "Some Medical Aspects of the History of Fort Sam Houston," *Military Medicine* 129 (November 1964): 1046, accessed September 2, 2017, http://www.dtic.mil /dtic/tr/fulltext/u2/454027.pdf.

34. Michie and Lull, "Measles," 422, 419, 417; Kiel, "Some Medical Aspects."

35. Kreidberg and Henry, *History of Military Mobilization*, 311, 314, 317.

36. Samuel T. Moore, *America and the World War* (New York: Greenberg Publisher, Inc., 1937), 97; Kreidberg and Henry, *History of Military Mobilization*, 229–234, 315, 318–319.

37. Love and Davenport, "Immunity of City-Bred Recruits," 129–130.

38. Love and Davenport, "Immunity of City-Bred Recruits," 130.

39. Michie and Lull, "Measles," 421.

40. Medical Association for the Advancement of Science, "Medical Inspection," 559.

41. F. T. Woodbury, "Model Barrack for Prevention of Respiratory Disease in the Army," *JAMA* 72, no. 17 (1919): 1212.

42. Woodbury, "Model Barrack," 1213–1214.

43. Michie and Lull, "Measles," 417, 446.

44. James G. Cumming, Charles B. Spruit, and Charles Lynch, "The Pneumonias: Streptococcus and Pneumonococcus Groups," *Journal of the American Medical Association (JAMA)* 70, no. 15 (1918): 1066.

45. Rufus Cole and W. G. MacCallum, "Pneumonia at Base Hospital," *JAMA* 70, no. 16 (1918): 1146–1156, accessed September 2, 2017, https://babel.hathitrust.org/cgi/pt?id =mdp.39015082605612;view=2up;seq=6.

46. Logan Clendening, "Reinfection with Streptococcus Hemolyticus in Lobar Pneumonia, Measles and Scarlet Fever and Its Prevents," *American Journal of the Medical Sciences* 156 (Philadelphia and New York: Lea & Febiger, 1918): 575–576, 580, 584–586.

47. Greenway, Boettiger, and Colwell, "Pneumonia and Some of Its Complications."

48. Vaughan and Schnabel, "Pneumonia and Empyema," 465; Michie and Lull, "Measles," 419.

49. Michie and Lull, "Measles," 442.

50. Robert L. Levy and H. L. Alexander, "The Predisposition of Streptococcus Carriers to the complications of Measles: Results of Separation of Carriers from Non-Carriers at a Base Hospital," *JAMA* 70, no. 20 (1919): 1827–1830.

51. Joseph A. Capps, "A New Adaptation of the Face Mask in Control of Contagious Disease," *JAMA* 70, no. 13 (1918): 910.

52. Capps, "A New Adaptation," 910–911.

53. Michie and Lull, "Measles," 419, 444.

54. Victor C. Vaughan, "Communicable Diseases in the National Guard and National Army of the United States during the Six Months from September 29, 1917 to March 29, 1918," *Journal of Laboratory and Clinical Medicine* 3, no. 11 (August 1918): 644.

55. Michie and Lull, "Measles," 419.

56. Kreidberg and Henry, *History of Military Mobilization*, 334.

57. Michie and Lull, "Measles," 425.

58. "Medical Mobilization and the War," *JAMA* 71, no. 1 (September 14, 1918): 910.

59. Michie and Lull, "Measles," 425.

60. Following the Twenty-Second, "Sickness & Disease: The Impact of Non-Combat Casualties on Fighting Strength in the AIF," accessed September 2, 2017, https:// anzac-22nd-battalion.com/sickness-disease-the-impact-of-non-combat-casualties-on -fighting-strength-in-the-aif.

61. Love and Davenport, "Immunity of City-Bred Recruits," 130–142.

62. Michie and Lull, "Measles," 419.

63. Michie and Lull, "Measles," 414.

Chapter 13

Influenza during World War I: The Great Flu Pandemic, 1916–1919

Jillion Becker

It stalked into camp when the day was damp; And chilly and cold. It crept by the guards; And murdered my pards, With a hand that was clammy and bony and bold, And its breath was icy, and mouldy, and dank. And it killed so speedy, And gloatingly greedy, That it took away men from each company rank.[1]

—Pvt. Josh Lee

World War I, or the Great War, became an all-encompassing event that accounted in the public mind-set for many of the social anomalies that occurred from 1914 to 1920. Among these anomalies was a major influenza pandemic that killed millions in a short span of time; yet, it had escaped long-term historical notice until the past two decades. The memories of survivors, those who were infected and those who escaped infection, were tucked away with elements of their other wartime experiences. Not surprisingly, the memories of those directly affected were connected to personal loss rather than the collective episode of isolation and panic. Reconciling the two memories, of personal loss and association with the war, provides a clearer picture of the great influenza pandemic of 1918. One essential element of the pandemic that has surfaced in recent research is that, were it not for the unique circumstances created by a world at war, the conditions would not have existed for the virus to become so widespread and peculiarly virulent, nor would it have erupted three times in such rapid sequence.

Identification and Transmission of Influenza Virus

Influenza is a viral infection that is often associated with subsequent bacterial infections such as pneumonia. The definitive differentiation between bacteria and viruses is less than 100 years old. Viruses were first named in the 1890s, but they were not conclusively identified in the lab until the 1930s.[2] Because there was no means of isolating viruses, many diseases caused by them were given incorrect etiologies. Influenza was no exception. Robert Friedrich Pfeiffer isolated bacillus bacteria from influenza patients; thus, he thought he had identified the causative agent of influenza. As a result of his identification of *Bacillus influenza*, Pfeiffer's *Bacillus* became universally accepted.[3] Unfortunately, the medical protocol for combating this secondary bacterial infection did not address the infection caused by the virus. Nonetheless, the disease, now identified as a virus, is sometimes still referred to as bacterial influenza.

Typical symptoms of influenza include cough, fever, chills, sore throat, congestion, muscle aches, headaches, and extreme fatigue. Flu can often be accompanied by secondary infections, including streptococcus and pneumonia. Bacterial pneumonia is one of the most common complications of influenza, resulting in high mortality rates. Secondary infections during World War I were caused by any number of bacteria. Even today, it is difficult to determine whether the respiratory symptoms presented by a patient are caused by influenza. Only by testing specifically for the virus can doctors give a positive diagnosis. What became evident from studying the 1918 pandemic was the realization that higher infection and mortality rates occurred in people from lower socioeconomic classes.[4] This realization, while helpful in understanding the role of disease diffusion and the impact of overall health in influenza patients, did little to assist in the initial diagnosis and treatment of influenza during the war.

In addition to the difficulty of making a historically correct diagnosis of influenza, the disease was easily transmitted from host to host. The flu was spread from person to person via the droplet mode of transmission—coughing, sneezing, or even speaking within six feet of an infected person puts an individual at risk. Additionally, the virus survived on inanimate surfaces, providing another mode of transmission. The populations most susceptible to infection typically included those individuals with chronic health conditions, those over the age of 65, pregnant women, and young children. The best prevention was for susceptible populations to avoid those who are or may be sick.

Constant Adaptation of Influenza as a Cause of Pandemics

The adaptability of flu viruses makes matters worse. The constantly changing nature of flu viruses means there is always a risk of epidemic. Antigenic drifts typically occur slowly as a virus replicates over time, leaving closely related viruses and building immunity in exposed populations. More significant changes are the product of antigenic shifts. A shift is an abrupt change that typically occurs when the infected population changes from one specific animal to another. Historically, pandemic flu occurred as a result of a dramatic antigenic shift.[5] Of the four types of influenza viruses (A, B, C, and D), type A is the most likely to be altered by antigenic shift and, therefore, is the most likely causative agent for pandemic flu. Of the four documented influenza pandemics of the last century (1918, 1957, 1968, 2009), each was caused by a different strain of influenza A.[6] Of these, the most virulent and fatal was the pandemic of 1918.

The misnamed "Spanish flu" recently became a topic of fascination for researchers from a vast scope of fields. Scientists had never stopped investigating the virus, and modern epidemiology was partly founded as a legacy of this pandemic. None-theless, the disease missed detection for decades as the focus of researchers targeted the setting of the disease, World War I. Only recently have historians, anthro-pologists, and others brought a previously marginalized event out of obscurity. Formerly considered insignificant, researchers began to uncover the full impact of the pandemic on history, particularly as it related to the Great War. Treated as a postscript to the war, for decades little mention was made to the worldwide pandemic.

Extreme Virulence and High Death Toll of the "Spanish Flu"

The great influenza outbreak spread across the world from March 1918 to May 1919. Estimates of upward to 650,000 people were killed in the United States alone in less than one year. The number of American servicemen killed by this dis-ease matched the number of Americans killed on the battlefield during the Great War. Conservative estimates of the number of deaths worldwide directly resulting from this strain of influenza are 40–50 million, four times that of the number who "died in combat on all fronts in the entire four years of the War."[7] Less conserva-tive estimates go as high as 100 million deaths globally. In Philadelphia alone, the number of deaths in just over a month was 12,162 between September 29 and November 2, 1918.[8] American troops on American soil accounted for 14, 616 deaths between September 12 and October 18.[9]

Deaths from disease in 1918 were not only due to influenza but also to subse-quent secondary infections such as pneumonia. History is riddled with statistics of those who died, the morbidity and mortality demographics, and other similar figures. Excluding military casualties, proportionally, more people died in Amer-ica in 1918 than in any other year. Included in those calculations are potentially flu-related deaths from starvation, malnourishment, and similar casualties that resulted from the loss of caregivers. These latter figures alone were certainly higher than in any other year, though the numbers were not directly attributed to influ-enza.[10] The numbers do not account for adjustments to include unborn children of mothers who died before they carried to full term.[11]

Historical Analysis of Memory and Reality in Studying the Great Flu Pandemic

Despite the extreme toll on human life, history books today rarely make mention of the 1918 pandemic. The most likely explanation is found in an understanding of the collective public opinion. In 1920, a *Public Health Report* released on Feb-ruary 6 compared the then-current influenza outbreak to one that took place in 1918. The main purpose of the report was to assure the public that the mortality figures were significantly lower than those in 1918 and that the 1920 outbreak was "decidedly less serious" and following more closely to "normal" flu statistics. From this report, it is clear that the 1918 Spanish flu pandemic had a great impact on the average American's opinion of influenza and also corroborated with the theory that it was held in collective memory.[12] Further evidence of collective memory of the event was seen in the 1930s as the discovery of viruses spurred renewed literary interest in the long-forgotten event.[13]

The collective memory of civilization tends to be fickle, and the pandemic of 1918 was no exception to this. Historian Alfred Crosby attempted to explain the phenomenon of what seemed to be an entire population forgetting the greatest single cause of death in an approximated three-month period. World War I was taking place at this time, and there was a certain amount of expected death. It was also significant that the age group most frequently cited in the mortality statistics, 20–40 years of age, was the same as those who were already expected to be lost in battle on the front lines.[14] Furthermore, the initial emergence of the disease in military encampments helped to explain the natural correlation in the American consciousness between the war and the epidemic.[15]

Crosby discovered during his research that interviewing individuals, rather than groups, tended to provide a fuller understanding of the attitude of Americans toward the events of 1918. In general, contemporaries remembered many details about the pandemic and how it became "one of the most influential experiences of their lives."[16] Many children lost siblings, friends, extended family members, or parents. To these individuals, the great influenza pandemic became their first encounter with death, particularly with death of such a great magnitude. Recollections were shared about the number of bodies stacked in morgues, in back alleys, and in mass graves. Francis Russell, an eyewitness to the events, described his experience of realizing the mortal nature of humanity: that "[he] too must one day die."[17] In autobiographies, individuals who lost family members remembered them within those pages. Despite these horrific memories, or maybe because of them, many writers chose to leave the significance of the influenza pandemic out of their recollections. Others, especially the very young, recalled memories of illness in their communities but failed to connect those childhood experiences to a specific disease until much later in their lives.

Recollections of the event and period also appear in the writings of fiction writers. The group of writers known throughout the decades following the Great War as the "Lost Generation" was composed of individuals who felt a need to portray elements of their life experiences in text. Their works were commentaries on the state of society and of America as a whole in relation to politics and public-opinion-shaping media. However, the pandemic of 1918 rarely received any mention in their works, even those that directly covered the war and the general time period. Many mentioned some epidemic as a player in the plot line, but it was generally of a more "sensational" nature, such as "spinal meningitis."[18] At this time of few medical advances, there were a great number of epidemics that rotated through populations. Any epidemic would fill the role in the story; disease was expected.[19] *Pale Horse, Pale Rider* was one of the only works from a writer who lived through the pandemic that directly addressed the influenza pandemic. This short story was written by Katherine Anne Porter, who herself was stricken with influenza and came close to death. The power of the story comes from her emotion at losing her lover to the same infection.[20]

In the last 10–15 years, a renewed focus on researching and writing about the "Spanish flu" has emerged. Historian Howard Phillips fittingly dubbed this recent revival of scholarly and public interest as the "second wave."[21] In his historiography of the topic, Phillips asserted that the more traditional research (prior to the 1990s) treated the pandemic as high drama, a public health crisis, scientific exploration, and "an epidemiological episode." The most current wave of research, spurred on by the 1999 outbreak of avian flu in Hong Kong and furthered by the 2009 swine flu epidemic in Mexico, has sparked widespread calls for studies into possible pandemics and responses. The expansion of terrorism and fears of potential bioterrorism have furthered public demand for information. Many of the recent works on the great influenza pandemic have been disseminated in popular culture formats, such as feature films, documentaries, TV dramas, and even novels.[22]

Tracing the Origins and Diffusion of Influenza during World War I

As more interest has been directed to pandemics in general and the Spanish flu specifically, trends have appeared in the focus of research. One avenue of research on the 1918 pandemic is for scholars to track the diffusion of the disease as it spread from place to place and region to region. The purpose of this spatial analysis was to identify the source of the disease's origin. Unfortunately, the almost simultaneous outbreaks of influenza in places as far apart as China, Africa, and North America make the task of discerning an origin point difficult. A second approach to quantify the morbidity and mortality of the disease impact has also been undertaken with distinctly different outcomes. Part of the difficulty with this approach is the lack of proper diagnosis of the virus in 1918. As a result, some historians utilize numbers for any similar reports of disease, while others restrict their numbers to those with relatively clear diagnoses. Scholarly research on quantification of the 1918 outbreak often treats the pandemic "as universal in scope and similar in response," according to Matthew Heaton and Toyin Falola. Their assertion was based on their historiographical study of the pandemic in Africa, which generated different responses and accounting for morbidity from port cities to rural regions.[23] Wherever the pandemic spread, and whatever approach was used in researching its diffusion, the simultaneous occurrence of World War I and the outbreak combined to accelerate morbidity and mortality.

In 1918, the conditions inherent to war made the risk of disease greater. The overcrowding of military camps and trenches, the use of chemical gas as a form of warfare, the fact that most of the troops received inadequate rest and nutrition, and the greatest movement of men across the globe ever witnessed in history made the Great War ripe for epidemic. Influenza spread between people in close proximity. The conditions of overcrowding at military posts, in transport ships, and in the trenches of European combat made this transmission that much easier.[24] Flu struck those in ill health hardest. It has been speculated that trench diseases and chemical gases weakened the health of troops even more than normal exhaustion from fighting an extended war.[25] Additionally, the vast deployment and mobilization of men across almost every continent allowed the disease to become pandemic in a relatively short period of time, often with outbreaks seeming to be simultaneous. This has made finding the foci that much more difficult for modern-day epidemiologists.[26]

Not only did war conditions affect the health of the soldiers, these conditions also affected civilians, both by interactions with soldiers and by the limited access to health care.[27] Certainly, port cities such as New York that attracted large immigrant populations that crowded into substandard housing created optimal conditions for infection to spread. Poverty ensured that some ethnic clusters had little access to health care. Additionally, a large percentage of the physicians from around the world worked in the war effort to address the ongoing medical conditions of war and the emerging pandemic. They either supported troops clinically or worked in laboratories to help fight whatever diseases affected the soldiers. This reduced the number of physicians available to treat civilians. In many communities, the ratio of physician to patient was 1 to 5,000.[28]

One problem encountered by physicians who attempted to diagnose and treat the flu was that there was no previous wartime influenza pandemic to reference. Much of what contemporary physicians knew they had learned from the "Russian flu" pandemic of 1889, which had had a much lower fatality rate.[29] The flu of 1918 was pathologically similar to previous flu outbreaks; yet, there were some marked differences, namely, the mortality rates of the pandemic. Contemporaries examining the excessive mortality rates questioned whether the environment and circumstances of the population had changed so dramatically from earlier years to account for heavier incidence of the flu in the healthiest sectors of the population. However, at least one commentator found it easier to explain the change as a modification of the "infecting organism" rather than a variation in circumstances.[30] It is more likely that a combination of the two aspects occurred. The unique environment of 1918, after four years of global war, provided a significant enough impetus to create a pandemic. Although not understood at the time, it is likely that enough of a modification to the virus was possible to create three successive waves, the latter two being far more deadly than the original widespread wave.

Guy Carleton Jones, the future surgeon general of Canada, upon the onset of World War I, had warned "that a global war might bring new diseases home to civilian populations."[31] The 1918 pandemic came in three waves. The first primarily infected armies, and though it was highly contagious, it was relatively mild and had a low mortality rate. The second wave reached soldiers and civilians together.[32] This wave was the most fatal influenza pandemic yet known. The disease spread just as Jones had warned: "'the trail of infected armies leaves a sad tale of sickness amongst the women and children and non-combatants.'"[33] The "roles of military camps [were as] 'kindling and acceleration and spatial transmission of epidemic events.'"[34] Jones also reported that "the pandemic's progress [could] be tracked simply by plotting where soldiers [had] disembarked from troop trains and troopships."[35] The soldiers were infected, and as they mobilized and deployed across the globe, they spread the disease. The Brazilian naval fleet exemplifies this with their ships deployed to the West African coast. Not only did they become infected because of interaction with a British ship, but they also spread the infection to Dakar.[36] Many such anecdotes exist in the war and epidemic narrative.

While modern analysis of the great flu pandemic accounts for three waves of contagion, confusion still surrounds its origin. Some theorize the virus initially emerged in France during the war. A purulent bronchitis outbreak at the British army base in Etaples, France, in 1916 was typified by heliotrope cyanosis, a condition in which the patient would literally "turn [a shade of] blue from lack of oxygen."[37] This was later considered one of the hallmark symptoms of the Spanish flu. English virologist J. S. Oxford et al. described this army base as having the "requisite conditions for cross species transfer" between an on-base piggery and a nearby geese market.[38] In addition to the cross-species contamination, the British base was home to at least 100,000 soldiers in overcrowded barracks that already suffered from "compromised respiratory system[s] from gas attacks."[39] In March 1917, the same purulent bronchitis with heliotrope cyanosis was documented at the Aldershot barracks in England.[40]

The presence of the piggery and geese market at the base is significant. Influenza pandemics are the result of a change in the original strain of the flu virus, in what is denoted as an "antigenic shift." Because the influenza virus is small and contains eight separate strands that each contain a complete genetic unit, it allows for great reproductive potential as well as the ability for the individual strands to be altered in their human—or other animal—host. Indeed, the original records of the 1918 pandemic among soldiers at Camp Funston, the largest training camp for World War I, built on Fort Riley, bore a particularly strong resemblance to swine flu. The presence of pigs or fowl (avian flu) in an affected population area opened up the possibility for the virus to continue to shift as it spread from human to human and from human to animal to human.[41] Recognizing the possible connection, the officials at the British army based in Etaples decided to experiment with moving the piggeries from the immediate proximity of the base in this earlier flu epidemic.[42] Later phylogenetic analysis of evidence from the 1918 pandemic confirmed a connection between the pandemic—known to be an H1N1 virus—and swine strains, with an additional avian ancestor.[43]

The unique symptoms of the 1918 flu included the heliotrope cyanosis observed at Etaples two years prior, which produced what was termed the "cytokine storm."[44] The cytokine storm caused a buildup of pus and blood in the lungs, which would cause the patient to begin to drown internally; the resulting lack of oxygen turned the patient blue. In essence, "the 1918 virus turned the body's immune system against itself, making it most deadly for those with particularly robust internal defenses."[45] Those individuals with the most "robust" immune systems were those aged 20–40 years old, hence the characteristic mortality curve of the Spanish flu. Traditional mortality curves showed peaks at younger ages and peaks at older ages, forming a sort of U shape. With the 1918 pandemic, a peak also occurred at the ages 20–40. The result chart for mortality formed a "crude W with its highest point in the middle, where both science and common sense declare it should not be."[46]

Other factors that contributed to this unusual fatality pattern included the fact that a vast number of men in this age range were soldiers living in the harsh conditions of war. Similarly, those not at war were likely the breadwinners of the family and could not afford sick days or to avoid working with others who might already be infected.[47] In both cases, infected individuals continued to work among their peers in the initial contagious period, thus spreading the disease to others.

Most scholars studying the great influenza pandemic agree that it began in earnest in March 1918. Yet, evidence suggests that another explanation for the flu's origin might be possible. The aforementioned outbreaks at Etaples, France, and the Aldershot barracks in England may have been forerunners to the great pandemic, but evidence suggests the origination of these two outbreaks may have occurred in China.

Chinese laborers from Canton, brought to work behind the lines by the French and British during World War I, might have served as carriers who unwittingly transferred the pandemic to France and subsequently to England, Canada, and even the United States. Unfortunately, the virological data needed to support such a conclusion is not available at this time.[48] However, there is evidence of a correlation between the importations of Chinese laborers to Canada, Kansas, West Africa, and France with emerging mild influenza outbreaks. The laborers originated from a region in China that had experienced a flu epidemic during World War I.

No matter what the origin of the virus, the epidemic spread across the United States at a time when public attention was directed toward the war overseas. The mild first wave from March to May did not have as many recorded deaths, nor was it officially reported as influenza in many cases. Historians often cite two locations as the origin point for the Spanish influenza in America: Camp Funston, Kansas, and Camp Devens, Massachusetts.[49] By the time the second wave hit in August 1918, the whole world had been affected by the first wave of the pandemic. In America, public authorities began to belatedly inform the public, going so far as to put out notices in multiple languages to inform relatively new communities of migrants.[50] But few countries had done anything to raise awareness or limit the spread of infection.[51]

The initial outbreak in the United States in 1918 was recorded in Kansas. As suggested, the seriousness of the outbreak was not initially realized. In its annual meeting, the Kansas State Board of Health reported in June 1918 the increased number of reported cases of communicable diseases. Yet, the analysis of this increase was attributed "to the fact that the reports are year after year becoming more complete under the able direction of the chief of the division."[52] Another problem with assessing the impact of the first wave of illness at places like Camp Funston was the failure of people to report to sick call or to hospitals. Those soldiers who had family nearby often stayed with them during the initial outbreak or remained in their barracks due to the mild symptoms. Without a clear distinction between the various forms of respiratory illnesses and with no means of providing a definitive diagnosis of influenza in 1918, documenting the extent of the early mild form of the outbreak was nearly impossible.

Even the severe secondary wave had similar difficulties. One soldier from Camp Funston, Kansas, wrote his family about a fellow soldier who was home when he got sick with the influenza. The underlying perception of the writer was that the professed illness might have been a means of extending leave time.[53] Whether that perception was true or not, the reality was that the crowded conditions at the camp provided excellent conditions for the spread of influenza, likely encouraging people to flee for the presumed safety of their homes. Such actions more than likely helped to spread the influenza from the military camps to the neighboring civilian communities.

As the secondary wave of influenza spread around the globe from August through November, the number of casualties escalated precipitously. Military statistics published in November 1918 showed over 14,000 deaths of personnel in America alone attributed to influenza and related pneumonia from September 12 to October 18. In 1918, reports of an epidemic in a military camp came from Camp Devens, Massachusetts, on September 16 and appeared in the journal *Science*.[54] Sailors docked in Boston had been ill, and that infection initially spread primarily among soldiers. Not realizing the potential threat, military activities, including public recruiting events, continued unchecked. After several parades and rallies in support of the war efforts, the first civilian in Boston was hospitalized with a reported case of the flu.[55] The general American population still had little concern for influenza, which was considered to be a real threat to only the very young and very old. It was not until much later in the course of the pandemic that state health boards realized the unique morbidity and mortality traits of the second wave and declared the disease reportable. Consequently, accurate numbers of the contagion were not recorded until toward the end of the outbreak.[56]

Public and Military Responses to Emerging Influenza Outbreaks

When examining the impact of the influenza pandemic of 1918, the state of Pennsylvania is often used as an example. Through study of the Pennsylvania outbreak, a pattern becomes clear of the epidemic as it occurred among American citizenry and how public officials responded. Thanks to Pennsylvania, many states received some advance warning about the potential extent of the epidemic. With many cases of influenza seen in Massachusetts, and other reports emerging in Pennsylvania (over 600 soldiers and some civilian cases), officials in Pennsylvania should have been able to make some preparations for what eventually arose there. However, without official warnings, few precautions were undertaken.[57]

It was not until September 21, 1918, that health officials in Pennsylvania made influenza a reportable disease.[58] Despite the official acknowledgment of the pandemic and the danger of its diffusion, on September 28, a liberty bond parade was still held in Philadelphia to encourage the buying of bonds in support of the war effort. Wilmer Krusen, the director of the Philadelphia Department of Public Health and Charities, refused to cancel the festivities, disregarding the threat of influenza and the likely close contact of individuals while at the parade.[59] Not surprisingly, over the next three days, the number of infections and deaths began to climb.

On October 3, Krusen and the Department of Public Health closed "all places of public amusement and assembly." However, many places of business, including public eating facilities, were left open.[60] Hospitals soon became crowded, and temporary hospitals in tents and closed schools were required to provide the necessary capacity to care for the number of ailing individuals. A rudimentary telephone hotline, Filbert 100, was implemented to allow those who fell ill to stay home until visited by a police officer to determine whether the sickness was even influenza and how urgently a doctor was needed. The concept was intended to save room in the hospitals. This emergency hotline was one of the only numbers residents of Philadelphia were able to dial because of the shortage of "hello girls"[61] to direct the calls for nonemergencies. This restriction on telephone usage was necessary, as on October 7 alone, 850 employees of the Bell Telephone Company in Pennsylvania stayed home due to illness.[62]

Telephone operators were not the only personnel in short supply for the pandemic. Dr. Isaac Starr described his experience as a medical student in Philadelphia. His classes were canceled because of the pandemic; he and all third- and fourth-year students were sent to the hospitals to help the overworked staff of physicians. The rapid nature of the infection's progression and the quick decline in health of those who became ill was described firsthand in his memoir. He told how "25% per night" died "during the peak of the epidemic." The bodies were then removed unceremoniously into trucks simply to make room for more dying patients.[63]

Information advising the population on how to fight the flu was published for weeks to "minimize the epidemic."[64] Krusen, hoping to avoid panic, nonetheless continued to issue statements that the pandemic was under control. For each day in early October, he claimed that the peak of infection and deaths had been reached; yet, with the passing of each day, the numbers continued to increase.[65] The people of Philadelphia, like elsewhere, quickly became disillusioned with the propaganda. Despite the lack of accurate newspaper coverage, they were able to discern that the claims of declining influenza impacts made by officials were contrary to the obvious heightened contagion and deaths as the pandemic continued to run its course.[66]

The aim of the local and national government during this time of chaos was to "preserve morale."[67] Instead, contradictory messages caused the people to stop trusting the papers and the officials. The population "became isolated"[68] as many public gathering places were closed and individuals were too afraid to visit their neighbors. With the mandated limitation on public contact and interactions, and with a prohibition on nonemergency calls, the government managed to heighten the capacity for fear in Pennsylvanians more than the flu did on its own.

As outbreaks spread across cities and the nation, the number of available physicians and nurses fell quickly from an already less-than-adequate ratio to patients. Not only were many medical personnel already serving at stateside military facilities or overseas during World War I, but many had also succumbed to the disease. In Spokane, Washington, the nursing shortage was so dire that officials requested the return of nurses previously sent to Fort Wright (Spokane) and Camp Lewis (Tacoma).[69] Physicians were called out of retirement, and anyone able to lend a hand was asked to volunteer to ease the burden on the nurses and raise the morale of the sick.

Because of the virulence of the disease and the number of ill, dying, or dead in the communities, the morale of healthy individuals had dwindled at an alarming rate. Morticians were unable to bury individuals in a timely fashion due to the substantial number of people dying and the shortage of help to bury the dead. Contributing to this bottleneck of effective internment was a lack of coffins and the limited number of workers available due to illness or a fear of contact with the deceased. The resulting dilemma raised alarm and became interwoven in the minds of citizens with war events abroad.[70]

In the United Kingdom, extreme efforts were made to discover the true etiology of the disease as the second wave of the pandemic hit British military forces. The Royal Army Medical Corps (RAMC) used the military system in place, but it was soon compelled to enlist physicians and other scientists to assist with the medical needs of the military during the war. As the pandemic numbers of influenza rose, so too did the efforts utilized by the RAMC to understand the pathology and biology of the causative agent, in hopes that some prevention or treatment could be implemented. The officials decided that almost all efforts would be redirected for this purpose, beginning in August 1918. Walter Fletcher, the secretary of the Medical Research Council, published a sort of call to arms in the *British Medical Journal*, advising his colleagues to make preparations for a second pandemic as news of revived outbreaks among British troops in France spread.[71]

Analyzing the Impact of the Deadly Second Wave of the 1918 Pandemic

With the extensive use of trench warfare in dire conditions on the Western Front for World War I, it is not surprising that disease impacted the effectiveness of militaries on both sides of the conflict. The highly fatal second wave of the 1918 influenza pandemic that struck the Western Front during the last eight weeks of the war brings into question which "battle" of the war was truly the most deadly. It is estimated that as many as 100,000 soldier fatalities can be traced to influenza, with millions left ineffective for weeks due to the effects of the disease.[72]

Near the end of the conflict, an all-out war effort on the part of both the Allied and Central powers was complicated and made far more deadly by another battle within. The Meuse-Argonne offensive began on September 26, 1918, and continued for the next 47 days. One of the largest commitments of troops in the war, the offensive understandably resulted in high casualties. A large portion of those deaths had resulted from the influenza pandemic that coincided with the offensive, emerging on September 15 and raging beyond the war's end. When comparing the impact of the pandemic on the forces, the American military had the highest incidence of infected soldiers, with over 1 million contracting the illness. The Germans also had a high level of morbidity, with approximately 700,000 cases. The English forces in France experienced only 313,000 reported cases.[73] Between these four combatant nations, approximately 200,000 cases of influenza were reported amid one of the last great offenses of the war.

The pandemic's second wave appears to have landed in Europe in July at the port of Brest, France, with the disembarkation of U.S. soldiers from Camp Pike, Arkansas. Reported cases of this virulent outbreak spiked in August and then spread outward with the movement of forces from the port city.[74] Influenza wormed its way into the ranks of the Argonne offensive, rendering noneffective large numbers of soldiers on both sides. The impact on this offensive, the largest for the Americans during World War I, was tremendous. Almost 70,000 soldiers were hospitalized in the First Army, with individual hospitals admitting over 1,000 cases a day. Three weeks into the conflict, mortality caused by a secondary infection of pneumonia increased to 45.3 percent of those suffering from influenza. By late October, the medical system was extremely overloaded, with 20,000 patients over the estimated capacity.

The impact of the disease combined with injuries from the offensive and caused a shift in the protocol for medical treatments. Medical personnel on the front lines were charged with screening injured and ill soldiers to determine those able to return to fighting within three days. Those more severely wounded or seriously ill were transported back to evacuation or base hospitals. As the reported cases stemmed from the numbers at the base hospitals, it is likely the total number of soldiers affected by the influenza exceeded those in the official records. German general Erich von Ludendorff reported that, "The enemy did not come on with his usual ardor. . . . At these points the fighting power of the Entente has not been up to its previous level. Further the Americans are suffering severely from influenza."[75] It is difficult to determine the full impact on the various forces, as censorship was employed to prevent knowledge of the pandemic from reaching and influencing military decisions of opposing forces. As the war came to an end on Armistice Day, November 11, 1918, the influenza pandemic was in decline but not gone. Soldiers continued to report for sick call, adding to the number of casualties from the disease, if not from the war.

Lasting Impacts of the 1918 Influenza Pandemic and World War I

The challenges faced by civilian and military officials during the pandemic included discrepancies in "proven" etiologies. While some physicians searched for Pfeiffer's bacillus in victims, others had already determined that influenza was caused by a filterable virus and could not be detected. Still others found some other common bacterium in the cases they observed. By November, when the War Office requested a vaccine for mass distribution among the troops, there was no agreement on what a vaccine should inoculate against. Aggregate vaccines were created that combined a variety of bacteria, predominantly Pfeiffer's bacillus, but also differing amounts of other isolated bacteria.[76] These vaccines were only successful in occasionally preventing secondary infections, which often prevented death, but not the initial influenza infection.[77]

One of the most significant reminders of the 1918 pandemic included the advancements made in medicine in understanding, finding, and treating this and other viral diseases. Even today, scientists attempt to discover what exactly composed this peculiarly virulent strain of influenza in 1918.[78] The pandemic fostered emerging efforts focused on the prevention of a future outbreak. The incidence of influenza on pandemic levels during World War I meant that during World War II the military recruited physicians at levels intended to prevent such an incident from occurring again. By 1939, there was still not a guaranteed vaccine against influenza, though two of the virus types had been isolated and researched.

In America, the Army Medical Corps conducted work on a promising flu vaccine under the supervision of Thomas Francis Jr. and Jonas Salk.[79] The continued advancements in technology and science blended into improvements in medicine and the application thereof. More preventative measures were made through vaccinations, immunity, and simply a much-improved quality of life for all people in the developed nations. Additionally, treatment options improved for those contracting influenza. There were more physicians per each individual and more opportunities to recognize diseases as soon as an infection took place. Another outcome of the deadly pandemic was the emergence of more abundant and efficient treatments to overcome the infectious agents, such as antiviral drugs. While the public memory of the pandemic faded or became convoluted with more prevalent memories of the war, scientists never stopped working to prevent a recurrence.[80]

Epidemiologists have studied this pandemic to more fully understand epidemics in general and how to prevent another influenza pandemic of this magnitude. More recently, historians have researched the pandemic to determine whether the pandemic directly affected the outcome of World War I. Some claimed that the German troops were slowed in their advance because of the flu, leading to their eventual loss. Another report revealed that President Wilson succumbed to the disease while in the Paris Peace talks, possibly contributing to his inability to enact his Fourteen Points plan, whether as a symptom of encephalitis lethargica or from the general malaise that often followed recovery from this version of influenza. Contemporary sources have noted a distinct change in his personality after his bout with flu, and his acceptance of the terms of the treaty that countered his original intentions was quite out of character.[81]

Though much of what happened in 1918 is not quantified, enough personal accounts exist to provide a fairly clear depiction of what life was like during the pandemic. Poor record keeping prevented reliable final counts of those infected and who died. The potential secondary infections that affected people years after the initial infection further complicated a thorough accounting of the pandemic's overall impact. Nevertheless, it is safe to assert that over 50 million people were affected by the influenza pandemic of 1918–1920. We may never know definitively the clinical identity of the second wave of the pandemic, including whether it was the same infection as the precursor outbreak in Etables, France, in 1916 or the first and third wave of the 1918–1919 pandemic. Also still unknown is the reason for its peculiar virulence and why in each wave the population age group that traditionally was least affected by influenza became the most likely to die. Definitive answers may soon be available, as research into the second wave of the pandemic is rapidly spreading and new theories emerging. What is sure is that the "Spanish flu" spread rapidly and fatally, and while the conditions of World War I helped to fuel this rapidity, the organization of physicians and scientists in the war effort ensured that much was done to try to understand the disease and how future influenza pandemics could be prevented.

NOTES

1. Pvt. Josh Lee, "The Flu" (1919), in Peter C. Wever and Leo van Bergen, "Death from 1918 Pandemic Influenza during the First Word War: A Perspective from Personal and Anecdotal Evidence," *Influenza and Other Respiratory Viruses* 8, no. 5 (September 2014): 538.

2. Ann H. Reid, Jeffery K. Taubenberger, and Thomas G. Fanning, "The 1918 Spanish Influenza: Integrating History and Biology," *Microbes and Infection* 3 (2001): 81.

3. Jeffery K. Taubenberger, Johan V. Hultin, and David M. Morens, "Discovery and Characterization of the 1918 Pandemic Influenza Virus in Historical Context," *Antiviral Therapy* 12, no. 4, Pt. B (2007): 581–591.

4. Mark L. Metersky et al., "Epidemiology, Microbiology, and Treatment Considerations for Bacterial Pneumonia Complicating Influenza," *International Journal of Infectious Diseases* 16, no. 5 (May 2012): e321–e331.

5. Centers for Disease Control and Prevention, "How the Flu Virus Can Change: 'Drift' and 'Shift,'" accessed September 2, 2017, https://www.cdc.gov/flu/about/viruses/change.htm.

6. Centers for Disease Control and Prevention, "Types of Influenza Viruses," accessed September 2, 2017, https://www.cdc.gov/flu/about/viruses/types.htm.

7. N. P. Johnson and J. Mueller, "Updating the Accounts," *Bulletin of the History of Medicine* 76, no. 1 (Spring 2002): 105; Jeffrey Anderson, "When We Have a Few More Epidemics the City Officials Will Awake: Philadelphia and the Influenza Epidemic of 1918–1919," *Maryland Historian* 27, no. 1-2 (1996): 1–26; and Alfred W. Crosby, *America's Forgotten Pandemic: The Influenza of 1918* (Cambridge, UK: Cambridge University Press, 2003), 11.

8. Crosby, *America's Forgotten Pandemic*, 86.

9. George A. Soper, "The Influenza Pneumonia Pandemic in the American Army Camps during September and October, 1918," *Science* 48, no. 1245 (November 1918): 451–456.

10. John M. Barry, *The Great Influenza: The Story of the Deadliest Pandemic in History* (New York: Penguin Books, 2004), 396–397; Jeffery K. Taubenberger and David M. Morens, "1918 Influenza: The Mother of All Pandemics," *History* 12, no. 1 (January 2006), accessed September 2, 2017, https://wwwnc.cdc.gov/eid/article/12/1/05-0979_article.

11. Howard Phillips, "The Recent Wave of 'Spanish' Flu Historiography," *Social History of Medicine* 27, no. 4 (2014): 798.

12. "Influenza—Prevalence in the United States," *Public Health Reports* 35, no. 6 (February 6, 1920): 269–275.
13. Caroline Hovanec, "The 1918 Influenza Pandemic in Literature and Memory" (master's thesis, Vanderbilt University, 2009), 1–2.
14. Crosby, *America's Forgotten Pandemic*, 311–328.
15. Crosby, *America's Forgotten Pandemic*.
16. Crosby, *America's Forgotten Pandemic*, 323.
17. Francis Russell, "Journal of the Plague: The 1918 Influenza," *Yale Review* 47 (1957): 223–224.
18. Crosby, *America's Forgotten Pandemic*, 315.
19. Crosby, *America's Forgotten Pandemic*.
20. Katherine Anne Porter, *Pale Horse, Pale Rider* (Orlando, FL: Harcourt Brace & Company, 1939); and Crosby, *America's Forgotten Pandemic*, 317–319, 323.
21. Phillips, "The Recent Wave," 789.
22. Phillips, "The Recent Wave," 790.
23. Matthew Heaton and Toyin Falola, "Global Explanations versus Local Interpretations: The Historiography of the Influenza Pandemic of 1918–19 in Africa," *History of Africa* 33 (2006): 209.
24. J. S. Oxford et al., "A Hypothesis: The Conjunction of Soldiers, Gas, Pigs, Ducks, Geese and Horses in Northern France during the Great War Provided the Conditions for the Emergence of the 'Spanish' Influenza Pandemic of 1918–1919," *Vaccine* 23 (2005): 941.
25. J. S. Oxford et al., "World War I May Have Allowed the Emergence of 'Spanish' Influenza," *The Lancet: Infectious Diseases* 2 (2002): 113; Oxford et al., "A Hypothesis," 942.
26. Phillips, "The Recent Wave," 803; and Jeffery K. Taubenberger, Ann H. Reid, Thomas A. Janczewski, and Thomas G. Fanning, "Integrating Historical, Clinical and Molecular Genetic Data in Order to Explain the Origin and Virulence of the 1918 Spanish Influenza Virus," *Philosophical Transactions: Biological Sciences* (2001): 1830.
27. Phillips, "The Recent Wave," 802.
28. Fred R. van Hartesveldt, "The Doctors and the 'Flu': The British Medical Profession's Response to the Influenza Pandemic of 1918–19," *International Social Science Review* 85, no. 1-2 (2010): 32.
29. Alain Gagnon et al., "Age-Specific Mortality during the 1918 Influenza Pandemic: Unraveling the Mystery of High Young Adult Mortality," *PLoS One* (2013): 2.
30. "The Epidemic of Influenza in England," *Science, New Series* 52, no. 1336 (1920): 124.
31. Mark Osborne Humphries, "Paths of Infection: The First World War and the Origins of the 1918 Influenza Pandemic," *War in History* 21, no. 1 (January 8, 2014): 56.
32. Humphries, "Paths of Infection."
33. Humphries, "Paths of Infection."
34. Phillips, "The Recent Wave," 801–802.
35. Phillips, "The Recent Wave," 803.
36. Cynthia Schuck-Paim, G. Dennis Shanks, Francisco E. A. Almeida, and Wladimir J. Alonso, "Exceptionally High Mortality Rate of the 1918 Influenza Pandemic in the Brazilian Naval Fleet," *Influenza and Other Respiratory Viruses* 7, no. 1 (2013): 31.
37. Humphries, "Paths of Infection," 57, 59–60.
38. Oxford et al., "A Hypothesis," 942.
39. Oxford et al., "A Hypothesis."
40. Humphries, "Paths of Infection," 59–60.

41. Geoffrey W. Rice and Edwina Palmer, "Pandemic Influenza in Japan, 1918–19: Mortality Patterns and Official Responses," *Journal of Japanese Studies* 19, no. 2 (Summer 1993): 392, accessed September 2, 2017, http://www.jstor.org/stable/132645.

42. Oxford et al., "A Hypothesis," 944.

43. Jeffery K. Taunbenber et al., "Initial Genetic Characterization of the 1918 'Spanish' Influenza Virus," *Science, New Series* 275, no. 5307 (March 21, 1997): 1795, accessed September 2, 2017, http://www.jstor.org/stable/2892709.

44. Milorad Radusin, "The Spanish Flu—Part II: The Second and Third Wave," *History of Medicine* 69, no. 10 (2012): 919.

45. Humphries, "Paths of Infection," 59.

46. Crosby, *America's Forgotten Pandemic*, 21; and Oxford et al., "The 1918 Spanish Influenza," 83.

47. Phillips, "The Recent Wave," 797.

48. Christopher Langford, "Did the 1918–19 Influenza Pandemic Originate in China?," *Population and Development Review* 31, no. 3 (September 2005): 474–475.

49. Barry, *The Great Influenza*, 95–7, 184–191; Crosby, *America's Forgotten Pandemic*, 4, 10, 19.

50. Julian A. Navarro, "Influenza in 1918: An Epidemic in Images," *Public Health Reports* 135, Supplement 3: The 1918–1919 Influenza Pandemic in the United States (April 2010): 13, accessed September 2, 2017, http://www.jstor.org/stable/41435295.

51. Michael Bresalier, "Fighting Flu: Military Pathology, Vaccines, and the Conflicted Identity of the 1918–19 Pandemic in Britain," *Journal of the History of Medicine and Allied Science* 68, no. 1 (2013): 15–28.

52. Kansas State Board of Health, "Ninth Biennial Report Being the Thirty-Third and Thirty-Fourth Annual Reports of the State Board of Health of the State of Kansas, June 30, 1916, to June 30, 1918," *Influenza Encyclopedia: The American Influenza Epidemic of 1918–1919, a Digital Encyclopedia*, University of Michigan Center for the History of Medicine and Michigan Publishing, accessed September 2, 2017, http://quod.lib.umich.edu/f/flu/7740flu.0013.477/17/--ninth-biennial-report-being-the-thirty-third-and-thirty?page=root;rgn=full+text;size=150;view=image;q1=Fort+Riley.

53. Carol R. Byerly, "The U.S. Military and the Influenza Pandemic of 1918–1919," *Public Health Reports (1974–)* 125, Supplement 3, "The 1918–1919 Influenza Pandemic in the United States" (April 2010): 90, accessed September 2, 2017, http://www.jstor.org/stable/41435302.

54. Soper, 451–452.

55. Crosby, *America's Forgotten Pandemic*, 40.

56. *Public Health Reports (1896–1970)* 33 (1918).

57. Crosby, *America's Forgotten Pandemic*, 73–75.

58. Crosby, *America's Forgotten Pandemic*.

59. Barry, *The Great Influenza*, 205.

60. Anderson, "When We Have a Few More Epidemics," 11.

61. A. A. Hoehling, *The Great Epidemic* (Boston: Little Brown and Company, 1961). 71.

62. Barry, *The Great Influenza*, 325; Crosby, *America's Forgotten Pandemic*, 75; Hoehling, *The Great Epidemic*.

63. Isaac Starr, "Influenza in 1918: Recollections of the Epidemic in Philadelphia," *Annals of Internal Medicine* 145, no. 2 (July 2006): 138–140.

64. Barry, *The Great Influenza*, 221.

65. Crosby, *America's Forgotten Pandemic*, 71, 75, 84–85.

66. Crosby, *America's Forgotten Pandemic*.
67. Barry, *The Great Influenza*, 331.
68. Barry, *The Great Influenza*, 331, 225.
69. "Spokane, Washington," *Influenza Encyclopedia: The American Influenza Epidemic of 1918–1919, a Digital Encyclopedia*, University of Michigan Center for the History of Medicine and Michigan Publishing, accessed September 2, 2017, http://www.influenza archive.org/cities/city-spokane.html#.
70. Barry, *The Great Influenza*, 327–328; Crosby, *America's Forgotten Pandemic*, 82–83; and Hoehling, *The Great Epidemic*, 71–75.
71. Bresalier, "Fighting Influenza in Britain," 111.
72. Wever and Bergen, "Death from 1918 Pandemic Influenza," 538.
73. Wever and Bergen, "Death from 1918 Pandemic Influenza."
74. Barry, *The Great Influenza*, 182.
75. Jonathan H. Jaffin, "Medical Support for the American Expeditionary Forces in France during the First Word War" (master's thesis, U.S. Army Command and General Staff College, 1991), 163, 176, 155–156.
76. Bresalier, "Fighting Influenza in Britain," 114.
77. Bresalier, "Fighting Influenza in Britain," 121.
78. Reid, Taubenberger, and Fanning, "The 1918 Spanish Influenza," 81–86.
79. Thomas Francis and Jonas Salk, "A Simplified Procedure for the Concentration and Purification of Influenza Virus," *Science, New Series* 96, no. 2500 (1942): 499–500; and Thomas Francis, Jonas Salk, Harold Pearson, and Philip Brown, "Protective Effect of Vaccination against Induced Influenza A," *Journal of Clinical Investigation* 24, no. 4 (1945): 536–546.
80. Barry, *The Great Influenza*, 457–459; Crosby, *America's Forgotten Pandemic*, 264–290.
81. Crosby, *America's Forgotten Pandemic*, 189–196; Radusin, "The Spanish Flu," 926.

Chapter 14

Colonialism and War as Drivers of HIV/AIDS in Sub-Saharan Africa, 1990–2003

Wesley Renfro

Although the history of wars and conflicts is replete with massive and systematic sexual violence against vulnerable women, modern-day wars in African nations and elsewhere are increasingly characterized by the use of rape as a weapon of war, the intentional or willful transmission of the HIV to innocent victims, and the neglect of these victims in post-conflict reconstruction programmes.[1]

—Obijiofor Aginam

HIV/AIDS is a global pandemic that currently infects nearly 40 million people. The human immunodeficiency virus (HIV) is a disease that attacks the immune system in humans. The acquired immune deficiency syndrome (AIDS) refers to a cluster of symptoms, as well as illnesses, that typically occur in the end stages of an HIV-infected person's life. Since the 'pandemic surfaced in the early 1980s, HIV/AIDS has killed or been associated with the deaths of roughly 30 million people, mostly in Sub-Saharan Africa. While HIV/AIDs deaths have steadily declined since a peak in 2005, the pandemic still claimed 1 million lives in 2015.[2] Medical personnel and even the general public in developed regions are familiar with the basic biological mechanisms that account for HIV/AIDS transmission, that is, contact with blood, semen, or other bodily fluids. Despite this, many are unaware of the role that social and political forces played in helping facilitate the pandemic. In particular, there has been a comparative lack of public and scholarly attention on the special roles that colonialism and warfare played in bringing the disease into the human population and causing it to become such a scourge in Africa.

In the United States and most of the rest of the developed world, men having sex with men (MSM) were the common perceived vectors for transmitting the HIV infection.[3] As a result, the public tended to conceive of HIV/AIDS as a gay health care issue. This perception extended into the realm of public health. Unfortunately, this focus tended to obscure the fact that globally the most common method of transferring HIV/AIDS was heterosexual sex. Indeed, the story of HIV/AIDS in the developing world is one of the most important but least understood social, political, and medical processes of the past century. This chapter attempts to partially fill this gap by exploring the ways in which social and political factors, especially colonialism and war, influenced the progression of HIV/AIDS in Sub-Saharan Africa.

Colonialism Context for Wars and HIV Virus

Colonialism, which is often coterminous with war, contributed to the making of the HIV/AIDS pandemic in multiple ways. Examples included the disruption of traditional economies, which increased reliance on bushmeat; the practice of offering political, social, and economic incentives that produced a population shift from rural to urban areas; the common practice of European men frequenting sex workers in colonial holdings (those colonies with negligible populations of European women); and the perpetuation of dubious medical practices among subjugated peoples. Wars in the Sub-African region further exacerbated these trends through the disruption of populations, the instigation of migrations, and the normalization and even encouragement of rape as a weapon of war. Additionally, wars often increased reliance on sex workers among fighters and undermined the state's capacity to provide public information and public health measures intended to help mitigate the epidemic once it was identified.

Identification of HIV/AIDS required a major shift of the disease from its source of origin. Beginning in late 1980, physicians in several American cities began to notice unusual rises in several diseases, including *Pneumocystis carinii* pneumonia (PCP) and Kaposi's sarcoma, among populations of otherwise healthy men.[4] This was odd given that these diseases typically struck older and less healthy individuals. Kaposi sarcoma was especially vexing, as it most often afflicted people who lived in areas surrounding or adjacent to the Mediterranean Sea. These initial reports caused alarm and gained the attention of some government health researchers. On June 5, 1981, the Centers for Disease Control (CDC) published its *Morbidity and Mortality Weekly Report* that contained the first report of what is now called HIV/AIDS.[5]

Although HIV/AIDS is an indiscriminate killer, it first emerged as a public health crisis in the MSM population and continued to be disproportionally common among MSM, trans populations, sex workers, intravenous drug users, and, in the earliest years of the crises, hemophiliacs. Indeed, nearly four decades after the CDC's first reports on the "new" disease, the MSM population still accounted for a clear majority of new infections in the United States despite only constituting around 3 percent of the overall population.[6] This stands in stark contrast in Sub-Saharan Africa, where heterosexual sex is the primary method of transmission. This chapter is useful for several reasons, including drawing attention to the causes and consequences of an HIV/AIDS crisis that is primarily heterosexual in its origins.[7]

Identifying and Understanding the HIV Virus

HIV, specifically HIV-1 Group M, is responsible for the AIDS pandemic. HIV is a zoonotic disease (transferred at one point from animals to humans) that attacks the immune system. Untreated, HIV weakens the immune system so that it is unable to fend off illness, and the infected person dies of opportunistic diseases. Immediately after infection, the body attempts to fight the infection by developing antibodies. The initial phase, known as *seroconversion*, usually produces a mild sickness similar to influenza, though some do not display symptoms. Most HIV-positive individuals seroconvert within a month of infection, though it can take up to six months. After this flu-like illness, HIV-positive individuals enter a period of asymptomatic infection in which they have no outward signs of infection, but HIV is slowly eroding the body's immune system. The asymptomatic period is crucial to understanding the HIV/AIDS epidemic because the asymptotic phase may last up to a decade. In other words, HIV-positive individuals may feel perfectly healthy for a very long time. Although they appear to be healthy, they are capable of transmitting the disease. Eventually, the degradation of the immune system does produce symptoms. Once this occurs, the infected individuals enter the symptomatic infection stage. A range of acute illness marks this period as individuals begin to suffer from opportunistic ailments such as pneumocystis pneumonia (PCP). The final stage of the sickness is alternately called advanced HIV disease or AIDS. In a clinical sense, AIDS occurs when an HIV-positive person's CD4 (immune system) cells are less than 200 cells per cubic millimeter of blood.[8]

The AIDS pandemic is of comparatively recent vintage, but the history of humans and HIV is considerably longer. The literature on HIV conclusively demonstrates that HIV is a zoonotic disease, indicating a disease that jumped the species barrier. Put simply, simian immunodeficiency virus (SIV) was transmitted from a nonhuman primate to a human and produced HIV in the human host. Although it is impossible to know the exact mechanism that caused the zoonotic incident that produced HIV in humans, many scholars subscribe to the natural transfer hypothesis that suggests that a hunter became infected while butchering a primate for bushmeat.[9] Consuming primates for food is not common, but it is not unusual during periods when food production is limited.[10] Zoonosis is common and includes well-known diseases, including anthrax, avian influenza, salmonella, hantavirus, Lyme disease, Marburg virus, Ebola, and toxoplasmosis. Untreated, HV/AIDS produces 100 percent lethality, though it is somewhat difficult to transmit, as it requires contact with blood, semen, preseminal fluid, rectal fluid, vaginal fluid, or breast milk. The difficulty of transmission effectively rules out casual routes of infection between primates and humans, and thus supports the hunter-cutter hypothesis.

It is important to note that while many conceive of HIV as a singular virus, in reality, there are many different kinds of HIV. HIV is divided into two types. HIV-1 is responsible for the global pandemic. HIV-2 is similar to HIV-1 in most respects, but it is less virulent and more difficult to transmit. It is most common in West Africa and is only rarely found outside of the region. France and Portugal, however, sometimes see cases, mostly because of their colonial involvement in West Africa. Portugal, in particular, has dealt with cases of HV-2, as a number of Portuguese soldiers fighting in colonial wars acquired the disease.[11] Both HIV-1 and HIV-2 are further subdivided into groups. There is a near consensus that HIV-1 Group M "spilled over" from chimpanzees or western lowland gorillas in modern-day Cameroon at the close of the 19th century or beginning part of the 20th century. Some research suggests that the zoonotic episode occurred in 1908, though this dating is not universally accepted.[12] Most research suggests that HIV-2 broke the species barrier in the same fashion and came from sooty mangabeys or Old World monkeys.

SIV has been present in primate populations for thousands of years. During that long period, it is likely that there were multiple spillovers in which humans butchering bushmeat became infected. One fascinating question is why HIV took hold and spread during the 20th century but not in earlier periods. After all, if butchering bushmeat produced HIV infection in humans circa 1908, and this turned into a massive pandemic, it is logical to wonder why hunters butchering bushmeat in 1650 or 1770 or some other year failed to cause a pandemic. Indeed, the empirical record suggests that there were many previous spillovers, but only the most recent caused a pandemic.[13] Colonial practices and warfare during the 19th and 20th centuries account for the comparatively easy process of HIV taking root in human populations, which in turn caused the current global pandemic.[14] Warfare, especially the series of interconnected wars that played out in Central Africa during the 1990s, greatly amplified the scale of the pandemic in that region.

In the vernacular of epidemiology, colonialism helped increase the reproductive ratio of HIV so that it exceeded 1, ensuring that the disease would not hit a dead end and die out in humans. The basic reproductive ratio is also called the *r naught* (R_0) and refers to the number of new cases caused by a single case. If a disease has an R_0 of less than 1, the disease will eventually disappear. Higher R_0 means that an infection is spreading more quickly and more widely than infections with a lower R_0. Compared with other kinds of infections, HIV is somewhat more difficult to acquire because it requires intimate contact and not every sexual act with an HIV-positive person will cause a new case.

It is entirely possible that, in the past, many people became HIV positive via zoonosis, but because the R_0 remained less than 1, the virus failed to find a sustainable foothold in humans. In other words, although HIV would have spilled over from primates into the human population, the virus quickly died out. For example, a hunter who butchered bushmeat could have become infected with HIV, but if no one else was infected because he lacked a sexual partner, or he did infect his partner but both died before producing any new cases, the virus died with them. There are many variants of this dead-end scenario, especially in times and spaces characterized by low population density. Given that SIV has been present in primates for thousands of years and humans butchered bushmeat during this period, it is likely that HIV was introduced to humans many times, but the social conditions were not correct for these spillovers to produce a pandemic.

Colonial practices changed the social conditions and unwittingly encouraged a higher R_0 for HIV.[15] Although multiple reinforcing colonial practices helped raise the R_0, research suggests that the most important practices involved raising the population density. Africa has always had urban centers, but European colonialism dramatically increased the number of cities in Africa as outside powers created new infrastructures to help them obtain and administer their newfound possessions. Existing cities became more populous during the colonial era.

This urbanization affected the spread of HIV in several critically important ways. First, the new urban areas were considerably wealthier than the surrounding rural areas. They naturally became a lure for rural peoples seeking commerce; specialized services, such as medicine, that were limited to urban areas; and other services. Some, though not all, then returned to their villages. Others permanently settled in these urban centers. Gender imbalances were pervasive, and most cities had many more men than women. Most of the Africans coming to the cities for commerce or for other purposes were male, working as traders. Many European powers sent considerable numbers of men to African colonies, but they were generally reluctant to send European women to these same colonial areas.[16]

Given this gender imbalance, it is not surprising that prostitution and the sex trade flourished in colonial cities. For Europeans, the most common type of sex work involved an arrangement whereby an African woman helped provide domestic and sexual services. Unlike street prostitution, in which sex workers typically had many sexual encounters in a short period of time, the combination of domestic and sexual work meant that women were able to have sexual encounters with fewer men.[17] This helped raise the R_0 of HIV in colonial Africa but was somewhat limited because the women, while not monogamous, typically had just a few sexual partners. In short, colonialism produced a rise in population density, and the imbalanced ratio of women to men encouraged the rise in sex work. This combination helped ensure that HIV did not hit a dead end in this instance.

Factors Common to Diffusion of HIV

Other colonial practices also helped HIV spread. Some scholars argue that the presence of Europeans also caused a spike in bushmeat consumption, which may have produced more incidents of spillover. Colonialism also produced many military encounters. Many conflicts were small and not properly considered wars, as most scholars of war adhere to a definition that entails at least 1,000 battlefield deaths per year, but the "Scramble for Africa" had produced a general militarization of the continent. The literature clearly demonstrates that wars, great and small, are amplifiers of disease, including HIV/AIDS, as they often include increases in the sex trade and rape.[18]

There is rich extant literature that suggests that colonialism, including the wars associated with European colonialism in Africa, helped raise the R_0 to greater than 1, thus ensuring that HIV stayed in the human population.[19] It is possible, and perhaps even likely, that absent these colonial conditions, the R_0 would have remained too low to permanently lodge HIV in humans. However, although colonialism may have created the conditions that allowed HIV to survive in humans, later wars in Africa greatly expanded the severity of the epidemic and help to explain why Africa is the epicenter of the pandemic today.

Before the developed world's discovery of HIV/AIDS in the early 1980s, HIV was slowly circulating through the population in Africa (and elsewhere). The long asymptomatic period in most HIV infections meant that there was a considerable period during which many new infections occurred but there was no accompanying public health crisis. Moreover, because HIV opened the door for many opportunistic infections, it was difficult to diagnose HIV. It was not uncommon for seemingly healthy people to die from tropical diseases and infections, and the capacity of most African nations to spot diseases and mount effective public health bureaus was extremely limited in most places. The first part of this story was not unique to Africa, as HIV spread unrecognized around the globe.

Historical Analysis of the Spread of HIV

Since the 1980s, HIV/AIDS has emerged as a major global epidemic and one of the most vexing public health challenges in the modern era. Nonetheless, the distribution of HIV/AIDs cases remains very uneven. By the late 1990s, Sub-Saharan Africa surged past other regions in the globe in terms of new HIV infections and deaths. There were multiple overlapping reasons for the emergence of Sub-Saharan Africa as the epicenter of the pandemic. These include the limited state capacity to fund public health and education campaigns, cultural practices and mores that made education campaigns on sexual and reproductive health more challenging, and the cost and availability of condoms and medicines to fight HIV/AIDs, among other factors.[20] The series of wars in Sub-Saharan Africa during the 1990s and early 2000s also exacerbated the pandemic in the region.

Although the topic has received some attention in research on HIV/AIDs and epidemics, and in the literature available on war and conflict, it is important to note that these literatures have not often "spoken" to one another. Gaps in knowledge and the lack of interdisciplinary collaboration between scholars of war and scholars of health should not surprise anyone. This gap is beginning to shrink with the growing recognition that public health and war are inherently connected. In recent years, scholarship on war and conflict shifted away from a strict focus on politics and states to a more inclusive approach that acknowledges the need to study the intersection of war with other causal forces, including disease and public health.[21] The rise of this "human security" paradigm has revitalized the study of conflict in many respects. The effort is not yet fully developed, and many findings are tentative, especially in the study of complex multicausal events. Although key debates on this topic remain, it can be demonstrated that an understanding of HIV/AIDS as it played out in Sub-Saharan Africa cannot be achieved without accounting for the causal role of war and conflict.

As Buve, Bishikwabo-Nsarhaza, and Mutangadura note in their discussion of the socioeconomic and cultural contexts of the HIV/AIDS pandemic in Sub-Saharan Africa, "no less than 28 of 53 African states have been at war" since 1980.[22] Stefan Elbe similarly concluded that, "Armed conflicts are increasingly occurring in environments of widespread HIV/AIDS prevalence."[23] Because HIV/AIDS and war are both complex and multicausal, they are difficult topics to study. Nonetheless, scholars increasingly investigated the possible connections between the two, and there was a near consensus in the literature that these two concepts were closely related. There are now a number of hypothesized causal connections linking the high levels of war in Sub-Saharan Africa and the prevalence of the pandemic. These mechanisms include soldiers having multiple sexual partners during conflicts; the rise of rape as a weapon of war; changes in migratory patterns (i.e., refugees); and the degradation of states and nonstate actors capable of effectively mounting public health campaigns that could otherwise arrest the spread of HIV.

Origins of Three Related Sub-Saharan African Conflicts

A full investigation of all the wars in Sub-Saharan Africa between the discovery of HIV/AIDS in the 1980s and the peak of the pandemic in 2005 is beyond the scope of this chapter. Instead, this work provides an overview of three related conflicts between 1990 and 2008: the Rwandan Civil War (inclusive of the infamous Rwandan genocide in 1994), from 1990 to 1994; the First Congo War, from 1996 to 1997; and the Second Congo War, from 1998 to 2003. Although often presented separately, many scholars consider these wars to be closely related, and some lump them together as part of the same massive war.

The Rwandan Civil War was fought between the Hutu and Tutsi ethnic groups between 1990 and 1994, though there was a longer history of tension in the country. In precolonial times, the Tutsi state pursued anti-Hutu policies. During the colonial era, the Germans and Belgians continued to favor the Tutsi at the expense of the Hutu. The Hutu revolted in 1959, and during the next four years, there were periodic bouts of violence between the two groups. After decades of simmering tensions and occasional violence, a civil war began in 1990. The war quickly stalemated and produced an uneasy peace agreement in the form of the 1993 Arusha Accords.

Before the accords were implemented, someone shot down the plane containing Rwanda's dictatorial president, Juvenal Habyarimana, and the Burundian president, Cyprien Ntarymira, in April 1994. Although no one knows for sure who ordered the attack, several credible reports suggest that parts of the Hutu military establishment orchestrated the attack. Regardless of who had planned the attack, the assassination presaged the better-known Rwanda genocide of 1994, in which the Hutu killed at least 800,000 Tutsi in a 100-day orgy of mass killing.[24] This death toll is even more staggering when one considers that the total number of deaths in the civil war before the genocide did not exceed 10,000.

The Rwandan genocide is well-known because of the pace of the killing and the general failure of the international community to do anything to curb or stop the violence—despite ample evidence that their actions could have prevented or minimized the mass murders. In many accounts, however, the genocide is treated as a singular event, divorced from the civil war that had preceded it and the Congo Wars that followed it. More recent analysis suggests that connecting the genocide and civil war provides clarity on a number of issues, including the spread of HIV/AIDS in the region.

Although wartime sexual violence is not uncommon in conflict zones, the use of rape as a tool of war during the Rwandan genocide was noteworthy. Members of the Rwandan military and other irregular forces raped at least 500,000 women during the genocide. Some Hutu women were targeted, but the vast majority of women raped were Tutsi. The rapes were often carefully orchestrated and intended to further demoralize and damage the Tutsi population and their remaining Hutu allies. There are reports that HIV-positive soldiers and militia members deliberately sought to infect women with HIV. This represents one of the first, and most significant, attempts to weaponize the HIV virus in a bid to achieve war-related aims. Françoise Nduwimana, when testifying about a Rwandan rape survivor, reported that the victim said,

> For 60 days, my body was used as a thoroughfare for all the hoodlums, militia men and soldiers in the district. . . . Those men completely destroyed me so much pain. They raped me in front of my six children. . . . Three years ago, I discovered that I had HIV/AIDS. There is no doubt in my mind that I was infected during these rapes.[25]

This story is commonplace among female survivors. Donovan commented about the intentional infection of victims: "Among the weapons of choice calculated to destroy while inflicting maximum pain and suffering was HIV."[26] Verwimp concluded that men were encouraged and rewarded for such behavior.[27] One problem that continued to vex researchers about this conflict was the difficulty of systematically demonstrating the number of new cases of HIV infection that resulted from the mass raping of women during the genocide. Given the long asymptomatic period, the general scarcity of public health infrastructure, and the stigma associated with being a rape victim, it was impossible to know with certainly how many of the documented infections in Rwanda were caused by wartime rape. Verwimp critiqued the ways in which scholars and others collected data: "Another deficiency of the data collection is the absence of rape as a weapon used in the genocide. When a woman died of AIDS after 1994 and the disease was contracted because of rape in 1994, the woman is not registered as a casualty in the data."[28] Despite these limitations in accountability, there was a sharp spike in reported HIV infections following the conclusion of the genocide. This is not surprising, given that some estimates placed the number of woman and girls raped as high as 500,000.[29]

The Rwandan Civil War also produced many refugees, with most ending up in camps close to the borders in neighboring countries. Some of the literature on refugee camps suggests that they posed a number of threats to security and served as incubators and amplifiers for disease. In this case, the refugee population set in motion a chain of events that contributed directly the Congo Wars that followed the Rwandan Civil War. These camps also helped exacerbate the budding HIV/AIDs crises in the region.

The Rwandan Patriotic Front (RPF), a mostly Tutsi militia, finally ended the genocide with its successful summer campaign that culminated in the capture of Kigali on July 4, 1994. While most consider this to be the conclusion of both the Rwandan

Civil War and the associated genocide, this is somewhat misleading because the conclusion of the genocide is largely indivisible from the subsequent Congo Wars. With the RPF rise to power, millions of Hutu fled the country, mostly seeking to evade prosecution or general retribution for Hutu-supported crimes during the conflict.[30] Neighboring Zaire, in particular, absorbed many fleeing Rwandans.

State capacity in this part of Africa was generally low, but Zaire was especially poorly prepared to deal with a refugee crisis. Led by a corrupt and increasingly ineffectual military dictator, Zaire was extremely fragile and ripe for ethnic conflict in the 1990s. While some international actors attempted to help coordinate a humanitarian response, the military in Zaire led the feeble response, which mostly involved housing refugees under terrible conditions in camps. The squalor created several public health crises and, on its own, helped contribute to the HIV epidemic in the country. On the political front, these camps quickly became staging areas from which Hutu militia fighters launched cross-border raids into Rwanda. These raids created many more refugees because populations along the border feared for their physical safety. The raids also caused the Tutsi government in Rwanda to launch a campaign into Zaire to stop the cross-border raids, and ultimately to seek the removal of the regime in Zaire as it was supporting the Hutu groups. This response is usually called the First Congo War. However, the First Congo War was part of a much bigger regional conflict that had its origins in the Rwandan Civil War.

The RPF, led by Paul Kagame, was the central actor in the First Congo War, though the conflict involved many states and nonstate actors, including Zaire, Uganda, Rwanda, Burundi, and Angola. The war also included irregular soldiers from the National Union for the Total Independence of Angola (UNITA), the Army for the Liberation of Rwanda (ALIR), the White Legion, the Alliance of Democratic Forces for the Liberation of Congo (AFDL), and the Hutu Interahamwe. Fought between 1996 and 1997, the war eventually led to the overthrow of Mobutu Seso Seko in Zaire. Although the conflict did achieve its main objective of removing Seso Seko from power, it did not produce a revitalization of Zaire. Laurent Desire-Kabila succeeded Seso Seko, but his leadership was equally disastrous; his ineptitude sparked the Second Congo War in 1998.

Although some scholars distinguish the First Congo War from the Second Congo War, many consider them to be one conflict generally known as the Great African War. The latter approach is more accurate, but it still fails to explicitly acknowledge that both conflicts are very much part of a chain of events that started with the Rwandan Civil War. The Second Congo War, like its predecessor, was mostly a contest over the leadership of the Democratic Republic of the Congo. Seso Seko dubbed the country Zaire in 1971, but after his ouster, the country reverted to the Democratic Republic of the Congo.

The Second Congo War was recognized as the deadliest conflict since the World War II, with estimated deaths numbering at least 5 million. The war also produced millions of refugees. At its peak, the Second Congo War involved a host of states and nonstate actors in the region, including the Democratic Republic of the Congo, Angola, Chad, Namibia, Zimbabwe, Uganda, Rwanda, and Burundi. Both

Congo Wars were fought over control of the Democratic Republic of the Congo and were exacerbated by endemic ethnic strife (itself influenced by the legacy of European colonialism). By 2002, things had begun to go badly for one major party in the war, Rwanda. South Africa, sensing an opportunity, orchestrated a peace deal. The Sun City Agreement was the first in a series of agreements that provided a fragile but general peace in 2003.[31]

Sexual Violence and the Congo Wars as a Means of Spreading HIV

As Kalonda-Kanyama demonstrates in his article on the civil war, HIV is more common in the parts of the region that were involved in the Congo Wars. In particular, his work makes it clear that sexual violence during the Congo Wars was a primary cause of the increased HIV prevalence rate in war-torn areas of the Congo. In a repeat of the violence that occurred in Rwanda, rape was used as a weapon of war on a massive scale, and HIV became a weapon that was used to further instill terror in civilian populations.[32] Although precise estimates of the number of rape victims are difficult to ascertain, most researchers concluded that there were hundreds of thousands of survivors. Some believed these numbers were much higher and that methodological problems such as victim reluctance to report assaults meant the total was significantly higher. As in the preceding Rwandan Civil War, rape was used by regular and irregular militia groups and was a hallmark of this conflict. These crimes had many repercussions, but it is important to note that they directly contributed to a rise in HIV/AIDS.

Peak HIV/AIDS prevalence in the Congo hovered around 5 percent during the early 2000s before declining somewhat. The HIV/AIDS prevalence rate in the regions immediately involved in the Congo Wars peaked at 20 percent.[33] In other words, the parts of the country that were home to the fighting forces and wartime rapes common during the conflict quadrupled the HIV/AIDS rates found in more peaceful parts of the Congo.

The causal relationship between HIV/AIDS and conflict is complicated and contested. Spiegel authored a well-respected analysis of the factors that inhibited simplistic assumptions that war and conflict universally led to increases in HIV/AIDS. Researchers have difficulty pinpointing the exact cause of HIV transmission. This problem is especially acute in situations where rape was commonplace and victims were unwilling to report or acknowledge their rape or HIV status. The long period between seroconversion and the onset of advanced HIV or AIDS makes it difficult to know when and how the disease was transmitted, even in societies with stable governments and health care facilities. Furthermore, the reliance on national-level data can mask significant regional variations.

In the case of the Congo, a cursory examination of the state's peak HIV-prevalence rate suggests that, although the country had a long and complicated history of warfare, its aggregate HIV-prevalence rate was comparable, and in some cases lower, than similarly placed neighbors in the region. This national-level analysis is often misleading—especially in the context of the wars that had bedeviled Sub-Saharan Africa since 1990. The Congo is massive, 2.35 million square kilometers, making it roughly twice as large as the combined area occupied by the United Kingdom, France, and Germany. Reliance on aggregated national-level data obscured the connections between HIV and conflict in the Congo because war did not rage in the entire country; instead, it was mostly localized to some of its eastern regions. The eastern parts of the Congo beset by the fighting, refugee populations, and mass rapes had HIV-prevalence rates that topped 20 percent. The fact that most of the rest of the country remained under 5 percent strongly suggests that war and its associated ills were a potent causal factor for the epidemic's spread.

Rwanda, too, demonstrated some of the methodical issues that made it difficult to tease out the exact causal relationship between war and HIV/AIDS. The record is clear that rape was widespread, and rape plus the threat of HIV infection was used with ruthless brutality as a weapon of war. Nonetheless, it is difficult to pinpoint the exact degree to which these factors caused a spike in HIV. Rwanda's aggregated national HIV-prevalence rate did not appear to increase after the civil war and genocide and has remained stable at approximately 3 percent.[34] Some might be tempted to conclude that, despite the conflict and systematic raping of women, there was no real surge in HIV infections. This conclusion does not account for the demographic turmoil in the state.

Before the genocide, Rwanda's population was 6 million. Roughly 800,000 were killed in the spring and summer of 1994, and several million fled the country. Indeed, many of the refugees settled in adjacent areas, like camps in Rwanda and border countries, and were reflected in the high rates of HIV there. Put plainly, the conflict probably contributed to a rise in HIV/AIDS prevalence rate in the region, but it did not automatically increase Rwanda's national prevalence rate, as many of the Rwandan victims immediately fled the country. Further compounding these issues is the long time between infection and advanced HIV/AIDS and increases in state capacity and public health efforts in the past 15 years.

Combined Impact of Wars, Violence, and HIV on the Emerging Modern Pandemic

Despite these methodological quibbles, there is a near consensus among scholars that some kinds of conflict were very likely to contribute to HIV/AIDS. Conflicts that involved significant numbers of irregular militia forces that utilized rape as a weapon of war were more likely to result in HIV/AIDS. The status of refugee camps was less clear, and some researchers do not believe that they caused spikes in HIV/AIDS.[35] Whatever the exact causal contribution of camps to HIV/AIDS prevalence, it is clear that HIV/AIDS inhibited recovery and rebuilding efforts in postconflict societies.

The detrimental effects of HIV/AIDS were magnified in countries that attempted to rebuild after a period of conflict. The cases of Rwanda and the Congo illustrated most of these perils. Because HIV/AIDS mostly struck individuals between 15 and 65 years old, any increase in the prevalence rate caused considerable economic strain, as it removed working-age individuals from the economy. This meant less consumption, lower revenues for the government, and significant opportunity costs, such as fewer individuals starting businesses and engaging in commerce. Cumulatively, this greatly impoverished state capacity. It meant that states were less able to provide for public goods, less capable of building institutions, and less likely to identify sustained economic development. Places with high mortality from HIV/AIDS experienced great complications, as large numbers of orphans further strained economies and state capacity. The increased opportunity costs from increased HIV/AIDS influenced security issues because the populations of the war-torn regions were especially vulnerable to radicalization. Today's disease orphans may well turn into militia fighters in the future.[36]

Although HIV may have entered the human population many times, it turned into a global pandemic of terrifying proportions in the latter half of the 20th century. European colonialism helped create a set of conditions that made it comparatively easy for HIV/AIDS to establish itself in the human population and to eventually turn into a pandemic. Not the only or even the most significant cause of HIV/AIDS, it is important to consider colonialism's comparatively understudied contexts to more fully understand the disease. Similarly, it is important to consider the role that conflicts played in helping exacerbate the pandemic. Research strongly suggests that the Rwandan Civil War and subsequent Congo Wars amplified the HIV/AIDS prevalence rate in areas affected by the conflict. This chapter spotlights the role of rape as a weapon of war in these conflicts. Not all conflicts increased the rate of HIV/AIDS or disease. However, data reinforces the findings that some kinds of conflict are likely to exacerbate the pandemic.

Research on the relationship between conflict, sexual violence, and the spread of HIV/AIDS is valuable to understanding past conflicts as well as to more fully consider future conflicts. Though the pandemic has stabilized in parts of the world, many places are susceptible to the sorts of conditions described herein. Indeed, the Congo remains chronically unstable; some researchers do not believe that the Second Congo War has actually ended, despite the official pronouncement otherwise. Other regions in Africa and beyond continue to experience the onset of violence that can likely replicate similar conditions necessary to accelerate the HIV/AIDS pandemic. The impacts of the HIV/AIDS pandemic on developed nations such as the United States were initially viewed through the lens of MSM activities and as a gay health care issue, but the vast majority of HIV/AIDS cases have occurred in developing nations, often in the context of war through heterosexual activities that included rape and typically as a result of postcolonial social and political upheaval.

NOTES

1. Obijiofor Aginam, "Rape and HIV as Weapons of War," United Nations University, last modified June 27, 2012, accessed September 2, 2017, https://unu.edu/publications /articles/rape-and-hiv-as-weapons-of-war.html.
2. Haidong Wang and the GBD 2015 Collaborators, "Estimates of Global, Regional, and National Incidence, Prevalence, and Mortality of HIV, 1980–2015: The Global Burden of Disease Study 2015," *The Lancet HIV* 3, no. 8 (2016): 361.
3. Centers for Disease Control and Prevention, "HIV among Gay and Bisexual Men," cdc. gov, last modified September 2016, https://www.cdc.gov/hiv/pdf/group/msm/cdc-hiv -msm.pdf. For more complete analyses of the role of MSM in the pandemic, see Chris

Beyrer et al., "Global Epidemiology of HIV Infection in Men Who Have Sex with Men," *The Lancet* 380, no. 9839 (2012): 367–377.

4. Randy Shilts, *And the Band Played On: Politics, People, and the AIDS Epidemic* (New York: St. Martin's Press, 1987), 80–81.

5. Centers for Disease Control and Prevention, "*Pneumocystis* Pneumonia—Los Angeles," *Morbidity and Mortality Weekly Report* 30, no. 21 (1981): 1–3.

6. It is very difficult to estimate the total size of the MSM population. See David W. Purcell et al., "Estimating the Population Size of Men Who Have Sex with Men in the United States to Obtain HIV and Syphilis Rates," *Open AIDS Journal* 6 (2012): 98–107.

7. Ayesha B. M. Kharsany and Quarraisha A. Karim, "HIV Infection and AIDS in Sub-Saharan Africa: Current Status, Challenges, and Opportunities," *Open AIDS Journal* 10 (2016): 34–48.

8. Centers for Disease Control and Prevention, "1993 Revised Classification System for HIV Infection and Expanded Surveillance Case Definition for AIDS among Adolescents and Adults," *Morbidity and Mortality Weekly Report* 41, no. 51 (1992), accessed December 12, 2017, https://www.cdc.gov/mmwr/preview/mmwrhtml/00018871.htm.

9. Nathan D. Wolfe, Peter Daszak, A. Marm Kilpatrick, and Donald S. Burke, "Bushmeat Hunting, Deforestation, and Prediction of Zoonotic Disease," *Emerging Infectious Disease* 11, no. 12 (2005): 1822–1827.

10. David Quammen, *Spillover: Animal Infections and the Next Human Pandemic* (New York: W. W. Norton & Company, 2012), 38–43, 85–86, 451–452.

11. Cliff A. Smallman-Raynor, "The Spread of Human Immunodeficiency Virus Type 2 into Europe: A Geographical Analysis," *International Journal of Epidemiology* 20, no. 2 (1991): 480–489.

12. Quammen, *Spillover*, 41–42. See also Heidi Ledford, "Tissue Sample Suggests HIV Has Been Infecting Humans for a Century," *Nature*, last modified October 1, 2008, accessed September 2, 2017, http://www.nature.com/news/2008/081001/full/news.2008.1143 .html.

13. Beatrice H. Hahn, George M. Shaw, Kevin M. De Cock, and Paul M. Sharp, "AIDS as a Zoonosis: Scientific and Public Health Implications," *Science* 28, no. 287 (2000): 607–614.

14. Recently, there has been more research that explores the origins for HIV that explicitly examines biological and social forces. See, for example, Stephanie Rupp, Phillipe Ambara, Victor Narat, and Tamara Giles-Vernick, "Beyond the Cut Hunter: A Historical Epidemiology of HIV Beginnings in Central Africa," *EcoHealth* 13, no. 4 (2016): 661–671.

15. Craig Timberg and Daniel Halperin, *Tinderbox: How the West Sparked the AIDS Epidemic and How the World Can Finally Overcome It* (New York: Penguin, 2012), 1–4, 49–51; and Amit Chitnis, Diana Rawls, and Jim Moore, "Origin of HIV Type 1 in Colonial French Equatorial Africa?," *AIDS Research and Human Retroviruses* 16, no. 1 (2004): 5–8. See also Tamara Giles-Vernick, Ch. Didier Gondola, Guillaume Lachenal, and William H. Schneider, "Social History, Biology, and the Emergence of HIV in Colonial Africa," *Journal of African History* 54, no. 1 (2013): 11–30.

16. Quammen, *Spillover*, 481–482.

17. Quammen, *Spillover*.

18. Nancy M. Mock et al., "Conflict and HIV: A Framework for Risk Assessment to Prevent HIV in Conflict-Affected Settings in Africa," *Emerging Themes in Epidemiology* 1, no. 6 (2004), accessed December 12, 2017, https://www.ncbi.nlm.nih.gov/pmc/articles

/PMC544944/. See also Stefan Elbe, "HIV/AIDS and the Changing Landscape of War in Africa," *International Security* 27, no. 2 (2002): 159–177.

19. Timberg and Halperin, *Tinderbox*, 1–4.

20. For a specialized discussion of HIV/AIDS and state capacity in Zimbabwe that contains generalizable points for other states in the region, see Andrew T. Price-Smith and John L. Daly, "Downward Spiral: HIV/AIDS, State Capacity, and Political Conflict in Zimbabwe," *Peaceworks* No. 53 (Washington, D.C.: United States Institute of Peace, 2004).

21. Sabina Alkire, "A Conceptual Framework for Human Security, Working Paper 2," Centre for Research on Inequality, Human Security, and Ethnicity, CRISE (2003): 3–5.

22. Anne Buve, Kizito Bishikwabo-Nsarhaza, and Gladys Mutangadura, "The Spread and Effect of HIV-1 Infection in Sub-Saharan Africa," *The Lancet* 359 (2002): 2013.

23. Stefan Elbe, "HIV/AIDS and the Changing Landscape of War in Africa," *International Security* 27, no. 2 (2002): 161.

24. See Samantha Power, *A Problem from Hell: America and the Age of Genocide* (New York: Basic Books, 2002); and Gerard Prunier, *Africa's World War: Congo, the Rwandan Genocide, and the Makings of a Continental Catastrophe* (New York: Oxford University Press, 2009).

25. Aginam, "Rape and HIV as Weapons of War."

26. Paula Donovan, "Rape and HIV/AIDS in Rwanda," *The Lancet Supplement* 360 (December 2002): 17.

27. Philip Verwimp, "Machetes and Firearms: The Organization of Massacres in Rwanda," *Journal of Peace Research* 43, no. 1 (2006): 8.

28. Verwimp, "Machetes and Firearms," 11.

29. Binaifer Nowrojee, *Shattered Lives: Sexual Violence during the Rwandan Genocide and Its Aftermath* (New York: Human Rights Watch, 1996).

30. Ray Wilkinson, "Heart of Darkness," www.unhcr.org, last modified December 1, 1997, accessed September 2, 2017, http://www.unhcr.org/3b6925384.html.

31. The preceding section is a broad synopsis of the very complicated Congo Wars. There are several excellent histories on the conflict, including Gerard Prunier, *Africa's World War: Congo, the Rwandan Genocide, and the Makings of a Continental Catastrophe* (New York: Oxford University Press, 2009); Fiilip Reyntjens, *The Great African War: Congo and Regional Geopolitics, 1996–2006* (New York: Cambridge University Press, 2009); and Rene Lemarchand, *The Dynamics of Violence in Central Africa* (State College, PA: University of Pennsylvania Press, 2009).

32. Isaac Kalonda-Kanyama, "Civil War, Sexual Violence and HIV Infections: Evidence from the Democratic Republic of the Congo," *Journal of African Development* 12, no. 2 (2010): 47–60.

33. Emily Wax, "Cycle of War Is Spreading AIDS and Fear in Africa," *Washington Post* (November 13, 2003), accessed September 2, 2017, https://www.washingtonpost .com/archive/politics/2003/11/13/cycle-of-war-is-spreading-aids-and-fear-in-africa /6736e773-5817-4cce-ab07-742a1c82f873/?utm_term=.852b9c6f6940.

34. United Nations, "HIV/AIDS, Malaria and other diseases," www.w.one.un.org, last modified 2017, accessed September 2, 2017, http://www.rw.one.un.org/mdg/mdg6.

35. Paul B. Spiegel, "HIV/AIDS among Conflict-Affected and Displaced Populations: Dispelling Myths and Taking Action," *Disasters* 28, no. 3 (2004): 322–339.

36. See Institute of Medicine and Committee on Envisioning a Strategy to Prepare for the Long-Term Burden of HIV/AIDS: African Needs and U.S. Interests, *Preparing for the Future of HIV/AIDS in Africa: A Shared Responsibility* (Washington, D.C.: The National Academies Press, 2011).

Chapter 15

Mumps: Lasting Remnant of the Bosnian War, 1992–2012

Rebecca M. Seaman

> Death as a result of wars is simply the "tip of the iceberg." Other conse-
> quences, besides death, are not well documented. They include endemic
> poverty, malnutrition, disability, economic/social decline and psychosocial
> illness, to mention only a few.[1]
> —R. Srinivasa Murthy and Rashimi Lakshminarayana

The relationship between wars and epidemics is complex. Some wars occur amid the traumas associated in part with massive epidemics or pandemics. Other epidemics arise during wars because of the conditions of conflict. Still others see the disruptions of war reach their tentacles across time, resulting in the delayed emergence of epidemics years or even decades later. Such was the case of the mumps epidemic that erupted in Bosnia approximately 15 years after the conclusion of the Bosnian War of the 1990s. The 2011–2012 outbreaks in Bosnia of mumps, and later measles, have direct relationships to the wartime disruption of medical services, access to vaccinations and boosters, and lasting economic upheaval and psychological traumas. The perpetuation of insufficient diets, lapses in health care, and heightened levels of stress that undermined immune systems also facilitated these viral epidemics, long after the war that had created the inhospitable and corrupt socioeconomic environment was brought to a close.

Understanding the Presentation and Transmission of the Mumps Virus

Mumps is a virus that invades lymphoid tissues, typically causing inflammation of the parotid or salivary glands. Mumps is a member of the paramyxovirus family, a group of three genera that includes *Paramyxovirus* (parainfluenza and mumps viruses), *Pneumovirus* (syncytial virus), and *Morbillivirus* (measles); all of these are considered respiratory viruses.[2] The mumps virus infects the respiratory track and is spread through droplets from sneezing or coughing as well as through contact. It is also found in infectious form in most body fluids for two weeks following the onset of symptoms. Once exposed, the incubation period lasts from two to four weeks. Depending on the age of patients, up to 30 percent of people demonstrate no symptoms or experience only mild fevers with aches and malaise. However, more common symptoms include low-grade fever, headache, body aches, tenderness, and swelling of the parotid glands as well as occasional swelling and tenderness of the submandibular glands. Swelling gradually diminishes after four days or up to a week. The disease is contagious about two days before the onset of symptoms, and it remains contagious for over a week after clinical presentation. Most people are inconvenienced by the acquisition of mumps (bedrest, extreme lethargy, quarantine), but rare complications do occur. Complications may include meningitis, deafness, orchitis (testicular swelling), pancreatitis, or myocarditis as well as other rare inflammatory complications.[3]

Typical of many viruses, there is no distinct treatment for mumps except for maintaining a quarantine to prevent further spread of the contagion. Humans are the only known natural hosts. Today, prevention is best accomplished through vaccinations of susceptible populations. Historically, people contracted mumps as one of the numerous childhood diseases, with most experiencing the virus by age 10. Typically emerging in the winter and spring months, mumps were endemic to urban areas where the population density allowed for the recurrence of epidemics on a regular basis. The advent of vaccination reduced the occurrence of the virus, but outbreaks still occurred, especially in early school-age children who were in close proximity to those who may not have received proper immunization protocols.[4]

Hippocrates provided the first historical record of mumps in the fifth century BCE. He accounted for an epidemic in the early spring, that resulted in

> swellings beside one ear, or both ears, in most cases unattended with fever. . . . [In] some cases there was slight heat, but the swellings subsided without causing harm. . . . Many had dry coughs which brought up nothing when they coughed, but their voices were hoarse. Soon after, though in some cases after some time, painful inflammations occurred either in one testicle or in both.[5]

As a highly contagious respiratory illness, it is not surprising that mumps epidemics historically experienced sharp increases during periods of military mobilizations. Prior to the development of a vaccine in 1967, mumps epidemics occurred every two to five years and were found globally. Those countries without vaccination programs still experience frequent epidemic peaks.[6] In World War I, reported cases of mumps represented the third highest of all communicable diseases, behind influenza and measles. Understandably, the worst outbreaks occurred at mobilization camps during the winter and early spring months. Like measles, the primary disruption was the lost duty time, especially due to the long incubation and contagion period. Unlike the influenza virus, mumps progressed very slowly throughout military camps. Later studies conducted during World War II demonstrated a consistent progression of about 17 weeks for the epidemic to peak at a single camp.[7] The combination of wartime conditions, the mobilization of large and divergent sections of the population with varying exposure and immunity to mumps, and the length of contagion period for the disease made mumps a force to be reckoned with during major wars of the past. The wars experienced throughout the Balkan region in the 1990s witnessed the same disruptions and epidemic susceptibility that negated the advancements in vaccinations and medical protocols.

Historical Origins of the Bosnian Wars

The Balkan region has historically been a shatter zone that experienced war in repeated waves, from as early as the Peloponnesian Wars of the fifth century BCE and throughout much of history. Contested by the Greeks, Romans, Goths, Turks, Slavs, and Austrians, the resulting internal mixture of ethnic and religious groups added to the turbulence of the geographically fragmented region. Indeed, Archduke Franz Ferdinand's assassination, the "spark" that ignited World War I, took place in the capital city of Sarajevo, Bosnia. Postwar efforts attempted to create stability through annexing multiple territories into the Kingdom of Serbs, Croats and Slovenes, later renamed Yugoslavia. These attempts tenuously unified diverse populations within the region until World War II.

Recent historical works tackle the internal issues of religion and secularism within Bosnia-Herzegovina and the nationalistic movements of the region during World War II. Marko Hoare's *The Bosnian Muslims in the Second World War: A History* (2013) takes a revolutionary approach that tries to highlight collaboration among historically disparate groups in the region for the purpose of opposing the Nazis and the Croatian Ustasha state. Hoare notes the political disagreements between communists and Muslims, but he determined that "ideological differences were often less important than family bonds, childhood friendships and momentary tactical choices." Hoare concludes that any convergence or collaboration of the various groups was short-lived and tactical in nature, as the Muslims remained anticommunist and the Bosnian-Serbs that comprised most partisan groups sought a unified Yugoslavia, but under Serbian rule.

Meanwhile, Emily Greble's *Sarajevo 1941–1945: Muslims, Christians and Jews in Hitler's Europe* delved into the local dynamics of religious and civic groups and leaders. In doing so, she revealed that the collaboration between typically opposed local groups allowed them to adapt to the wartime conditions and resist common foes, despite the continued nationalist and racist ideologies of the Ustasha state and between the various opposition groups.[8]

Balkan nationalism, or Balkanization, played a role in the attempts to unify the divergent groups as well as creating divisions within the populations. As early as the 1830s, the Illyrian movement attempted a pan-Slavic political and cultural unification of southern Slavic peoples along the lines of language, which was later appropriated by Ante Starčević into a somewhat racial policy of Greater Croatia that troubled Croatian politics thereafter. In the mid-19th century, the Strossmayer Party built upon this concept of nationalism but pushed for a united Yugoslavia through a Croatian-Serbian coalition.[9] Another regional attempt at unification was the Croatian Peasant Party, seeking Croatian unity along cultural lines in the period between the two world wars. However, underlying religious affiliations often thwarted unification efforts based on cultural lines and political ideologies.[10]

Religion also sometimes united divergent ethnic groups, but it also divided ethnic and cultural groups internally. The long history of Balkanization brought about the occupation of the region by peoples of different religious backgrounds: western Roman Catholic (with Latin script), Eastern Orthodox (with Cyrillic script), and Muslim (some with Semitic script) were the dominant groups. The blend of religious intransigence with the political dominance of a particular cultural, ethnic group, or extra-national group exacerbated the divisions, resulting in such distinctions as Croat-Catholics and Orthodox-Serbs by 1940. Efforts of external religious authorities, such as requiring their religious adherents to remain apolitical, were thwarted by some of the extremist leaders within the region who sought to connect political, ethnic, and religious identities. Local clergy often gave their support to this convergence of religion and politics. This further divided the population, as some clergy supported one political party or ideology while others of the same faith supported an opposing party or ideology. The confusion was complete, for the local population and for historians trying to make sense of the alignments through the lens of time. To better understand the internal divisions that helped precipitate the 1990s conflicts and eventually resulted in preventable epidemics over the next two decades, it helps to start with examining the status of these core themes, beginning with World War II.

During World War II, the historic antagonisms of the Balkans erupted into a civil war under the guise of resisting German Nazi and Italian Fascist occupation. Bosnian partisans fought Croatian Fascist troops that, in turn, used the Nazi invasion to seize power. The alignments presaged similar conflicts in the late 20th century. The artificial Croatian borders drawn by Hitler and Mussolini created an Ustasha state that was approximately 50 percent Croat, with the remainder composed of Serbs (Orthodox), Jews, Roma (gypsies), and Muslims. According to Balkan historian Emily Greble Balić, the predominately Catholic Croats considered the Croat Muslims to have been forced into conversion during the previous Ottoman rule. The Muslims were incorporated into the Croatian nationalist rule, giving Catholic Croats a stronger hold on the artificial state. The Muslim Croats received some autonomy and even secured some appointments within the new government.

Together, the Catholic and Muslim Croat alliance attempted to reverse the trend of prewar centralization. Some hoped for a degree of political and religious autonomy, others hoped to stem the Serb influence, and still others sought complete ethnic cleansing of Serbs, Jews, and Roma. The Croatian Ustasha leadership claimed to represent all combined interests, despite inherent ideological and religious conflicts. Within days of gaining power, they put forth an agenda that rescinded the rights, confiscated the properties, and ultimately perpetuated policies of genocide against the Serbs, Jews, and Roma of the new Ustasha state.[11]

Orthodox Serbs, Jews, Roma, and even some Muslims coalesced around their opposition of the Croatian Catholic-Muslim alliance, but they diverged on the aforementioned issues of religion and on their ultimate political goals. Many (but not all) partisans supported communist ideologies. The material shortages and daily hardships during the war necessitated some collaboration but simultaneously exacerbated the conflicts between divergent groups. Nonetheless, the ultimate Axis powers' loss at the end of the war left the partisans with a strong communist backing and in the position of ascendency.

Yugoslavian Structure and Cultural Discord

Yugoslavia was reestablished after the war as a communist state under Josip Broz Tito. Despite the Cold War politics of containment, Tito managed to secure Marshall Plan funds from the West to rebuild the six republics redrawn from the expanded Croatian claims of the Nazi-Fascist era. The six republics retained sovereignty in name only, with local cultural and political institutions under their control, but they had to relinquish all political power to the Yugoslavian government.[12] Under Tito, the Croat-Catholics and Orthodox-Serbs continued to assert dominance in their respective regions, with Bosnia experiencing struggles between the two groups as they vied for influence in the ethnically diverse republic. The decision to report Muslims as either "undetermined," Serb, or Croat in the 1948 census began a shift that introduced a new contestant for political dominance in Bosnia, one that reached full status as a "nation" within Yugoslavia in 1969.[13] Whether it was the result of the Yugoslavian economic resurgence or his authoritarian policies, Tito managed to hold the fragmented country together by playing the various sides against each other amid increasing ethnic and political tensions. This semblance of unity lasted until his death in 1980.

The death of Tito and the ensuing breakdown of Soviet Communism witnessed the collapse of totalitarianism and created a void in effective political leadership and unification of the Balkan region. This was most obvious in Bosnia, the territory identified as "Serbian and Croatian and Muslim" by Tito but was avidly sought after by each individual group.[14] Gen. Charles G. Boyd (Ret.), the former deputy commander in chief of the U.S. European Command, stated in a political analysis of Bosnia that the constant goal of factions in the region was to avoid "minority status in Yugoslavia or any successor state."[15] The combined influence of ethnic and cultural struggles for political and majority dominance, in a region historically beset by conflict, oppression, and geographic fragmentation, created the conditions that ensured a resurgence of civil war in the 1990s.

At the outset of hostilities within Bosnia, the preexisting religious and ethnic divisions still competed for influence. According to researchers Andrew Slack and Roy Doyon, the conflict existed at three levels. The highest-level conflicts included the expansionist goals of Tudjman (Greater Croatia) and Milosevic (Greater Serbia). At the Bosnian republic level were the political struggles of Izetbegovic and the Bosnian Muslims, Boban and the Bosnian Croats, and Karadzic and the Bosnian Serbs. The local-level conflict consisted of latent ethnic nationalist sentiments of the individual population clusters, which awaited inspiration and leadership from others. The war consequently developed from a combination of two forces: the strategic interests of the local, national, and external stakeholders and the "demographic histories that disposed local populations to support the military effort."[16]

When considering the war from outside the region, the usage of ethnic terms or religious alignments add to the confusion instead of helping people to understand the local interests. The use of such terms as "Serbs" and "Croats" were meant to clarify a particular side in the fray, but strict division along ethnic lines ignored historical religious ties in a religiously diverse region. Muslims, Macedonians, Slovenes, and others existed in small numbers, and they survived by shifting their alliances between whichever dominant group provided them some sense of political voice.[17] As previously mentioned, during the Ottoman occupation of the region, many Catholic Croats were converted from Catholicism to Islam. During World War II, this reality was viewed through the lens of expediency, with the Ustasha Catholic Croats accepting the necessity of such historic conversions in an effort to align the Muslims to their cause in rooting out Jews, Orthodox Serbs, and Roma.

During the conflict of the 1990s, the Orthodox Serbs viewed the Muslims, whether Serbs or Croats, as complicit in the atrocities perpetuated during World War II. Tracing the history of their region back to the Ottoman invasion and Battle of Kosovo (1389), these Orthodox Serbs commemorated their attempts to reject Turkish rule and actively sought to root out any elements of "Turkification." Indeed, Muslim Slavs were viewed racially as Turks and therefore as responsible for not only claiming what rightfully belonged to Christian Serbs but deemed genocidal by nature (a reference to the Nazi-Ustasha atrocities laid at the feet of the Croats and Muslims). When this religious and historical mythology was coupled with years of the nationalist propaganda of Serbian leader Slobodan Milošević, the violence became ingrained and eventually drove killings based on perceived religious identities. Many people thus classified did not even identify themselves as religious. Nonetheless, they were given labels because their religious identity "was handed down through the family."[18]

The resurgence of conflict in the Balkans emerged when Milošević revoked the autonomy of two provinces, Vojvodina and Kosovo. He miscalculated how internal and external interests would receive this act. Instead of addressing their concerns, Tito had alienated them and ensured any transition of power would be beset by troubles. Most importantly, his government incited rebellion among Serbs in the region by fomenting rumors of Croat and Muslim massacre conspiracies. With the Croatian president Franjo Tudjman asserting a fascist threat from Serbs in Croatia, Milošević asserting a Muslim and Croatian threat in Serbia, Muslims hoping for their own independent nation, and the fanning of Serbian emotions via the myth of the 14th-century loss to the Muslim Turks, the stage was set for a civil war. The depth of historical grudges combined with fears fed by recent propaganda to ensure that the violence escalated and resulted in attempts of ethnic cleansing on the part of Croats and Serbs.

The United Nations sought to end the violence through the insertion of peacekeeping forces. Sarajevo became the sight of the UN forces' headquarters. Hoping to end the internal strife, these external diplomats failed to provide military, economic, or political leadership for the new nation, leaving the antagonists within to fight for dominance. Within a year, the cost in lives and displaced peoples demonstrated the depth of the unleashed violence.[19] By 1993, the United Nations had declared three towns as "safe havens." But by 1995, these were under the control of the Bosnian government, and the UN peacekeeping forces were unable or unwilling to stop the ensuing Serbian policies that resulted in mass rape, massacres, and genocide. According to Gen. Boyd,

> It [the United States, the United Nations, and NATO] has supported the creation of safe areas and demanded their protection even when they have been used by one warring faction to mount attacks against another. . . . It has pushed for more humanitarian aid even as it became clear that this was subsidizing conflict and protecting the warring factions from the natural consequences of continuing the fighting. It has supported the legitimacy of leadership that has become increasingly ethnocentric in its makeup, single-party in its rule, and manipulative in its diplomacy.[20]

The very forces that claimed to enforce peace instead facilitated further violence and the complete breakdown of Bosnia society. It was only after the explosion of a bomb in a crowded Sarajevo market that NATO finally joined military assaults on Bosnian Serb locations. The conflict finally came to a close in late 1995, but only after the widespread destruction of the nation's infrastructure and the extensive loss of civilian and military lives.

The analysis of data in 2010 revealed that of the almost 2 million Muslim Bosniaks, 3.1 percent were killed in direct combat, as targeted victims, or as collateral damage. The Serbs experienced the second-highest rate of casualties, with the loss of 1.4 percent of their total population of 1,361,814. The lowest casualties were for the Croats (1 percent of 758,585) and the "other" category (1.2 percent of 352,106).[21] These figures only convey part of the trauma. When testifying before The Hague tribunal, the Polish demographer Ewa Tabeau indicated that out of 481,109 Muslims living in 27 Bosnian municipalities in 1991, more than half were no longer there by 1997; they were either killed or fled as refugees internally or abroad. The worst-case scenario was for the Bosnian city of Prijedor, where the Muslim population accounted for 42.6 percent of the population before the war but only 1 percent of the population by 1997. Meanwhile, Tabeau testified that the Serbian population had grown from 43 percent to 89 percent in the same time frame.[22]

The causes of these drastic demographic changes were many. Mass executions accounted for some losses, as in the 8,000 Muslim Bosniaks killed in Srebrenica in July 1995. Additional casualties affecting shifting demographics included the killing of citizens via snipers and bombings as well as casualties from actual combat. When speaking of the siege of Sarajevo, Tabeau indicated that "more civilians were killed every day than soldiers, which made us conclude that civilians were systemically targeted."[23]

The military also targeted public facilities. The Sarajevo State Hospital was bombed repeatedly, destroying it floor by floor, disrupting the electrical power and leaving it with "little food, scarce medical and surgical supplies, and no heating."[24] Similarly, the Koševo Hospital in Sarajevo was targeted, with bullets shattering windows and artillery leaving shell holes throughout the complex. Doctors at Koševo Hospital reported depending completely on humanitarian aid from foreign countries and living off diets of bread and milk when not on duty. Additional reported conditions included no heat for the first two winters of the war, no beds, lice infestations, and health problems.[25]

Within Bosnia-Hercegovina, the total loss of health care facilities was estimated at over 35 percent destroyed or damaged beyond effective use.[26] With the conflict vastly increasing the number of injuries of military personnel and civilians, the remaining hospitals were overcrowded and strapped for resources. Infrastructure damage often left the medical facilities without electricity and forced doctors to operate with makeshift lighting. The lack of medical supplies exacerbated efforts to treat the injured and ill during the worst hostilities of the war.

Lasting Impact of Bosnian War on Medical Care

Medical supply shortages and electrical outages had immediate and lasting impacts on the people of Bosnia. The disruptions of wars often hinder the flow of needed supplies and also redirect funds toward medical or military services deemed far more strategic at the time. The war in Bosnia lasted from 1992 to 1995 and included a 44-month siege of the capital city of Sarajevo. During the siege, the city experienced shortages of food, electricity, medicine, and other necessities. Not surprisingly, immunization protocols practiced prior to the war were abandoned in Sarajevo and in most war-torn areas of Bosnia. Those children that had received initial vaccinations for infectious diseases such as mumps, measles, and rubella (MMRs) often did not receive the later booster shots needed to guarantee immunity.

Additionally, those who lived in municipalities where hostilities were less common still felt the indirect impact of the war's disruptions through the improper handling of vaccines. MMR vaccines require constant temperatures, or maintenance of "cold chain," to remain viable.[27] The irregular supply lines servicing the military, government, medical clinics, and general population were increasingly run by black marketers, who were successful entrepreneurs but not knowledgeable about vaccine storage requirements. These black-market supply chains were less than efficient in maintaining environmental controls. Once vaccines were in the hands of medical personnel, the erratic power supplies created disruptions that still allowed for temperatures to fluctuate beyond the narrow parameters needed to maintain quality vaccines.

The shortages of vaccines and problems with maintaining cold chain storage requirements were further compounded by the violence in Bosnian society. Parents hesitated to take their children into the surviving medical facilities due to the violence on the streets and the obvious targeting of hospitals and medical clinics. Additionally, the hostilities left increased numbers of children orphaned, with no guardians to ensure vaccinations were administered at the appropriate age levels. The upheaval in society also provided daily distractions that led to the neglect of vaccination schedules by parents and medical personnel alike.

The results of the failure to vaccinate and the use of vaccines that were not properly maintained were not immediate. The last major mumps, measles, and rubella epidemics hit Sarajevo, Bosnia, in 1996–1997, just after the end of the war. Rubella did not resurface until 2010, with 951 reported cases. In 2014, 780 cases of measles were recorded. However, it was the back-to-back mumps epidemics of 2011 and 2012 that drew attention due to the consistently high numbers, with over 15,000 cases in Central Bosnia. In Sarajevo alone, 1,313 cases were recorded in 2011, and an additional 554 were reported in 2012.[28] While the disruptions of wars often result in similar outbreaks years later, the longevity of the Bosnian War and the displacement of citizens for sometimes over a decade made the resulting mumps epidemics in Bosnia more widespread. Astoundingly, the failure to vaccinate did not end with the war itself.

The breakdown of society during the war accounts for the initial failure to vaccinate children who were either born during that time or eligible for their booster vaccines during the war. According to a study on the intergenerational effects of war on children, during the Bosnian War, "immunization rates fell from approximately 95 percent pre-conflict to around 30 percent."[29] This accounts for 72 percent of mumps patients falling in the age groups of 15–19 or 20–29 in 2011 and 2012. However, it does not account to the continued failure to vaccinate or administer booster shots after the war. Of the 15,600 reported mump cases during the two epidemics in Bosnia, 5,677 occurred primarily in Central Bosnia, Zenica-Doboj, Sarajevo, and Herzegovina-Neretva, where the hostilities were concentrated during the war and where reconstruction took years to affect. However, the second wave also saw cases in Una-Sana and Tuzla cantons. These cantons experienced high levels of migration out of the war-torn regions, but they did not have the same breakdown of infrastructure as the cantons that were hit by the first wave.[30]

A report by Hukic et al. on the "Mumps Outbreak in the Federation of Bosnia and Herzegovina" reveals that deficiencies in vaccination programs extended well beyond the 1992–1995 hostilities. Periodic disruptions to supplies and cold chain interruptions continued for several years.[31] The size of the outbreak and the successive epidemics in two consecutive years indicate the susceptibility of a large sector of the population. The failure to maintain cold chain storage and the failure of timely vaccinations accounted for the largest number of cases among patients aged 15–19 and 20–29. The spread of mumps, measles, and rubella among the younger population groups from 2010 to 2014 is a clear indication that the disruptions of the 1992–1995 conflict and continued disruptions in society following the war resulted in failures to vaccinate, inadequate vaccination applications, and inferior vaccines.

Yet, another reality of postwar Bosnia needs to be factored into any study involving health care—that of corruption. The black market that helped maintain Bosnia during the siege of Sarajevo did not disappear at the end of the war. Indeed, the leaders of the black market became the new elite in Bosnia. Not surprisingly, crime found its way into the medical system. By 2011, amid the mumps epidemic, a report revealed that more than half of the citizens paid bribes to doctors to gain access to services in a timely fashion. In a study conducted of returning Bosnian refugees, over 60 percent reported corruption in the public hospitals. Returning refugees especially reported problems in accessing medical care.[32] The control of black marketers over supplies drove up the costs for medical goods, including vaccines. Meanwhile, the corruption and bribes in the hospitals is more likely connected to the perceptions of poor pay for medical personnel in the public health care system of a society still rebuilding from a devastating war.

Stress and Health during and after War

Finally, as is true of almost any epidemic, the underlying health of society, specifically those who contract infectious diseases, plays a role in the dynamics of an outbreak. The public infrastructure of transportation, power, and sanitation is crucial to the stability of a healthy society, as is the availability and efficiency of health care services. Yet, physical health is also related to levels of stress, and Bosnian populations boasted extreme levels of stress, even two decades after the war of the 1990s. The violence associated with the civil war explains some of the posttraumatic stress disorder (PTSD) levels in the society. As a civil war, not just military personnel were affected. Women living in high-conflict areas around Bosnia experienced PTSD seven times higher than the control group in a study by Devakumar et al. in 2014. The study also discovered that the increased stress levels affected unborn children, "leading to an increased susceptibility to mental illness in the child."[33] Another study by the Ministry of Health published in 2012 revealed that more than 60 percent of the Sarajevo population suffered from PTSD.[34] While mothers and children who experienced heightened anxiety and rapes during the Bosnian War would seem to have little connection to mumps epidemics, these experiences produced effects in offspring, such as increased risk of immune system modulation and infections.[35] This underlying lasting impact of the Bosnian War, combined with wartime malnutrition and delays in postwar recovery, helps to explain the widespread epidemic outbreaks of respiratory viruses, especially the back-to-back outbreaks of mumps in 2011 and 2012. The epidemics affected not only those who received inadequate or no vaccinations during the war, but also those born well after the war who received recommended vaccinations but suffered from intergenerational impacts and continued social and economic upheavals.

PTSD is not the only form of stress encountered across post–civil war Bosnian society. The displacement of approximately 2 million people, almost half the Bosnian population, affected those displaced persons, their families, and their societies. Dislocation resulted in high rates of poverty as well as limited access to services intended to balance the traumas associated with forced relocation. As the dislocation was often of people from minority groups, the resulting change in the ethnic composition in their places of origin, as well as their new destinations, created demographic upheavals that contributed to increased stress levels. Returning refugees often discovered that their homes had been designated "abandoned" and claimed by others, forcing the returning refugees to find new housing on shoestring budgets.

Meanwhile, fears of a resurgence of ethnic conflict led to the segregation of ethnic and religious groups, creating two distinct governing districts in Bosnia. Instead of solving the age-old problems, this approach entrenched the distrust between cultural and ethnic groups.[36] With this knowledge, it is not surprising to learn that the Ministry of Health study from 2012 discovered that 73 percent of the Sarajevo population suffered from stress-related problems.[37] The cycle of distrust and violence seemed to repeat itself and further undermined the health of the citizenry of Sarajevo and Bosnia-Herzegovina.

The impact of stress on the health of the affected population is often overlooked. As a study on stress and immunity indicated, "Chronic stress impedes the immune response to infection, increasing risks for catching contagious diseases and having prolonged illness episodes."[38] The combination of insufficient, missing, or compromised vaccination for mumps with long-term socioeconomic disruption left the majority of the Bosnian population in the war-torn areas affected by stress, opening them up to inhibited immune responses when finally exposed to the virus in 2011 and 2012.

Disruptions of War as a Lasting Impact on Heath—Mumps in Postwar Bosnia

The 1992–1995 civil war in Bosnia, built upon ethnic, religious, and political animosities, tore the society apart and took a considerable toll on human life. The accompanying corruption and disorder of government and the damage to infrastructure and social and medical services set the stage for long-term societal upheavals. The targeting of medical facilities during the war and the ineffective handling and distribution of medical supplies—specifically vaccinations against infectious diseases—presaged the eruption of later epidemics. Meanwhile, the delayed reconstruction of Bosnian society and continued corruption over the next decade further interrupted necessary social and health care services, including emotional and psychological services for the large numbers of people suffering from emotional stress and PTSD. These factors combined to extend the impact of the disastrous war well beyond the early 1990s and into the 21st century.

As is often true, the circumstances of war created the conditions for infectious epidemics. But in the case of Bosnia and its civil war, the path toward two consecutive mumps epidemics was cleared and maintained for almost two decades, affecting not only the participants and witnesses of the war, but the following generation of Serbs, Croats, and Muslim Bosniaks.

NOTES

1. R. Srinivasa Murthy and Rashmi Lakshminarayana, "Mental Health Consequences of War: A Brief Review of Research Findings," *World Psychology* 5, no. 1 (February 2006): 25.

2. S. Baron, ed., *Medical Microbiology*, 4th ed. (Galveston: University of Texas Medical Branch at Galveston, 1996), chapter 59, accessed August 25, 2017, https://www.ncbi.nlm .nih.gov/books/NBK8461.

3. Margaret Hunt, "Virology, Chapter Fourteen: Measles (Rubeola) and Mumps Viruses," *Microbiology and Immunology On-line*, University of South Carolina School of Medicine, accessed August 7, 2017, http://microbiologybook.org/mhunt/mump-meas.htm.

4. Hunt, "Virology."

5. Hippocrates, "Epidemics I: First Constitution," *Hippocrates*, Vol. 1, trans. W. H. S. Jones (London: William Heinemann, LTD, 1957), 147–149.

6. A. M. Galazka, S. E. Robertson, and A. Kraigher, "Mumps and Mumps Vaccine: A Global Review," *Bulletin of the World Health Organization* 77, no. 1 (1999): 4.

7. Joseph Stokes, "Mumps," in *Preventive Medicine in World War II*, Vol. 4, *Communicable Diseases Transmitted Chiefly through Respiratory and Alimentary Tracts*, eds. Ebbe Curtis Hoff and Phebe M. Hoff (Washington, D.C.: U.S. Army Medical Department, Office of Medical History, 1958), 135–136, 138.

8. Xavier Bougarel, "Review Essay," *Southeast European and Black Sea Studies* 15, no. 4 (2015): 683–688.

9. Dusko Doder, "Yugoslavia: New War, Old Hatreds," *Foreign Policy* 91 (Summer 1993): 8.

10. Irina Ognyanova, "Religion and Church in the Ustasha Ideology (1941–1945), *CCP* 64 (2009): 157–158.

11. Emily Greble Balić, "When Croatia Needed Serbs: Nationalism and Genocide in Sarajevo 1941–1942," *Slavic Review* 68, no. 1 (Spring 2009): 120–121, accessed August 12, 2017, http://www.jstor.org/stable/20453271.

12. Doder, "Yugoslavia," 11.

13. J. Andrew Slack and Roy R. Doyon, "Population Dynamics and Susceptibility for Ethnic Conflict: The Case of Bosnia and Herzegovina," *Journal of Peace Research* 38, no. 2 (March 2001): 142, accessed August 12, 2017, ww.jstor.org/stable/425492.

14. Doder, "Yugoslavia."

15. Charles G. Boyd, "Making Peace with the Guilty: The Truth about Bosnia," *Foreign Affairs* 74, no. 5 (September–October 1995): 24, accessed August 12, 2017, http://www.jstor.org/stable/20047298.

16. Slack and Doyon, "Population Dynamics," 156.

17. Doder, "Yugoslavia," 9.

18. Michael Sells, "Crosses of Blood: Sacred Space, Religion, and Violence in Bosnia-Hercegovina," 2002 Paul Hanly Furfey Lecture, *Sociology of Religion* 64, no. 3 (2003): 310–314, accessed August 12, 2017, http://www.jstor.org/stable/3712487.

19. Doder, "Yugoslavia," 19–20.

20. Boyd, "Making Peace with the Guilty," 23.

21. Jan Zwierzchowski and Ewa Tabeau, "The 1992–1995 War in Bosnia and Herzegovina: Census-Based Multiple System Estimation of Casualties' Undercount," Conference Paper for the International Research Workshop on "The Global Costs of Conflict," Households in Conflict Network and German Institute for Economic Research, February 1–2, 2010, Berlin.

22. Velma Šarić, "Demographics of Bosnian War Set Out," *Institute for War and Peace Reporting*, TRI, no. 739 (May 4, 2012), accessed August 13, 2017, https://iwpr.net/global-voices/demographics-bosnian-war-set-out.

23. Šarić, "Demographics of Bosnian War."

24. Mary E. Black, "Abdullah Nakas, Bosnia and Hercegovina's Most Famous War Surgeon," *British Medical Journal* 332, no. 7545 (April 8, 2006): 856, accessed August 14, 2017, http://www.jstor.org/stable/25456613.

25. Lynne Jones, "On a Front Line," *British Medical Journal* 310, no. 6986 (April 22, 1995): 1052, accessed August 14, 2017, http://www.jstor.org/stable/29727045.

26. Sanjay Kinra, Mary E. Black, Sanja Mandic, and Nora Selimovic, "Impact of the Bosnian Conflict on the Health of Women and Children," *Bulletin of the World Health Organization* 80, no. 1 (2002): 75–76, accessed August 14, 2017, http://www.who.int/bulletin/archives/80(1)75.pdf.

27. Zarema Obradovic, Snjezana Balta, Amina Obradovic, and Salih Mesic, "The Impact of War on Vaccine Preventable Diseases," *Mater Sociomed* 26, no. 6 (December 2014): 382, accessed August 14, 2017, https://www.ncbi.nlm.nih.gov/pmc/articles/PMC4314173/pdf/MSM-26-382.pdf.

28. Obradovic, Balta, Obradovic, and Mesic, "The Impact of War," 383.

29. Delan Devakumar et al., "The Intergenerational Effects of War on the Health of Children," *BMC Medicine* 12, no. 1 (April 2014): 4–7, accessed August 13, 2017, https://www.researchgate.net/publication/261325728_The_Intergenerational_Effects_of_War_on_the_Health_of_Children.

30. M. Hukic et al., "Mumps Outbreak in the Federation of Bosnia and Herzegovina with Large Cohorts of Susceptibles and Genetically Diverse Strains of Genotype G, Bosnia and Herzegovina, December 2010 to September 2012," *European Surveillance* 19, no 33 (2014), accessed August 13, 2017, http://www.eurosurveillance.org/ViewArticle.aspx?ArticleId=20879.

31. Hukic et al., "Mumps Outbreak," 2.

32. Line Neerup Handlos, Karen Fog Olwig, Ib Christian Bygbjerg, and Marie Norredam, "Return Migrants' Experience of Access to Care in Corrupt Healthcare Systems: The Bosnian Example," *International Journal of Environmental Research and Public Health* 13, no. 9 (September 2016): 2–3, accessed August 13, 2017, www.mdpi.com/1660-4601/13/9/924/pdf.

33. Devakumar, et al., "The Intergenerational Effects of War," 5.

34. Denis Dzidic, "Bosnia Still Living with Consequences of War," *Balkan Transitional Justice* (April 2012), accessed August 13, 2017, http://www.balkaninsight.com/en/article/bosnia-still-living-with-consequences-of-war.

35. Devakumar, et al., "The Intergenerational Effects of War," 8–10.

36. Lana Pašić, "Political and Social Consequences of Continuing Displacement in Bosnia and Herzegovina," *Forced Migration Review* 50 (September 2015): 7–8, accessed August 13, 2017, http://www.fmreview.org/dayton20/pasic.html.

37. Dzidic, "Bosnia Still Living with Consequences of War."

38. Theodore F. Robles, Ronald Glaser, and Janice K. Kiecolt-Glaser, "Out of Balance: A New Look at Chronic Stress, Depression, and Immunity," *Current Directions in Psychological Science* 14, no. 2 (April 2005): 113, accessed September 6, 2017, http://www.jstor.org/stable/20182999.

Part IV

Epidemics of Mixed Origins during Wartime: Introduction

Rebecca M. Seaman

> With epidemics, people have been standing on the shore, waiting for the gusher to hit the ocean. But to prevent epidemics, you have to look at the various little sources that feed into the river.[1]
>
> —Nathan Wolfe

Part IV of *Epidemics and War* clusters together three chapters dealing with epidemics from diverse origins. Unlike the chapters in previous sections, these particular infectious diseases originate and spread through a variety of vectors and causal agents: protozoa, virus, bacteria, fungi, and even the inhalation fumes. The unique versatility of these diseases facilitated the widespread undermining of the health in broad sectors of the military and society and caused some of the highest rates of mortality typically seen in wars.

The infections can be transferred by parasites—such as the protozoan parasites of the genus *Plasmodium* responsible for malaria. However, arthropods can also convey diseases, and in the case of malaria, mosquitoes are the vectors for the *Plasmodium* species that infect humans. The complex vector process for malaria is explored in the chapter on the malaria in the Vietnam War. This chapter investigates how prevention and treatment was developed. Included in this study is an analysis of why malaria continues to emerge during some wars, despite medical advancements and preventative precautions. Although the Vietnam War did not see as many cases or fatalities from malaria as World War II, it posed interesting dilemmas for the U.S. military abroad and at home, as preventative medications produced side effects that discouraged proper adherence to the prescribed protocols.

The chapter on dysentery during the American Civil War examines the spread and extensive impact of the disease on combatants from both sides of the conflict. Often contracted through exposure to the bacteria *Shigellae* or *Samonellae*, dysentery can also spread through amoebas, parasitic worms, viruses and other protozoa. An ancient disease, dysentery often accompanies warfare and is categorized as one of the camp diseases commonly found with the mobilization of troops. This chapter looks at the conditions associated with the spread of dysentery and the prevalence of the infection in military camps as well as in prisoner of war camps in the North and the South. In particular, the chapter examines how and why dysentery became the leading killer during the Civil War, accounting for over one-half of the total deaths from the war.

Finally, pneumonia is covered in part IV in this book. Like dysentery, pneumonia can be contracted through various vectors and through contact, from viruses and bacteria to fungi and inhalation of irritating fumes. Pneumonia is studied in this section through the lens of the American Civil War. Outbreaks of pneumonia in its various forms occurred repeatedly throughout the war, but cases were far less evident than the devastation cause by dysentery, the high death tolls of typhoid, and even the occasional high-impact measles epidemics during the war. Often spreading to patients with wounds or those suffering from other diseases, the secondary nature of pneumonia made this disease easy to overlook by doctors of the era, by record keepers, and consequently by researchers studying the impact of disease during the Civil War. Despite such oversights, pneumonia is noted as the third-deadliest disease of the war, affecting officers and soldiers from the Union and Confederacy, African Americans fighting or living in contraband camps, and volunteers and medical staff in the military and civilian hospitals.

Each chapter in this section follows an epidemic that spread through various causal agents and opportunities for increased diffusion. As a consequence, they impacted more victims than typically encountered during periods of war. Two chapters focus on 19th-century epidemics, specifically during the American Civil War, and account for well over 50 percent of the deaths during the war. The remaining chapter covers malaria in World War II, with its massive 20th-century impact, especially in the Pacific, African, and Indian Ocean regions, and traces the occurrence and impact of malaria forward into the Vietnam War. Although the wars selected for these chapters fall in the last century and a half, all three diseases and their impacts can be traced through wars across the ages.

NOTE

1. Elizabeth Svoboda, "Deep in the Rain Forest, Stalking the Next Pandemic," *The New York Times* (October 20, 2008), accessed February 19, 2018, https://mobile.nytimes.com/2008/10/21/health/research/21prof.html.

Chapter 16

Malaria: Continuing Pestilence from World War II to the Vietnam War, 1939–1975

Larry Grant

> The history of malaria in war might almost be taken to be the history of war itself, certainly the history of war in the Christian Era.[1]
> —Col. C. H. Melville, Royal Army Medical Corps

In late June 1956, the World Health Organization's (WHO) Expert Committee on Malaria met to discuss an agenda largely devoted to the eradication of malaria. The committee's conference report concluded that, "Parasites, anophelines and men are the three factors that maintain malaria." The significant sticking points to eradicating malaria lay primarily in the areas of "management, method and money."[2] According to the report, the technical means to eradicate malaria were available. Completing the task required only the creation of an organization with capable administration, the necessary technical expertise, and experience treating the disease. These reforms would enable WHO to carry out a last campaign against the scourge of malaria.[3] Much of the optimism evident in the 1956 report was based on the successes of the massive World War II program—sometimes called the "malaria Manhattan project"—undertaken by America and its allies. This project attempted to reduce the great manpower losses caused by malaria, particularly in the Pacific theater, where repeated outbreaks occurred. Inevitably, despite wartime advances, the reality of malaria proved more complicated than WHO had anticipated, and attempts to suppress it remained less successful than hoped.

Protozoan Origins of Malaria

Malaria in humans is caused by protozoan parasites of the genus *Plasmodium*. Of the many species in the genus, the classic parasites infecting humans are *Plasmodium falciparum*, *P. vivax*, *P. malariae*, and *P. ovale*. Researchers have recently used polymerase chain reaction (PCR) techniques[4] to identify a fifth *Plasmodium* species, *P. knowlesi*,[5] and two subspecies of *P. ovale* with different genetic structures, *P. ovale curtisi* and *P. ovale wallikeri*.[6] Globally, *P. falciparum* causes the most serious forms of malaria and a significant mortality rate. *P. vivax* inhabits the widest geographic distribution, causing nearly half of the malaria infections that occur outside of Africa. *P. ovale* and *P. malariae* occur chiefly in Sub-Saharan Africa (*P. ovale*) and in South America, Asia, and Africa (*P. malariae*), though they represent only a small percentage of all infections. *P. knowlesi*, a zoonotic species found in Southeast Asia that normally infects the Southeast Asian macaque monkey, was first reported in humans in 1965.[7]

An understanding of the epidemiology of malaria requires knowledge of human genetics and behavior. It also requires some knowledge of such environmental factors as temperature, vegetation, and water features that influence the size, extent, and longevity of mosquito populations, in particular populations of female *Anopheles* mosquitoes. Infection risk varies within these mosquito-infested regions, as species' distributions often overlap and other conditions vary throughout any geographic area. However, marshes and swamps provide many of the necessary ingredients. It is not surprising, therefore, that before the development of modern germ theory, physicians historically associated malaria and other fevers with marshes and swamps. The miasma theory posited that malaria—deriving from *mal'aria*, the Italian term for "bad air"—and similar diseases resulted from exposure to air polluted with invisible particles of decomposing matter called *miasmata*.[8] The frequent appearance of malaria near swampy regions marked by an odor of decay suggested to early physicians a significant connection between disease and environment. In 1834, Doctor Alfred T. Magill wrote, "The subject of malaria, or marsh effluvium, has for a long time attracted much of the attention of the medical profession." He added, "None of all the many 'ills which flesh is heir to,' has probably been so prolific of destruction and misery to the race of mankind, as miasmatic exhalation."[9]

Though expanding, 19th-century doctors' understanding of the variables relating to malaria remained incomplete before the development of microbiology. Treatments, therefore, were dependent on the information doctors gathered by observing patients, and what they distinguished most readily were fevers. In modern medicine, a fever is a physiological condition in which the body's temperature rises above normal in response to infection. Early doctors, being unable to ascertain the underlying causes, diagnosed and treated diseases based on the type of fever they observed. The deadliest fevers were malarial fevers, which they identified as intermittent, remittent, or relapsing fevers. By this scheme, relapsing fevers recurred after long intervals, days or weeks, of normal temperature. In patients with remittent fevers, the patient's temperature rose and fell but always remained above normal. Intermittent fevers reappeared after regular periods without fever—quartan occurring every third day, tertian every other day, and quotidian every day.[10]

Historical Connection of Malaria to Environment and Mosquitos

In 1876, following the discovery of the anthrax pathogen, *Bacillus anthracis*, scientists began to search for the microorganisms responsible for other diseases, leading to the rejection of the miasma explanation for malaria. In 1878, Scottish parasitologist Patrick Manson found evidence of a parasitic disease, *filariasis*, that was passed between human hosts by mosquitoes. When French army doctor Charles Louis Alphonse Laveran observed active parasites in the blood of a patient in 1880, he concluded that he had discovered the parasite responsible for malaria. British medical researcher Ronald Ross further advanced the study of malaria transmission in 1897 and 1898, when he determined the complete life cycle of the malarial parasite, including its development in the mosquito.

Even before the biological relationship between mosquito, man, and parasite was known, the miasma theory provided a paradigm for disease control. Reducing human exposure to low-lying wetlands where malaria occurred could be achieved by draining stagnant marshy areas; by warning people to avoid such regions; particularly at night; and by closing openings in dwellings.[11] In the 17th century, cinchona bark was introduced to Europe as an effective treatment for malaria. The occupation of Cuba following the Spanish-American War exposed U.S. soldiers to mosquito-borne disease. Considerable efforts in vector control followed, particularly during the construction of the Panama Canal, when the need to control malaria and yellow fever was crucial to the success of the project. U.S. Army physician and major general William C. Gorgas and others, such as Col. Joseph A. A. LePrince, worked to eliminate or reduce the effect of the diseases with a systematic program of mosquito control.[12]

In the southern United States, similar public health measures were undertaken in the 1930s as part of the Tennessee Valley project. Nearly a third of the population suffered from malaria when President Franklin D. Roosevelt authorized the project, but by 1947, the use of insecticides and elimination of breeding locations virtually eliminated the disease.[13] In Germany at the same time, chemists developed several compounds, in particular atabrine, which was used extensively during World War II, and chloroquine, which was widely used after the war. Swiss chemist Paul H. Müller added another tool in 1939 to existing oil and arsenical insecticides. He discovered that dichloro-diphenyl-trichloroethane (DDT), created in 1874, was so effective against mosquito adults and larvae that it eradicated the disease in many locations where it was applied. Within two years of this discovery, the United States was at war and forced to fight an expanded war with malaria in addition to the war against the Axis powers.

Writing on war, Carl von Clausewitz asserted, "Everything is very simple in war, but the simplest thing is difficult."[14] This applies equally to medical issues. Disease transmission becomes harder as medical facilities are destroyed and personnel killed, wounded, or scattered. Sources of water and food are disrupted. Combat forces populations into regions that harbor diseases to which they are exposed.[15] In wartime, soldiers who might never have encountered a tropical disease at home find themselves transported halfway around the globe to fight in areas where disease is endemic. Armies try to prepare for these circumstances, but despite advances in tropical medicine during World War II, they could not prevent the infection of soldiers who carelessly exposed themselves or were too engaged in the basic task of staying alive to worry about infection.

Nevertheless, the malaria Manhattan project advanced knowledge of disease vectors and doctors' ability to diagnose, treat, and even prevent malaria. Every expectation was that after the mid-20th century there should have been a corresponding decline in malarial outbreaks. Yet, with the escalation of the Vietnam conflict in the 1950s–1970s, malaria again had a major impact on military forces arrayed against each other in Southeast Asia. Additionally, the hoped-for medical solutions came with side effects. Chloroquine commonly produced deafness, tinnitus, anorexia, nausea, vomiting, and diarrhea. Atabrine produced similar effects, adding headaches, stomach cramps, and loss of appetite while simultaneously producing yellow skin tones and providing ineffective protection from malaria in its initial-dosage protocol. Both also had a history of producing hallucinations in some patients. These side effects discouraged soldiers and sailors from following the protocols for administration and led to continued outbreaks of malaria. Despite the optimism of the 1956 WHO report, malaria continued to impact military forces and even to spread among civilian populations when soldiers returned home.

History of Malaria during Wars

One of the earliest references to malaria in the context of American military operations was the Continental Congress's allocation of $300 during the Revolutionary War to purchase cinchona bark—the source of quinine—from South American sources to treat soldiers who had contracted the disease.[16] Malaria was a recognized problem for Continental units and likely an even greater concern for the short-term militia units with limited access to similar assistance. Both sides in the Revolutionary War suffered losses to diseases that were significantly higher than their losses in combat. Despite its impact, malaria may have provided a small benefit to Americans in their drive for independence when comparing their losses to the disease's effect on British forces. Historian J. R. McNeill argues that "differential immunities" to malaria favored the American formations and "put Cornwallis' forces at a systematic disadvantage. . . . Mosquitoes and malaria helped drive Cornwallis from the Carolinas and then sickened his army at Yorktown to the point where he lacked the manpower to conduct counter-siege operations properly. American resistance to the British Army had been made more effective by American resistance to malaria."[17]

Malaria peaked in the United States in the mid-19th century, reaching hyperendemic levels in the southeastern states. A few years later, this region became the main theater of the Civil War and the scene of the U.S. military's most significant experience with malaria during the 19th century.[18] The effect of disease on Civil War armies was, according to doctor and medical historian Jeffrey S. Sartin, "numbing in its enormity." Malaria, he wrote, accounted "for 1,316,000 episodes and 10,000 deaths. Similar data for Southern casualties are lacking because of the destruction of records by the invading troops, but incidence and death rates were probably similar."[19]

The Spanish-American War saw its share of malaria victims. *The Report of the Secretary of War*, dated November 29, 1898 (based on information reported through October 25, 1898), listed malarial diseases as the most significant contributor to the sick report with 38,833 cases. As Surgeon General Sternberg reported in his annual report to the secretary of war at the end of 1899, malarial fevers "are held accountable for 476 deaths. . . . The rate of death from these fevers was highest in Cuba, 10.80 [per thousand]; lowest in Luzon, 0.65—222 deaths having occurred in the former island and only 15 in the latter."[20] Diarrheal disease and yellow fever accounted for most of the remaining deaths from infection during the war. According to the secretary's report, malaria cases continued to rise from July to August, even as troop strengths started to fall. It is likely that some infected soldiers discharged in July did not appear in the infection data, instead carrying the disease home with them at war's end.

During World War I, around 20,000 cases were reported in all armies on both sides of the Western Front over the course of the war. The vast majority of malarial infections in the U.S. Army occurred in the continental United States. "Of the total 15,555 primary admissions for malaria in the United States Army, no less than 10,510 were in troops serving in the United States. Only 950 admissions are recorded as occurring in our troops serving in Europe."[21] Infection in the training camps was more prevalent during the summer and fall months, precisely the period during which the first recruits arrived at the training camps.[22] Aside from the physical shortcomings of the camps with respect to billeting, dining, and general hygiene, the training and information available to officers and NCOs was insufficient to combat ensuing epidemics. Another 4,094 cases were recorded in the Philippines, Panama, Puerto Rico, Hawaii, and in other countries not specified. Only 2 of the 36 deaths attributed to malaria occurred in Europe. U.S. naval forces, sailors and Marines stationed outside of Europe also suffered from malaria infections.[23] Nearly 5,000 cases and 7 deaths from malaria occurred during the war years. "During 1917 and 1918, malaria accounted for 4,746 new hospital admissions among naval forces. . . . Most of the cases occurred in the Western Hemisphere, including the Americas and the Caribbean region."[24]

Development of Medical Treatments for Malaria

The search for other drugs to treat malaria advanced during the interwar period. The first successful synthetic malaria drug was plasmochin, produced in 1924 by Wilhelm Roehl, a chemist working for the German pharmaceutical firm Bayer. In 1932, Bayer, by then one of the companies in the IG Farben cartel, marketed another synthetic antimalarial drug, atabrine. The cartel's American partner, the Winthrop Chemical Corporation, sold atabrine in the United States.[25] The development of plasmochin and atabrine did not result in the displacement of quinine in the treatment of malaria for several reasons. First, patients taking both synthetic drugs suffered from significant side effects, such as severe blood disorders in the case of plasmochin, and other less severe but undesirable effects in the case of atabrine. Second, despite artificially high prices caused by the Dutch growers' near-monopoly control of quinine's principal source, the Dutch colony of Java in the Southwest, the synthetics were too expensive to justify widespread use in peacetime.[26]

Two events, however, ended ready access to quinine for the Allied forces during World War II. The German invasion of the Netherlands in 1940 and the Japanese occupation of Java in 1941 gave those two Axis powers control of the existing stockpiles of the drug and the plantations where much of the world's quinine was grown.[27] As the military forces of the United States faced a sizeable threat from malaria in every theater of war during World War II except Western Europe, this circumstance forced the United States to search for alternatives to prevent large numbers of soldiers from being rendered ineffective for combat operations. The most significant impact was felt in two theaters, the Mediterranean and the Pacific. Soldiers, sailors, and airmen elsewhere were exposed to the disease on a regular basis, but efforts to control the disease in those areas were seldom interrupted—where materials were available—by combat operations.[28]

The initial operations of U.S. personnel, after the Operation Torch landings in North Africa in November 1942, were not much troubled by malaria. "Antimalaria units had accompanied British and American Forces in their long trek across the southern coast of the Mediterranean into Tunisia and had successfully controlled malaria among those forces." Later operations in Sicily, "which was known to be highly malarious," and Italy in 1943 saw the highest levels of infection in that theater for the war.[29] U.S. Army medical reports recorded 731 malaria cases in 1942 in the Mediterranean theater. The number soared to 32,811 in 1943, dropped by one-third to 23,985 in 1944, and fell to 5,765 in 1945. Dr. Justin Andrews, an authority who worked on malaria control in the Mediterranean theater and later served as director of the agency now known as the Centers for Disease Control and Prevention, wrote that "the high rate in 1943 was due to poor malaria discipline, imperfect Atabrine (quinacrine hydrochloride) supply, and inadequate malaria organization."[30] The 1945 decline demonstrates the importance of corrective efforts.

Great energy was also expended on more traditional methods to control mosquitos in combat theaters. Dr. Andrews wrote,

> In Africa and Sicily, main reliance was placed on the physical improvement of streams, oil larviciding, and spray killing with pyrethrum. In Sardinia, Corsica, and Italy, these measures were supplemented and finally overshadowed by the aerial application of paris green and DDT. . . . Insect-proofing of buildings was practiced as screening supplies permitted.[31]

The army relied on these techniques early in the war to allow time for the expansion of atabrine production. When the pharmaceutical industry began to fill the shortage in 1943, the army successfully treated personnel in the Mediterranean with atabrine, using large doses to control infection.[32]

Malaria's Impact during World War II and Korea

The pattern seen in the Mediterranean repeated itself in the Pacific, where malaria's effect on U.S. Army operations was evident from Gen. Douglas MacArthur's famous comment to Col. Paul F. Russell, M.C., in May 1943. MacArthur told

Russell, "Doctor, this will be a long war if for every division I have facing the enemy I must count on a second division in the hospital with malaria and a third division convalescing from this debilitating disease!"[33] Roughly one-third of the 75,000 American and Filipino soldiers defending the Philippines suffered from malaria, and equally high infection rates were observed elsewhere in the Southwest Pacific.[34] The U.S. Navy and Marine Corps also suffered seriously from malaria infection. Beginning in 1942, the number of new cases among naval personnel shot up and remained high for the balance of the war years. During World War II, there were a total of "113,256 new cases of malaria resulting in 90 deaths and 3,310,800 lost man-days" among U.S. Navy and U.S. Marine Corps personnel. In 1942, malaria outbreaks among U.S. Navy and Marine Corps forces "reached crippling, epidemic proportions."[35]

Organizationally, 1943 proved a pivotal year in the fight against malaria in the Pacific and elsewhere. In March, MacArthur created a Combined Advisory Committee on Tropical Medicine, Hygiene, and Sanitation. Staffed by military specialists from the United States and Australia, the committee advised MacArthur on the prevention and treatment of tropical diseases. The following month, Col. Howard F. Smith, a U.S. Public Health officer and MacArthur's aide-de-camp, was appointed as the Southwest Pacific Area malariologist. His first job was to find effective ways to treat infected soldiers, to prevent future infections, and to attack the disease in Australia, Borneo, and New Guinea.[36] Also in 1943, the end of legal restrictions on the manufacture of atabrine made the drug available in large quantities. Further, scientific and medical organizations, universities, hospitals, industries, and the armed forces joined in the U.S. government–subsidized Cooperative Wartime Program to undertake systematic exploration of chemical compounds in search of effective drugs.[37] Over the next decade, primaquine, chloroquine, pyrimethamine, and proguanil were introduced as a result.[38]

As alternative paths to securing antimalarial drugs increased, the United States sought other sources for quinine in South America with mixed results. Missions sent to South America were able to provide some 12.5 million pounds of cinchona bark to the Allies. In the parallel laboratory search for a solution, William E. Doering and Robert B. Woodward created synthetic quinine in 1944. Although the method they employed to create the synthetic was not suitable for commercial manufacture, it sparked the development of other drugs that contributed to control of the disease.[39]

In the initial three-year period of the Korean conflict, more than 2 million Americans deployed to the Korean Peninsula. Malaria was a constant threat to U.S. personnel in Korea because of a large civilian reservoir of the disease and the presence of anopheline mosquitoes, primarily infected with *P. vivax*. Despite the recent advances made by the U.S. Army by the end of World War II, 311 cases of malaria and 29 deaths occurred among U.S. troops in 1950 alone.[40] Still, annual in-theater malaria admission rates in Korea remained below 20 per 1,000 during the war, a figure much lower than the overall rate (70.3 per 1,000 per year) for World War II.[41] The threat malaria presented, however, was not limited to the region. Soldiers returning to the United States from Korea brought malaria home with them. More than 10,000 cases were diagnosed in the United States from 1950 to 1954.[42] Later, American soldiers who were posted to South Korea continued to be exposed, and another outbreak in the United States caused by returning service members occurred in the mid-1960s. Seven cases were eventually diagnosed at Fort Benning, Georgia.[43] Soldiers later returning from Vietnam caused similar outbreaks.

America, the Vietnam War, and the Spread of Malaria

American involvement in Vietnam was initially small. In September 1950, the United States dispatched a 35-man Military Assistance Advisory Group (MAAG) to Saigon to coordinate aid and advice to the southern Vietnamese government.[44] The number of Americans dispatched to Vietnam remained small until 1954, when the French withdrew from the country after their defeat by the Viet Minh communist forces. The Geneva Agreements ended France's colonial rule in the region and partitioned Vietnam at the 17th parallel. Soon after, Americans began to trickle into South Vietnam to bolster the noncommunist government there. The contingent of U.S. military advisers posted to the country grew slowly during the Eisenhower administration. In 1955, there were 427 Americans in country and about 750–800 from 1956 to 1960. The number of Americans in the country increased to almost 1,000 in the first year of the Kennedy administration and then jumped to 8,500 in 1962. Following the Tonkin Gulf incident, President Lyndon B. Johnson expanded American military operations in Vietnam.[45] After peaking at 543,400 Americans in April 1969, the new administration of President Richard M. Nixon reevaluated U.S. involvement and began a drawdown of American personnel in South Vietnam. Following the Paris Peace Accords (January 27, 1973), the number of Americans continued to decline until all had been withdrawn in 1975.[46] South Vietnam collapsed under the weight of a North Vietnamese attack in the spring of 1975.

South Vietnam has three well-defined geographic areas that include the Mekong Delta region, the Annamese Cordillera mountain range, and a narrow coastal plain. The Mekong Delta, covering an area of about 65,000 square kilometers, forms where the Mekong River empties into the South China Sea, about 120 kilometers south of Ho Chi Minh City (previously Saigon). The delta experiences heavy rainfall, and as a rice-producing area, the ground is regularly covered with standing water. The Annamese Cordillera parallels the Vietnamese coastline along the border between Laos and Vietnam in a northwest-southeast direction. At its southern end, the range curves to the southwest before ending near Ho Chi Minh City. Several high plateaus, the Kontum, Lam Vien, and Dac Lac plateaus—known to Americans as the Central Highlands—form the south end of the range. Only a few places in the highland areas reached elevations above 2,000 meters. This means that most of the region is accessible to common mosquito vectors that prefer elevations under 1,500 meters. Heavy rainfall in the monsoon season and the dense vegetation on the plateaus ensure many breeding sites. The Vietnamese coastal plain lies between the Annamese Cordillera and the South China Sea. The region of interest for this chapter on malaria lies south of the 17th parallel; this coastal plain continues north to the delta of the Red River. In this coastal strip, rice and sugarcane are the major crops.

In Vietnam, the predominant malaria parasites and associated vectors infecting humans are the *Plasmodium* species, *P. falciparum* and *P. vivax*, and the mosquito species *Anopheles minimus*, *A. dirus*, and *A. sundaicus*.[47] Americans in South Vietnam also encountered the parasite *P. malariae*. *P. falciparum* is prevalent in the Central Highlands region, and *P. vivax* and *P. malariae* are widespread in the coastal and delta regions. The density of the vectors carrying the parasites also varies according to region and the seasonal climate, wet or dry. For example, *Anopheles minimus* is an important vector throughout Vietnam; but as the rainy season lengthens, conditions became less favorable for *A. minimus*, and the vector's population-density drops. Meanwhile, *A. jeyporiensis*, another highland vector, breeds effectively even during heavier rainfall. Consequently, the potential for exposure during the war was continuous whether the season was rainy or dry.[48]

As the U.S. commitment in Vietnam grew, the optimism of the 1950s malaria fighters collided with the reality of an evolving disease. Chloroquine-resistant malaria appeared among U.S. forces stationed in South Vietnam.[49] In response, in 1964, the army renewed its research into new antimalarial drugs to deal with the resistance threat.[50] Extensive medical support and disease control programs were introduced in Vietnam alongside American troop formations.[51] To ensure an early return to duty by as many personnel as possible, hospitals and a convalescent center were established. Major facilities in Vietnam included three 500-bed hospitals (two at Qui Nhon and one at Vung Tau), a mobile surgical hospital (An Khe), and a convalescent hospital with initially 1,000 beds, which were later doubled (Cam Ranh Bay). Smaller facilities and field hospitals were built throughout South Vietnam at most major troop concentrations.[52] Consequently, almost all patients diagnosed with *falciparum* were treated and returned to duty in Vietnam.[53]

An effective system of medical care, however, did not mean that malaria was eliminated as a concern. During the Vietnam War, malaria was the single most important infectious disease disrupting the health and effectiveness of the American military personnel deployed to Southeast Asia. In Vietnam, malaria was the third most frequent medical cause of hospitalization of army personnel, behind respiratory and diarrheal diseases. However, the extended time required for treatment and recuperation made malaria the major cause of medical disability.[54] By late 1965, nearly 10 percent of soldiers deployed in South Vietnam had contracted the disease. Deputy Surgeon General Spurgeon Neel wrote, "In December 1965, the over-all Army rate in Vietnam reached a peak of 98.4 per 1,000 per year; during that period, rates for certain units operating in the Ia Drang valley were as high as 600 per 1,000 per year, and at least two maneuver battalions were rendered ineffective by malaria."[55] More than 80,000 malaria cases were diagnosed in American soldiers from 1965 to 1971, though the low overall mortality rate (1.7 per 1,000) reflected the army's ability to diagnosis and treat new cases quickly.[56]

In addition to its effects on U.S. personnel, malaria was also a problem for the North Vietnamese Army (NVA) and its Viet Cong allies. Information from a captured medical report shows that, in late 1965, 6 percent of VC Detachment 204, Inter Detachment 200, was stricken with malaria—one-half of the unit's total sick list. The "incidence of malaria for all VC/NVA forces in South Vietnam during 1965," the analysis states, "was 15.5% per month. 66.9 % of these individuals were non-effective . . . because of malaria. If we assume that all of the non-effectives were hospitalized, 10.4% (15.5% × 66.9%) of the enemy were hospitalized each month with malaria."[57] Despite the use of antimalarial drugs, 80–100 percent of the Viet Cong troops were reported to have contracted malaria.[58]

To combat malaria that had infected as many as 50 percent of U.S. soldiers, the U.S. Air Force ordered the modification of the first of two UC-123 Provider military transports, previously engaged in herbicide spraying, to attack the mosquito vector through aerial spraying of insecticide. The 12th Air Commando Squadron aircraft began operations in late 1966 and formally began Operation FLYSWATTER in March 1967.[59] By mid-1967, the squadron was flying 20 sorties monthly, covering 15,000 acres per sortie. Flights took place shortly after dawn and shortly before sunset to coincide with the times when the mosquitos were most active. "The 'mosquito war' required over 1,300 individual missions and dispensed approximately 1.76 million liters of malathion concentrate. Operation FLYSWATTER was a significant part of the overall United States' preventative medicine program to reduce the number of man-days lost to ground forces due to malaria."[60]

The U.S. Army's surgeon general documented the varying effects of malaria on U.S. forces in Vietnam. The number of hospital admissions peaked near 100 per 1,000 in mid-1965, when troop formations first arrived. During the following year, the number of cases admitted oscillated from about 20–60 per 1,000. By 1969, the situation, if not entirely under control, had at least stabilized and remained consistently below about 30 cases per 1,000. The total number of cases and the number of deaths suffered by the U.S. Army during the five-year period, 1965–1970, tells the same story. Statistical analysis indicates that, while the total magnitude of the number of cases fell slowly, the rate of infection decreased more quickly due to the larger total population against which it is measured. For example, during 1967, the year with the highest total number of cases, the percentage rate of infection declined over the two previous years despite the increase in personnel, from about 130,000 in 1965 to four times that number, a total of 451,752, in 1967.[61]

Malaria on the Homefront in America

Rather than ending the malarial threat as U.S. troops were withdrawn from Vietnam, the return of large numbers of infected soldiers brought a new malaria danger to American shores. From 1966 to 1973, imported malaria caused more than 13,000 cases of *P. vivax* malaria in the United States, "the vast majority being imported infections related to service in Vietnam."[62] The downward trend in infections among returning military personnel continued in 1974, "but the incidence of malaria among civilians increased significantly."[63] Though not as pronounced as the increase in military cases, the rise in civilian cases is documented in a WHO 1974 report.[64]

Various pathways existed to spread the infection among the civilian neighbors of returned soldiers. Though malaria was no longer endemic in the United States, the mosquito vectors still existed in many parts of the country. As mentioned above, seven cases of malaria resulted at Fort Benning, Georgia, when sick soldiers returning from Korea passed the disease to local mosquitoes that infected military dependents.[65] The potential for the same mechanism to carry infection to the civilian population continued to exist, as was shown by the diagnosis of *P. vivax* infection in a group of Rangers long after their return to base following deployments to Afghanistan and Iraq.[66]

In addition to the natural vectors in the environment, malaria can be transmitted through other means. From 1972 to 1981, the Centers for Disease Control and Prevention (CDC) received reports of 26 cases of malaria that had resulted from blood transfusions. Of these cases, three donors were former military personnel who had acquired the disease while in Southeast Asia.[67] Intravenous drug use offered yet another method of transmission. From December 1970 through March of the following year, 48 cases of malaria were diagnosed in Kern County, California. In each case, the individual admitted to sharing drug paraphernalia, and authorities identified a Vietnam veteran as the probable source of infection. The veteran had not taken the prescribed medications to ensure against infection. The editors of the report noted that this was the third outbreak in the past six months.[68]

Combination of War, Malaria, and Failed Medical Protocols

Public health investigators who "researched this problem in detail . . . concluded that non-adherence to the recommended chemoprophylaxis regimen was widespread."[69] A study conducted at Fort Bragg, North Carolina, in 1970 found that "only 7.5% of individuals who completed a supervised 14-day regimen suffered a relapse, confirming primaquine's efficacy when used properly. In contrast, 22.3% of individuals who were given the unsupervised and self-administered 8-week regimen suffered a relapse." The researchers concluded that well-supplied and well-informed servicemen simply failed to comply with the recommend malaria countermeasures, contributing to their own relapses and to the potential spread of the disease among the civilian population.[70]

Malaria has seen a dramatic increase in public understanding of the origin, spread, and prevention of the disease, especially over the last few decades. Yet, the continued presence of geographic conditions and vectors, combined with the deployment of military personnel to regions with endemic malaria, provides a pathway for more outbreaks while the side effects of countermeasures discourage strict administration of antimalarial regimens. In 2011, after over nearly a decade of fighting in Afghanistan, 91 cases of malaria were contracted, "the highest number recorded among U.S. military members serving in that country in the last nine years; moreover, the Afghanistan-acquired cases constituted 73 percent of all documented malaria cases last year." As Col. Mark M. Fukuda noted, "After ten years of U.S. military presence in Afghanistan, and despite the availability of effective prevention measures and a long organizational history of fighting the disease, malaria remains a threat to U.S. forces and their operations in Afghanistan."[71] As the Ranger case cited above shows—where only 41 percent of the soldiers complied fully with medical direction—malaria will likely continue to impact military and civilian populations well into the future.

NOTES

1. Ronald Ross, *The Prevention of Malaria* (New York: E. P. Dutton & Co., 1910), 577.
2. World Health Organization, *Expert Committee on Malaria*, Sixth Report (WHO/Mal/180, June 28, 1956), 21–22.
3. World Health Organization, *Expert Committee on Malaria*.
4. The polymerase chain reaction is a technique used by molecular biologists when dealing with very small DNA samples to create additional copies of a DNA sequence of interest (even many millions) for easier analysis.
5. Anu Kantele and T. Sakari Jokiranta, "Review of Cases with the Emerging Fifth Human Malaria Parasite, *Plasmodium knowlesi*," *Clinical Infectious Diseases* 52, no. 11 (2011): 1356–1362, accessed September 2, 2017, http://cid.oxfordjournals.org/content/52/11/1356.full; and N. W. Lucchi et al., "A New Single-Step PCR Assay for the Detection of the Zoonotic Malaria Parasite *Plasmodium knowlesi*," *PLoS One* 7, no. 2 (2012): e31848, Epub February 20, 2012, accessed by September 2, 2017, http://www.ncbi.nlm.nih.gov/pubmed/22363751.
6. Adriana Calderaro et al., "Accurate Identification of the Six Human *Plasmodium* Spp. Causing Imported Malaria, including *Plasmodium ovale wallikeri* and *Plasmodium knowlesi*," *Malaria Journal* 12, no. 321 (2013), accessed September 2, 2017, https://malaria journal.biomedcentral.com/articles/10.1186/1475-2875-12-321.
7. William Chin, Peter G. Contacos, G. Robert Coatney, and Harry R. Kimball. "A Naturally Acquired Quotidian-Type Malaria in Man Transferable to Monkeys," *Science* 149, no. 3686 (August 1965): 865, doi:10.1126/science.149.3686.865.
8. Malaria is also called marsh or swamp fever because of its historical association with such areas. Steven R. Meshnick and Mary J. Dobson, "The History of Antimalarial Drugs," in *Antimalarial Chemotherapy: Mechanisms of Action, Resistance, and New Directions in Drug Discovery*, ed. Philip J. Rosenthal (Totowa, NJ: Humana Press Inc., 2001), 15.
9. Edmund Ruffin, ed., "On Malaria: Extracts from Three Lectures on the Origin and Properties of Malaria and Marsh Miasma," *The Farmer's Register* 2, no. 1 (June 1834): 20.
10. H. K. Walker, W. D. Hall, and J. W. Hurst, eds., *Clinical Methods: The History, Physical, and Laboratory Examinations*, 3rd ed. (Boston: Butterworths, 1990). Modern doctors believe that historical reports of patients with remittent fevers were ill with typhoid infections instead of malaria, while intermittent and relapsing fevers indicate patients with one or another variant of malaria. Though fever as an indicator can be misleading, modern medical techniques have linked intermittent tertian fevers to infection by the *P. falciparum*, *P. vivax*, and *P. ovale* parasites, and quartan fevers have been linked to the *P. malariae* parasite.

11. Ka-che Yip, *Disease, Colonialism, and the State: Malaria in Modern East Asian History* (Hong Kong: Hong Kong University Press, 2009), 3.

12. "LePrince, Malaria Fighter," *Public Health Reports* 71, no. 8 (August 1956): 756–758.

13. Kenneth J. Arrow, Claire B. Panosian, and Hellen Gelband, eds., *Saving Lives, Buying Time: Economics of Malaria Drugs in an Age* (Washington, D.C.: National Academies Press, 2004), 127.

14. Carl von Clausewitz, *On War*, eds. Michael Howard and Peter Paret (New York: Oxford University Press, 2006), 65.

15. Kenrad E. Nelson et al., *Infectious Disease Epidemiology: Theory and Practice* (Sudbury, MA: Jones and Bartlett Pub., 2005), 685.

16. Edgar Erskine, *Victories of Army Medicine; Scientific Accomplishments of the Medical Department of the United States Army* (Philadelphia: J. B. Lippincott Co., 1943), 160.

17. J. R. McNeill, *Mosquito Empires: Ecology and War in the Greater Caribbean, 1620–1914* (New York: Cambridge University Press, 2010), 233.

18. O'Neill Barrett Jr., "Malaria: Epidemiology," in *Internal Medicine in Vietnam*, eds. Andre Ognibene and O'Neill Barrett Jr., Vol. 2, *General Medicine and Infectious Disease* (Washington, D.C.: Office of the Surgeon General & Center for Military History, 1982), 286.

19. Jeffrey S. Sartin, "Infectious Diseases during the Civil War: The Triumph of the 'Third Army,'" *Clinical Infectious Diseases* 16, no. 4 (April 1993): 580–534, accessed September 7, 2017, http://www.jstor.org/stable/4457020.

20. U.S. Army, Surgeon-General's Office, *Report of the Surgeon-General of the Army to the Secretary of War for the Fiscal Year Ending June 30, 1899* (Washington, D.C.: U.S. Government Printing Office, 1899), 239.

21. Joseph F. Siler, *The Medical Department of the United States Army in the World War*, Vol. 9, *Communicable and Other Diseases* (Washington, D.C.: GPO, 1928), 513.

22. Siler, *The Medical Department of the United States Army*, 519; Roger K. Spickelmier, *Training of the American Soldier during World War I and World War II* (Fort Leavenworth, KS: U.S. Army Command and General Staff College, 1987), 28, 30.

23. Siler, *The Medical Department of the United States Army*, 512.

24. Christine Beadle and Stephen L. Hoffman, "History of Malaria in the United States Naval Forces at War: World War I through the Vietnam Conflict," *Clinical Infectious Diseases* 16, no. 2 (February 1993): 320–329, 322.

25. Leo Barney Slater, *War and Disease: Biomedical Research on Malaria in the Twentieth Century* (New Brunswick, NJ: Rutgers University Press, 2009), 48, 70.

26. Slater, *War and Disease*, 82.

27. Sonia Shah, *The Fever: How Malaria Has Ruled Humankind for 500,000 Years* (New York: Sarah Crichton Books, 2010), 99.

28. U.S. Army Medical Department, *Preventive Medicine in World War II*, Vol. 8, *Civil Affairs /Military Government Public Health Activities*, Part 3, *The Mediterranean* (Washington, D.C., 1976), 231–232.

29. U.S. Army Medical Department, *Preventive Medicine*, 232–234.

30. Justin M. Andrews, "North Africa, Italy, and the Islands of the Mediterranean," U.S. Army Medical Department, *Preventive Medicine in World War II*, ed. John Boyd Coates, Vol. 6, *Communicable Diseases, Malaria* (Washington, D.C., 1963), 249, accessed September 7, 2017, http://history.amedd.army.mil/booksdocs/wwii/Malaria/chapterV.htm.

31. Andrews, "North Africa." Paris green is arsenical insecticide used in the late 19th and 20th centuries for mosquito abatement.

32. Andrews, "North Africa," 249–250.

33. John Boyd Coates, ed., *Preventive Medicine in World War II*, Vol. 6, *Communicable Diseases, Malaria* (Washington, D.C.: Office of the Surgeon General, U.S. Army Medical Department, 1963), 2.

34. Seth Paltzer, "The Other Foe: The U.S. Army's Fight against Malaria in the Pacific Theater, 1942–45," Army Historical Foundation, *On Point*, April 30, 2016, accessed September 7, 2017, https://armyhistory.org/on-point.

35. Beadle and Hoffman, "History of Malaria in the United States Naval Forces," 322.

36. Ralph Chester Williams, MD, *The United States Public Health Service, 1798–1950* (Washington, D.C.: Commissioned Officers Association of the United States Public Health Service, 1951), 712.

37. M. H. Bickel, "The American Malaria Program (1941–1946) and Its Sequelae for Biomedical Research after World War II," *Gesnerus* 56, no. 1–2 (1999): 107–119.

38. Stanley C. Oaks et al., eds., *Malaria: Obstacles and Opportunities* (Washington, D.C.: National Academies, 1991), 157.

39. Vassiliki Betty Smocovitis, "Desperately Seeking Quinine: The Malaria Threat Drove the Allies' WWII Cinchona Mission," *Modern Drug Discovery* 6, no. 5 (May 2003): 57–58.

40. Richard V. N. Ginn, *The History of the U.S. Army Medical Service Corps* (Washington, D.C.: GPO, 1996), 242.

41. Overall admissions for malaria during Korea were 11.2 per 1,000. Spurgeon Neel, *Medical Support of the U.S. Army in Vietnam 1965–1970* (Washington, D.C.: GPO, 1973), 37.

42. M. G. Schultz, "Imported Malaria," *Bull World Health Organ* 50 (1974): 329–336.

43. James P. Luby et al., "Introduced Malaria at Fort Benning, GA: 1964–1965," *American Journal of Tropical Medicine and Hygiene* 16 (1967): 146–153.

44. MAAG continued until 1964, when the Military Assistance Command Vietnam (MACV) assumed the unit's duties.

45. Tonkin Gulf Resolution, Public Law 88-408, 78 Stat. 384 (August 10, 1964).

46. Directorate for Information, Operations, and Reports, *Department of Defense Selected Manpower Statistics, Fiscal Year 1983* (Washington, D.C.: Department of Defense, 1984), 128.

47. World Health Organization, *World Malaria Report* (2015), 176.

48. O'Neill Barrett Jr., "Malaria: Epidemiology," in *Internal Medicine in Vietnam*, Vol. 2, ed. Andre J. Ognibene (Washington, D.C.: Center for Military History, 1982): 279.

49. Andre J. Ognibene and Nicholas F. Conte, "Malaria: Chemotherapy," in *Internal Medicine in Vietnam*, Vol. 2, ed. Andre J. Ognibene (Washington, D.C.: Center for Military History, 1982): 313.

50. Stanley C. Oaks Jr., et al., *Malaria: Obstacles and Opportunities* (Washington, D.C.: National Academies Press, 1991), 157–158.

51. Neel, *Medical Support of the U.S. Army*, 32.

52. Carroll H. Dunn, *Base Development in South Vietnam, 1965–1970* (Washington, D.C.: GPO, 1991), 75–77.

53. Andre J. Ognibene, ed., *Internal Medicine in Vietnam*, Vol. 2 (Washington, D.C.: Center for Military History, 1982), 55.

54. C. J. Canfield, "Malaria in U.S. Military Personnel 1965–1971," *Proceedings of the Helminthological Society of Washington* 39 (Special Issue, Basic Research in Malaria, 1972): 15–18.

55. Neel, *Medical Support of the U.S. Army*, 38.

56. Canfield, "Malaria in U.S. Military Personnel," 15.

57. Thomas C. Thayer, ed., *A Systems Analysis View of the Vietnam War 1965–1972, Casualties and Losses*, Vol. 8, AD A051613 (Washington, D.C.: Department of Defense, OASD (SA) RP Southeast Asia Intelligence Division, 1975): 10, 19–20.

58. Andre J. Ognibene and O'Neil Barrett, "Clinical Disorders: Malaria," in *Internal Medicine in Vietnam*, Vol. 2, ed. Andre J. Ognibene (Washington, D.C.: Center for Military History, 1982): 276–277.

59. Alvin Lee Young, *The History, Use, Disposition and Environmental Fate of Agent Orange* (New York: Springer, 2009), 112–113.

60. Paul F. Cecil Sr. and Alvin L. Young, "Operation FLYSWATTER: A War within a War," *Environmental Science and Pollution Research* 15, no. 1 (2007): 3–7.

61. Figure taken from Canfield, "Malaria in U.S. Military Personnel," 16.

62. William D. Porter, "Imported Malaria: 50 Years of U.S. Military Experience," *Military Medicine* 171 (October 2006): 926–927.

63. "News," *Journal of Infectious Diseases* 133, no. 1 (January 1976): 95.

64. Figure taken from Schultz, "Imported Malaria," 50, 329–336. Chart on 330.

65. Porter, "Imported Malaria," 926.

66. Russ S. Kotwal et al., "An Outbreak of Malaria in US Army Rangers Returning from Afghanistan," *JAMA* 293, no. 2 (January 12, 2005): 214.

67. Isabel C. Guerrero et al., "Transfusion Malaria in the United States, 1972–1981," *Annals of Internal Medicine* 99 (1983): 221–226.

68. Centers for Disease Control and Prevention, "Induced Malaria—California," *Morbidity and Mortality Weekly Report* (March 27, 1971), 99–100.

69. Porter, "Imported Malaria," 926–927.

70. Like atabrine and chloroquine, primaquine's common side effects include stomachaches, loss of appetite, tiredness, weakness, and fever.

71. Mark M. Fukuda, "Editorial: Malaria in the U.S. Armed Forces: A Persistent but Preventable Threat," *Medical Surveillance Monthly Report* 19, no.1 (January 2012): 12.

Chapter 17

Dysentery in the American Civil War: An Inverse Force Multiplier, 1861–1865

Joshua M. Seaman

Dysentery is one of the four great epidemic diseases of the world. . . . It has been more fatal to armies than powder and shot.[1]

—William Osler

Diseases in 21st-century wars rarely carry the same gravity as those of the 19th century. Military leaders of the 19th century were compelled to calculate disease into their decision-making process because of its immense impact on the number of effective troops. Seeking to ensure the greatest possible strength, the army sought ways to improve the individual and group effectiveness of its soldiers and armies, thus making them stronger despite static enlistments. Modern military theory refers to the improved effectiveness of units as force multiplies. Diseases, however, produced the inverse of that concept, reducing the effective strength of an army despite the maintenance of static numbers of troops; in effect, disease was a force divider. Fortunately, modern medicines and sanitary practices have largely eliminated the diseases that once plagued field commanders. Because of the potential for disease to still wreak havoc on military campaigns and strategies, historians and medical doctors alike expended a great deal of effort to explore disease and its impacts during the American Civil War.

Disease as the Leading Killer in the Civil War

When measuring the lives lost during the war, the clear front-runner for cause was disease. Jeffrey Sartin, a medical doctor specializing in infectious diseases, cleverly coined disease as the "Third Army" in his study that explored the extent to which disease reduced both the Union and Confederate Armies. This Third Army plagued commanders and reduced the fighting capacity of the two standing armies throughout the Civil War. Because germ theory was yet unknown to physicians, military, and government leaders, this Third Army had the distinct advantage of being invisible to the naked eye. This invisibility precluded physicians from combating it effectively. Frederick Law Olmsted, the secretary of the Sanitary Commission during the war, provided direction to military leaders that demonstrated the contemporary understanding of how disease worked and how to combat it:

> It is well known that when a considerable body of men have been living together in a camp a few weeks a peculiar subtle poison is generated, the effect of which is exhibited in stiffness of the muscles; sickness of the stomach in the morning; sudden and unusual looseness of the bowels; and subsequently by dysentery, and other endemic and epidemic diseases of a still more fatal character, such as camp fevers and cholera.
>
> The conditions under which men can successfully resist this danger of camp life are as well determined, and the establishment of them forms as much a part of a commander's duty as the means of guarding against a surprise by an enemy. They are—1.—Regular action of the bowels; 2.—Pure air; 3.—Keeping the pores of the skin open and clean.[2]

Although the directive focused on clean air and clean bodies, it still lacked any understanding of microorganisms. Unseen and misunderstood, these microorganisms had a visible and staggering impact upon both the Confederate and Union Armies.

Union Army records indicate that nearly 63 percent of Union deaths were somehow related to disease. Confederate medical records, which are unfortunately less complete, indicate a similar 64 percent of deaths related to disease.[3] The remaining deaths were associated with battlefield action or from wounds received. It is staggering to consider that two-thirds of all military lives lost during to the Civil War had virtually nothing to do with direct battlefield action, but rather were caused by non-combat-related activity. The number of deaths, however, is not the only important metric to consider. Many of the soldiers wounded on the battlefield and those who contracted some form of a disease did not die. These wounded and diseased were frequently removed from muster and drained the fighting capabilities of the Union and Confederate Armies.

Difficulty in Identifying Dysentery among Other Illnesses

One disease with high morbidity was dysentery. Not necessarily fatal, it nonetheless had a noteworthy impact on both armies in the Civil War. As an infectious disease, dysentery influenced military personnel and even strategies. The magnitude of its spread, its debilitating effects, recurrence in the same individuals, and its ability to kill its victims all contributed to its importance.[4] The origin and spread of dysentery epidemics among armies of the Union and Confederacy, and the consequent impact on the conduct and outcome of the Civil War, set the stage for later scientific discoveries that prompted significant medical and military reforms. These discoveries and reforms helped improve military health in subsequent wars.

The study of dysentery presented its own challenges. First, disease was so prevalent and multivariant during the American Civil War that dysentery was often accompanied by any number of other conditions. Typhoid, malaria, measles, smallpox, pneumonia, tuberculosis, scurvy, and many others were commonly reported. The diseases manifested themselves differently, but their contemporaneous existence in a single patient or their simultaneous outbreak in a single unit increased the difficulty for historians to isolate the individual impact of dysentery as a disease. Civil War medical records additionally confounded the study of dysentery. Dysentery and diarrhea were diagnosed and recorded together, and even referred to interchangeably. Both are very similar in symptoms and diagnosis, but they have specific causes that may be quite different. Regardless, their practical effects on the individuals presenting symptoms were quite similar. Because of their practical effects and Civil War medical records, both conditions are considered together in this chapter.

Finally, dysentery during the American Civil War also presents a particularly interesting case for historians because it easily and effectively conveys the deep and tragic relationship between conflict and disease. Despite having some rudimentary knowledge to prevent the spread of "camp diseases," as they were commonly known, the need to expeditiously carry out the war conflicted with and often outweighed the precautions known to reduce the spread of disease. Therefore, in carrying out the war, commanders often unwittingly fostered the growth and spread of disease; subsequently, disease severely reduced the commander's ability to fight the war.

Tracing the History of a Disease with Multiple Causes

Also known as the "bloody flux," dysentery has plagued human populations for millennia. The history of dysentery can be traced through Sanskrit documents as early as 1000 BCE. Unlike many diseases that have viral, bacterial, or protozoa origins, dysentery has numerous origins, including irritation caused by chemicals. Historically common contagion originates through a bacterial or amoebic infection. The two principal bacteria responsible include the *Shigellae* and *Samonellae* groups. The *Shigellae* form was most likely to result in epidemics.[5] The amoeba-based cause of dysentery was typically *Entamoeba histolytica*. This amoeba was responsible for the most virulent cases of dysentery that resulted in death. Instead of just irritating the colon and causing severe diarrhea, the amoebas were able to heavily infect the lungs, brains, and other bodily organs beyond the gastrointestinal system.[6] Long before scientific ability was present to discern bacterial or protozoan presence in human fecal matter, recognition of different impacts of the disease on the human body became evident. As early as the second century CE, physicians began to discern a difference between bacterial and amoebic dysentery by virtue of observing the effects upon the liver, even though they had no understanding of the microscopic bacteria or amoeba responsible for the divergent results.[7]

Dysentery commonly presented as any sort of diarrhea or loose stool with the presence of blood. Pus or mucus was often present in the blood and stool mixture.[8] Transmission of these microbes occurred solely through contact and ingestion. When a person came into contact with and ingested the bacteria or amoebas, the resulting contagion attacked the entirety of the gastrointestinal system. Dysentery principally affected the large intestine, which in turn caused the loose, frequent, and bloody stools. The microbes were subsequently transmitted from the affected person through his or her feces. If the feces were not disposed of properly or left exposed, the potential for further transmission to another person increased. Contamination of water sources by fecal matter typically helped spread the disease in its bacterial and protozoan forms.

Simple exposure to contaminated foods or fluids did not ensure the acquisition of dysentery. Diets lacking a complete nutritional profile encourage the susceptibility of individuals to dysentery-causing microbes.[9] Long campaigns, inadequate diets, and the general lack of hygienic routines set the stage for large numbers of military personnel to become infected. The lack of knowledge on the part of physicians and military officers perpetuated the very conditions that exposed soldiers to dysentery and helped to spread the disease in crowded camp conditions. The relatively novel formula provided by Secretary Olmsted's directions to regimental commanders at the beginning of the war was mostly based on theories of order and cleanliness, not on medical knowledge of germ theory or an understanding of protozoa contamination. Consequently, if carried out dutifully and to the letter, these instructions would improve health but not necessarily deter the spread of dysentery. His instructions failed to take into account the reality of microorganisms that were at the root cause of dysentery, namely, field sanitation and a balanced diet.

Mid-19th-century physicians, unlike their modern counterparts, lacked even the most basic understanding of bacteria and amoebae. The concept of nonvisible living entities was not widespread or understood, and certainly not adopted by the U.S. military. It was not until after the war had reached its conclusion that physicians came to broadly adopt and apply the knowledge of microorganisms.[10] Even then, it was only after the Spanish-American War that the Army Medical Corps made radical reforms based on the new medical knowledge. Nevertheless, the military and its medical officers did understand issues of sanitation and hygiene to a certain extent.

To better understand the causes of a variety of diseases, Civil War physicians observed the occurrence of diseases and their transmission to help determine dysentery's general cause—unsanitary conditions. William Hammond, the surgeon general of the U.S. Army, set out clear guidelines for field hygiene in his *Treatise on Hygiene* published in 1863. Hammond warned against mass encampments and provided detailed tables on healthy spacing for camps, stating, "Battalion camps are not unfrequently [sic] arranged in such a way that the tents touch each other, except where a narrow passage is left between the rows for access. A camp so arranged can never be clean nor healthy."[11] Unfortunately, these instructional guidelines did not pinpoint the issues completely and focused on less-conclusive and often conflicting evidence. Indeed, inspections found that some of the cleaner camps experienced a higher rate of diarrhea and dysentery, while other camps, where conditions were considered extremely poor for the time, had few incidences of dysentery or diarrhea.[12]

Medical Inadequacy and Military Urgency

Incidences of disease in soldiers from rural areas were higher than those from urban areas. This was a common factor for childhood diseases because of the lack of exposure. The apparent lower population density found in rural regions of the country, along with farming patterns of life, contributed to this disparity. It was not until the soldiers from rural areas physically adjusted to the crowded camp life that their rate of sickness decreased.[13] Poor training further compounded the specific occurrence of dysentery or diarrhea among new recruits. Volunteers and conscripts often received poor training on field sanitation and cleanliness. Latrines, when they were even established, were frequently placed too close to tents or water resources, increasing the likelihood of microbial transmission. This practice directly violated part of Hammond's directions:

> Latrines should be situated at least 150 yards from the tents. This is the distance required by the General Regulations of the Army, and is not at all too great. They should be situated to leeward of the camp. A deep and narrow trench should be dug for the purposes; if too wide it will require more earth to cover the excretes, and will, moreover, expose a greater surface from which the noxious effluvia will be given off than if it is narrow. Every evening the accumulations of the day should be covered with at least a foot of earth.[14]

Hammond's direction aligned well to modern medical standards and certainly would have acted as a preventative measure against the transmission of dysentery insofar as segregating populations from contaminated waste. However, Hammond, like many other physicians, incorrectly attributed the cause of dysentery to the "noxious effluvia," or smell—often characterized as miasmas in the 19th century—rather than the bacteria or protozoa amoeba in the feces coming in contact with food or drinking water. Some military commanders dismissed the idea of disease-causing smell, more out of repeated exposure to the odor than out of any sense of germ theory, stating that it was simply the smell of a military camp and therefore a part of life in the military.[15]

Still, the Union Army's sanitation program revolved around the idea that "mephitic effluvia" was the cause of many camp diseases. It warned regiments against the foul smells coming from dirty latrines, garbage, and from too many men in a single tent. The guidelines suggested that officers should ensure soldiers had access to fresh air, dry ground, and sunlight. Given the nature of dysentery, these specific actions did little to stem its spread among soldiers, though it helped with other conditions. Nonetheless, these recommendations often fell on deaf ears, possibly a reaction of experienced soldiers discounting the advice of civilians in new positions of leadership. Line officers rarely enforced the recommendations out of ignorance, laziness, or complacency.[16]

The worst failures around camp sanitation involved the lack of satisfactory latrines. Regiments were known to dig insufficient latrines, poor latrines, or no latrines at all. In the case of the latter, soldiers simply relieved themselves next to their tents.[17] The absence of latrines was most common on long campaigns, where the energy needed to comply with proper latrine design was lacking at the end of a long day's march. However, poor training of recruits, noncommissioned officers, and officers in implementing new standards also contributed to this breakdown in military discipline. With the constant movement of the military forces, it was likely the civilians in the area of a temporary military encampment were also the recipients of dysentery and other diarrheal diseases.

Inconsistent Diagnoses and Dangerous "Cures"

In terms of diagnosis, modern and mid-19th-century medicine recognized the symptoms of dysentery. However, diagnosis in the Union Army was not very consistent. Many physicians found bloody stools to be inconsequential, whereas others identified these symptoms as a warning of serious illness. Regardless of the different diagnostic procedures, civilian and military medical records for dysentery and diarrhea were maintained together.[18] As a result, retroactive studies of dysentery during the Civil War and other conflicts must use records that lump simple diarrhea with the data on dysentery. While this likely inflated the data on dysentery, the difference in severity between the two illnesses ensured that dysentery cases were usually reported, while diarrhea often went unreported. Collectively, dysentery and diarrhea "occurred with more frequency and produced more sickness and mortality than any other form of disease" in the Civil War.[19]

The practical effect of dysentery on the affected soldier was often very broad, making the retroactive analysis even more problematic. Some who contracted the condition had very mild symptoms of diarrhea or no symptoms at all. In these cases, the affected individuals still functioned as soldiers, to include marching, while they continued to unwittingly spread the contagion to fellow soldiers and local civilians. Conversely, many soldiers experienced extremely painful evacuations and watery diarrhea that occurred as frequently as half-hourly. The repeated evacuations not only further irritated the infected colon but also resulted in dehydration. These extreme cases had a material impact on how many soldiers an army could muster during a campaign. Extreme cases also impacted the rate of movement of military forces where large numbers of soldiers experienced dysentery. Interestingly, the presence of diarrhea and dysentery in epidemic proportions may have protected soldiers from death in combat. According to some historians, because of dysentery's common occurrence, there was an "unwritten gentlemen's agreement among the soldiers of both armies that they would not fire on any man who was squatting in the bushes."[20]

Treatment of dysentery in the military varied. Joseph Janvier Woodward, a civilian physician who volunteered in the war and was appointed assistant surgeon general of the U.S. Army, published his *Outlines of Chief Camp Diseases of the United States' Armies*. In this work, he recommended cathartics like "caster oil, with which a few drops of laudanum may be combined, is one of the best. But sulphate of magnesia, pills of podophyllin and extract of colocynth, or rhubarb, along or combined with podophyllin, will answer the indication." He believed "they act simply by relieving the alimentary canal of any contents which may serve to irritate the diseased mucous membrane," but he acknowledged that too extensive of application increased the incapacitation of dysentery patients.[21] Today, these would be regarded as extreme forms of treatment and are actually extremely dangerous.[22] His research and extensive use of photography to capture images from microscopic analysis of disease certainly contributed to reforms in military and civilian medicine.[23] Unfortunately, these reforms were not enacted for decades within the military structure, leaving the harsh treatments advocated in his initial military publication to guide physicians during the war.

More common remedies for dysentery and diarrhea included opium and "blue mass." The latter item was a combination of mercurous chloride and chalk that was administered to soldiers who complained of pain and bloating but who did not have watery bowel movements. The end result, in addition to unwittingly poisoning the victim's system, was a purging of the bowels with the hope of remedying the pain and ridding one of symptoms probably associated with amoeba-related dysentery. Opium use was typically prescribed for soldiers with extreme diarrhea symptoms. Due to the widespread prevalence of dysentery and diarrhea compounded with dosages of opium, it is no wonder that general consumption of opium increased after the Civil War, gaining the name of "army disease."[24]

At the onset of the war, dysentery was limited in its occurrences when compared to previous European conflicts and the later stages of the Civil War. By June 30, 1862, around 32,000 cases had been recorded, and only 347 had reportedly died from the disease.[25] As the war progressed and nutritional diets decreased, dysentery became an increasingly difficult problem to contend with, considering the requirements placed on both armies throughout the Civil War.

The Role of Nutrition for Soldiers Contracting Dysentery

As indicated, nutrition played a key role in preventing and treating dysentery and diarrhea. Both the Union and Confederate Armies suffered from poor nutrition throughout the Civil War. Providing fresh vegetables and fruit to whole regiments, much less multiple corps of soldiers, was a monumental task for armies. Instead, many were fed a standard diet of salt-pork, hardtack, and beans. Such a regimen served to provide calories, filled the bellies of hard-marching soldiers, and allowed the food supplies to survive hot summers. Yet, this diet lacked the necessary nutrients to support the immune systems and overall health of the men.

There were several instances where regiments came into the possession of a large amount of fresh fruit. Physicians found that immediately after diets were supplemented with fresh fruits, much of the regiment quickly recovered from their diarrhea. Yet, receiving vast amounts of fresh fruits and vegetables was a rarity. The summer months, when fresh fruits and vegetables were abundant, were the prime time for campaigning and thus prevented easy access to fresh produce.[26] Indeed, the movement of large forces back and forth across farmlands disrupted the production of crops and further hindered the provisioning of armies on both sides of the conflict. According to the Union's medical director, Jonathan Letterman, a lingering diarrhea-related disease that sapped the energy was directly related to the diet of the troops. Discovering that large quantities of potatoes provided to regiments had not been distributed, Letterman issued an advisory to the military leadership to ensure better diets to improve health conditions. Unfortunately, such advisories were often met with ambivalence on the part of military leadership during the war.[27]

The Confederate forces frequently faced food shortages throughout the Civil War. Gen. Lee lamented the shortage of proper rations and its impact on his Army of North Virginia. He feared that the poor quality and inadequate amount of food reduced the men "morally and physically." Lee believed that deserters from the ranks increased as a result of inadequate food supplies. Soldiers ate whatever they could scavenge from their surroundings, including cats and rats.[28] This diet of inferior and insufficient food was further complicated by the lack of clean drinking water. Both problems contributed to the spread of dysentery. The Confederate States Army, when under siege in Corinth, Mississippi, in the fall of 1862, ran out of running water. Desperate, the soldiers began using water from stagnant pools that were clearly contaminated with excrement.[29] The Union Army experienced similar issues with soldiers drinking standing water from pools and puddles of rain, later to discover the pools were created by runoff from hillsides covered in the excrement of fellow soldiers.[30]

Troop movement complicated the ability of the armies to provide sanitary conditions and quality food for its personnel. Rapid and frequent movement made preparing proper latrines a greater burden for armies, as previously mentioned. Poorly disciplined units quickly fell into complacency about these necessities, especially when it was known they would be moving again soon thereafter. Despite poorly dug latrines, or no latrines at all, the frequent movements actually helped keep soldiers from contracting illnesses like dysentery because it kept them on the move; any unsanitary conditions would quickly be left behind. Unfortunately, the local citizenry around these temporary sites suffered from contaminated drinking water.

Large Armies and Declining Hygiene

The massive number of troops involved in the ongoing conflicts was a major contributing factor to the repeated outbreaks of dysentery. The Civil War is often viewed as one of the last wars using old military strategies and one of the first wars to use new technologies and strategies. To ensure victory, both sides of the conflict employed large concentrations of military force. However, these large concentrations of people increased the propensity for transmission of disease, especially such diseases as typhoid and dysentery. A key element of Civil War battlefield theory was to mass forces at an enemy's weak point. Therefore, the creation of large armies and their concentration was necessary. Unfortunately, this basic military strategy had a negative outcome in terms of infection prevention.

The worst conditions involving dysentery for active military units occurred during sieges on forts or cities. Armies under siege were typically cut off from external resupply and generally confined in tight quarters. This intensified sanitation issues and increased the ability for infectious diseases to spread more readily. This was exemplified in the aforementioned Siege of Corinth. In April 1862, Gen. P. T. G. Beauregard occupied the town of Corinth, Mississippi. Corinth was an important location for Union and Confederate forces due to the railroad network it possessed. The Union Army, led by Gen. Halleck, intended to seize Corinth as a strategic position to launch further campaigning throughout the South. Halleck began his approach toward the small town at a conservative pace. Meanwhile, in Corinth, Beauregard's Confederate Army was quickly reduced in fighting strength as the summer approached. Dysentery and typhoid ran rampant throughout Corinth as the tight confines only encouraged rapid transmission between individuals. The epidemic reduced Beauregard's effective army strength below half its total population. Meanwhile, as Gen. Halleck's Union Army began its siege, it did so with greater effective strength. Despite Halleck's lack of battlefield experience to this point, Beauregard was compelled to make the difficult decision to withdraw from Corinth. Beauregard's beleaguered forces were far too ineffective to reasonably sustain a prolonged siege by Halleck. The more prudent choice was to retreat to a more tenable position and regain the health of his unit.[31]

Halleck faced the same issues as Beauregard after he occupied Corinth. Not only were there problems of diarrhea, dysentery, and typhoid, but malaria and scurvy broke out as well. One regiment arrived in Corinth that summer, and within a week, only 35 men reported for duty due to weakness from diarrhea.[32] In response, Halleck ordered hospitals constructed to handle the increasing number of sick. Halleck's forces (like Beauregard's) were rendered too ineffective by disease to continue a serious campaign throughout the South, despite their easily won victory a few weeks prior.[33] In effect, Beauregard's choice to withdraw from Corinth sacrificed a strategic position, but he later gained a strategic ally against his Union foe in the form of disease.

Similarly, the Peninsular Campaign of 1862 was deeply affected by disease. This campaign sought to place pressure on the Confederacy through an amphibious landing on the Chesapeake peninsula followed by a march northwest to Richmond. Led by Gen. George McClellan, the Union Army slowly marched up the peninsula toward Richmond, but it was set back in part by well-prepared Confederate defensive positions and an array of diseases that drained McClellan's forces and hampered his progress. In July, McClellan's army experienced 42,911 cases of sickness out of his recorded strength of 106,069; almost 20 percent, or a total of 19,776, were related to dysentery or diarrhea.[34] This represents an enormous drain on McClellan's fighting force. Confederate records of sick rolls were poorly documented; however, an analysis of the terrain and conditions suggests that the Federal Army was more affected by disease in the peninsula campaign than its Confederate counterparts.[35]

Ultimately, McClellan ended his offensive only miles from his goal of Richmond, unable to continue. McClellan requested an additional 35,000 soldiers from President Lincoln to successfully take Richmond, but Lincoln, troubled by McClellan's slow advance and unsuccessful prosecution of the campaign, denied the request. McClellan's records showed 16,644 soldiers were on the sick rolls, and another 38,420 were absent from fighting, most likely due to disease as well. If McClellan had been able to effectively control the outbreak of disease in his army, he might have had the manpower necessary to seize Richmond.[36]

It is clear that dysentery influenced multiple campaigns as an inverse force multiplier. Unfortunately, it is more difficult to isolate the impact of dysentery from that of other diseases prevalent in the ranks in the Civil War. Data indicates that the number of Union soldiers who died from dysentery over the course of the war was approximately 60,000; yet, hundreds of thousands more showed signs of infection. Federal records show over 1.7 million reported cases of diarrhea and dysentery alone. Over 200,000 soldiers reported chronic diarrhea or dysentery, and another nearly 20,000 received medical discharges due to their condition.[37] At any given point in time, 10 percent of the Union Army was afflicted by disease. The greatest impact was felt during the summer, which was not only the season when dysentery was most common but also the primary campaign season. Nevertheless, military leaders of the time took pride in the relative health of their units.[38] Disease was constantly present in the war and therefore became another variable that commanders dealt with on the battlefield.

Civil War Prisons—Breeding Grounds for Dysentery

Some of the most unsanitary conditions throughout the Civil War were not present on the battlefield but instead existed in prison camps. The most notorious of the Civil War prison camps was Andersonville, Georgia. This camp was approximately 10 acres in size, and it housed roughly 32,899 prisoners at its peak in August 1864. This amounted to 35.7 square feet of space per prisoner. A single small stream flowed through the middle of the camp, providing the sole source of water for virtually all needs, drinking and cleansing.[39] The limited space made it impossible to separate men from human waste. Unsurprisingly, given these conditions, dysentery was a constant presence in Andersonville. As men contracted the infection, any attempts at refraining from contact with human feces were abandoned. The dysentery epidemic reached its peak intensity between March and August of 1864. During that short period of time, over 4,000 of 7,712 Union prisoner deaths were attributed to dysentery or diarrhea.[40]

Union prisoner-of-war (POW) camps also had overcrowded conditions and became prime breeding grounds for epidemics. Camp Randall, in Madison, Wisconsin, provided a well-documented case of such a POW camp for Confederate prisoners. Because of the high rate of mortality reported in the newspapers, Lt. Col. William Hoffman, the U.S. commissary-general of prisoners, was sent to investigate conditions. In addition to the high rate of mortality, Hoffman discovered a high incidence of morbidity. His investigation also revealed evidence of corruption and frugality that contributed to camp morbidity rates. The combination of these latter two factors produced results that further undermined the health and exacerbated the impact of diseases such as dysentery. Specifically, Maj. Smith, Hoffman's designated representative at Camp Randall, and Hoffman agreed to reduce rations to the disease-ridden men and to use the money saved to buy furniture and combs for the prisoners. These well-intended choices served to undermine prisoner heath, and the selected purchases provided no improvement in medical support. Furthermore, evidence of missing medication indicated problems with corruption that prevented even the limited treatments normally available.[41]

Another POW camp that has been compared to Andersonville is the Union camp at Point Lookout, Maryland, officially known as Camp Hoffman. On 23 acres, the camp was more than twice the size of its Southern equivalent at Andersonville and held the most captives of any POW camp in the Civil War. Over 52,000 Confederate prisoners resided at the camp in just under two years' time. Certain conditions at Hoffman were considerably better than Andersonville, such as a commissary, the ability to fish for additional food, and drainage systems to maintain sanitation. However, other conditions continued to perpetuate the exchange of such diseases as diarrhea and dysentery. The camp was drained and sewage emptied into the bay, but the practice of allowing the prisoners to fish and exercise on the beach exposed them to human waste. "Sinks," or holes created for defecation or urination, were few in number, poorly covered, and sometimes located directly under prison tents. The prisoners were compelled to defecate in the open. Additionally, inadequate clothing and shelter undermined prisoner health, as did the limited quantities of brackish water. The most common disease recorded at this camp was chronic diarrhea—often the term collectively used for diarrhea and dysentery—with 20–30 prisoners admitted to the hospital daily.[42]

The environment in prisoner-of-war camps worsened as the war stretched on. The pivotal point for deteriorating conditions was the cessation of parole for captives. The process of exchanging prisoners from both sides was discontinued in 1863. Without the ability to exchange parolees, captured soldiers were held in increasingly overpopulated camps. Neither side desired to spend the amount of funds necessary to maintain healthy conditions. Instead, supplies were redirected, and prisoners suffered as a result. Despite the previously mentioned corruption, frugality, high morbidity, and mortality that were common to POW camps, only one incidence of war crimes was successfully prosecuted at the war's end. Not surprisingly, this was with the commander of the camp at Andersonville. The extreme number of deaths (nearly 40 percent imprisoned there died) and the short life span of prisoners (one-third died within seven months of imprisonment)[43] resulted in an investigation and ultimately the conviction and execution of the camp commander.

The Combination of Dysentery, Conditions of War, and Attempted Reforms

Dysentery's role in the Civil War extends far beyond the actions of armies clashing with one another on the battlefield, in military encampments, or prison camps. The many experiences gained by physicians in the Civil War led to medical developments and reforms. Doctors documented their experiences from numerous battlefield traumas and diseases. These observations in turn aided research and methods to combat future casualties of war as well as those facing similar traumas or conditions outside of war. This amassed knowledge was combined into a six-volume publication, *Medical and Surgical History of the War of the Rebellion*. Additionally, the journals of Union and Confederate doctors were published for fellow medical practitioners and researchers to learn about infectious diseases and surgical techniques.

European medical researchers in the late 19th century drew heavily on the experiences of physicians from the Civil War. Pathologists such as Rudolf Virchow and Edwin Klebs issued written praise for the detailed work of the American medical staff during the war years. Klebs issued accolades stating, "The greatest and most admirable success has been attained by the North Americans in military medical work. The history of the war of secession has to show a display of medical and scientific activities that leave anything that ever since has been achieved in Europe way in the background."[44]

The most notable discoveries of the post–Civil War era were the works of Joseph Lister, Robert Koch, and Louis Pasteur. All three were European pathologists whose work proved the causative relationship between bacteria and diseases.[45] Their accomplishments in the field of microbiology changed medicine irrevocably; this directly translated into improved care and prevention of disease in the U.S. military. Physicians like Lister, Koch, and Pasteur were immeasurably aided by the experience and documentation that came from the Civil War that helped them identify and connect microbiological organisms to such infectious diseases as dysentery. Rates of infection in subsequent wars plummeted significantly after their discoveries in the late 19th century. Consequently, the Civil War saw a 10.2 percent mortality rate from disease, while the incidence of disease declined precipitously for the Spanish-American War (0.92 percent), the Philippine War (2.2 percent), and World War I (1.4 percent).[46]

The influence of disease on the Civil War is clearly undisputed, and dysentery took first place among those diseases. At its mildest, dysentery was a constant, bothersome companion to hundreds of thousands of soldiers on both sides of the blue-gray divide. At its worst, the disease rendered tens of thousands of soldiers unfit for duty and even caused death. This forced commanders to abdicate strategic positions to their opponents that might very well have changed the course of the war. Dysentery also compelled military commanders to decline pressing an offensive that would have otherwise dealt their opponents a strategic blow. Yet, it is from dysentery and other diseases' impact on the Civil War, and the tragic number of lives lost, that tremendous breakthroughs in medicine and military reforms occurred.

NOTES

1. Emily Dollar and Lee A. Witters, "That Bourne from Whence No Traveler Returns," *Dartmouth Medicine* 39, no. 1 (Fall 2014): 38.
2. Frederick Law Olmsted, "Letter to Regimental Commanders on the Strict Observance of Camp Police Rules, Washington, D.C., 1861," Library of Congress, Printed Ephemera Collection; Portfolio 204, Folder 26, accessed June 20, 2017, https://www.loc.gov /item/rbpe.20402600.

3.   Michael R. Gilchrist, "Disease & Infection in the American Civil War," *American Biology Teacher* 60, no. 4 (April 1998): 258.

4.   Paul E. Steiner, *Disease in the Civil War: Natural Biological Warfare in 1861–1865* (Springfield, IL: Charles C Thomas), 16.

5.   "Dysentery," *Gale Encyclopedia of Medicine*, 3rd ed. (2006), accessed September 7, 2017, http://www.encyclopedia.com/medicine/diseases-and-conditions/pathology/dysentery #1G23451600534.

6.   Gilchrist, "Disease & Infection," 260.

7.   "Entamoeba Histolytica," Stanford University, accessed September 7, 2017, https:// web.stanford.edu/group/parasites/ParaSites2006/Amoebiasis/Agents&History.html.

8.   Fitzroy J. Henry, "The Epidemiologic Importance of Dysentery in Communities," *Reviews of Infectious Diseases* 13, no. 4 (April 1991): S238.

9.   Henry, "The Epidemiologic Importance of Dysentery," S240-1.

10. Gilchrist, "Disease & Infection," 258.

11. William A. Hammond, *A Treatise on Hygiene with Special Reference to the Military Service* (Philadelphia: J.B. Lippincott & Co.), 455.

12. Gilchrist, "Disease & Infection," 259.

13. Richard H. Shryock, "A Medical Perspective on the Civil War," *American Quarterly* 14, no. 2 (Summer 1962): 166.

14. Hammond, *A Treatise on Hygiene*, 459.

15. Steiner, *Disease in the Civil War*, 17.

16. George Worthington Adams, *Doctors in Blue: The Medical History of the Union Army in the Civil War* (New York: Henry Schuman), 196.

17. Adams, *Doctors in Blue*, 20

18. Adams, *Doctors in Blue*, 201.

19. Stanhope Bayne-Jones, ed., "The American Civil War (15 April 1861–30 June 1865)— Beginnings of Bacteriological Era and Scientific Preventive Medicine (1861–1898)," in *The Evolution of Preventive Medicine in the United States Army, 1607–1939* (Washington, D.C.: U.S. Government Printing Office), 99, accessed September 7, 2017, http://history .amedd.army.mil/booksdocs/misc/evprev/ch6.htm.

20. Jeremy Agnew, *Alcohol and Opium in the Old West: Use, Abuse and Influence* (Jefferson, NC and London: McFarland & Company, Inc., Publishers, 2014), 73.

21. Joseph Janvier Woodward, *Outlines of the Chief Camp Diseases of the United States Armies: As Observed during the Present War* (Philadelphia: J. B. Lippincott & Co., 1863), 228.

22. Gilchrist, "Disease & Infection," 259.

23. J. S. Billings, "Memoir of Joseph Janvier Woodward, 1833–1884," in *Biographical Memoirs*, Vol. 2. (Washington, D.C.: National Academy of Sciences, 1886), 298, accessed September 7, 2017, http://www.nasonline.org/publications/biographical-memoirs/memoir -pdfs/woodward-joseph-j.pdf.

24. Billings, "Memoir of Joseph Janvier Woodward," 73.

25. Woodward, *Outlines of the Chief Camp Diseases*, 223.

26. Adams, *Doctors in Blue*, 200.

27. Jonathan Letterman, MD, *Medical Recollections of the Army of the Potomac* (New York: D. Appleton & Company, 1866), 105–107, accessed September 7, 2017, http://history .amedd.army.mil/booksdocs/civil/lettermanmemoirs/medical_recollections.html# Letter_from_Letterman_to_Hooker_on_Layout_of_Unhealthy_Huts_by_Soldiers_on.

28. H. H. Cunningham, *Doctors in Gray: The Confederate Medical Service* (Baton Rouge: Louisiana State University Press, 1986), 178.

29. Cunningham, *Doctors in Gray*, 181.

30. Adams, *Doctors in Blue*, 205.

31. Steiner, *Disease in the Civil War*, 162–163.

32. Steiner, *Disease in the Civil War*, 169.

33. Steiner, *Disease in the Civil War*, 182.

34. Steiner, *Disease in the Civil War*, 124.

35. Steiner, *Disease in the Civil War*, 139.

36. Steiner, *Disease in the Civil War*, 142-151.

37. Steiner, *Disease in the Civil War*, 18.

38. Shryock, "A Medical Perspective," 164.

39. Austin Flint, MD, ed., *A Report of the Diseases, etc., among the Prisoners at Andersonville, GA* (New York: Published for the US Sanitary Commission by Kurd & Houghton, 1867), 502–503.

40. Flint, *A Report of the Diseases*, 531.

41. Tommy Thompson, "'Dying like Rotten Sheepe': Camp Randall as a Prisoner of War Facility during the Civil War," *Wisconsin Magazine of History* 92, no. 1 (Autumn 2008): 10–11, accessed September 7, 2017, http://www.jstor.org/stable/25482093.

42. Richard A. Blondo, "A View of Point Lookout Prison Camp for Confederates," *OAH Magazine of History* 8, no. 1, *The Civil War* (Fall 1993): 30–34, accessed September 7, 2017, http://www.jstor.org/stable/25162923?seq=1#page_scan_tab_contents.

43. Dora L. Costa and Matthew E. Kahn, "Surviving Andersonville: The Benefits of Social Networks in POW Camps," *American Economic Review* 97, no. 4 (September 2007): 1467, accessed September 7, 2017, http://www.jstor.org/stable/30034102.

44. Shryock, "A Medical Perspective," 169.

45. Gilchrist, "Disease & Infection," 261.

46. Vincent J. Cirillo, "Two Faces of Death: Fatalities from Disease and Combat in America's Principal Wars, 1775 to Present," *Perspectives in Biology and Medicine* 51, no. 1 (Winter 2008): 123.

Chapter 18

Pneumonia in the American Civil War: Death Knell of the Sick and Invalid, 1861–1865

Rebecca M. Seaman

If grippe condemns, the secondary infections execute.[1]

—Louis Cruveilhier

The American Civil War produced more deaths than all previous U.S. wars combined. Typical of pre-20th-century wars, deaths from combat lagged far behind those from disease. Disease accounted for two-thirds of the Civil War deaths, with white participants experiencing mortality rates on a two-to-one ratio from disease and combat, respectively, and African American participants experiencing significantly higher rates of death due to disease. The leading killers included dysentery and other diarrheal diseases, followed by typhoid, and then pneumonia as the third leading cause of death by disease.[2] The frequency that wounded soldiers experienced complications following their injuries and surgeries made pneumonia a significant killer. Due to the overcrowded and unsanitary conditions of camp life and hospitals, it was not uncommon for those suffering from another illness to contract infections such as pneumonia.

As a "secondary" infection, pneumonia found ample targets in military hospitals and the military ranks during the Civil War. The lack of medical knowledge necessary to identify the infection source, coupled with the inability or unwillingness (initially) of medical officers to quarantine patients with infectious diseases, facilitated the spread of disease. Ineffective medicines and the lack of antibiotics to treat or prevent infection contributed to the spread of pneumonia and its high mortality rates. When combined with poor hygiene; poor diets; the large number of hospitalized wounded and extreme number of people suffering from dysentery, typhoid, measles, malaria, and other epidemic diseases, pneumonia posed a clear danger as a deadly secondary infection in the Civil War.

Symptoms and Various Causes of Pneumonia

Pneumonia is a disease that refers to the inflammation of lung tissues in the lower respiratory tract. The severity of the disease depends on the causal factors of the infection and what portion of the lung is affected. *Lobar pneumonia* refers to the infection of a single lobe within one lung; *single pneumonia* is when the infection is found throughout one lung, and *double pneumonia* is when the infection is found throughout both lungs. During the Civil War, double pneumonia was usually fatal.

Pneumonia was caused by a variety of factors, unlike other epidemics invading military camps overs the ages whose source was often a single agent. Fungi, bacteria, viruses, and even inhalation of irritating fumes produced pneumonia infections. The first two causal factors were contagious and spread through a variety of methods, again depending on the causal agent. The most common method of spread was through contact, coughing, and sneezing. Fungal pneumonia was contracted through fungi present in the surrounding environment. The inhalation of irritating fumes,[3] while not documented separately during the war when pneumonia's etiology was still unknown, was likely a factor that worked in common with other agents, as the smoke fumes from gunpowder used in firing cannon and firearms covered battlefields of the Civil War.

The most common bacterial agents of pneumonia in the Civil War included *Streptococcuss pneumoniae*, *Diplococcus pneumoniae*, and *Mycoplasma pneumoniae*. Bacterium *Streptococcuss pneumoniae*, or pneumococcal infection, ranged from ear and sinus infections to pneumonia and bloodstream infections.[4] Easily contracted in the close confines of military life—tent barracks, winter quarters, and especially overcrowded camp life and hospitals—this bacterial form was the leading cause of pneumonia in the Civil War. *Diplococcus pneumoniae* spread through the military ranks via "carriers," usually healthy soldiers who could ward off the bacterium in their own systems. Forced marches and malnutrition undermined the health of these carrier soldiers, and overcrowding facilitated the spread of infections through military camps.[5] In the context of the Civil War, this transference of bacterial pneumonia occurred repeatedly as new recruits joined the ranks of ill-fed veterans whose health was poor from exposure, insufficient diet, contaminated water, and inferior hygiene.

A common form of community-acquired pneumonia was from the bacterium *Mycoplasma pneumoniae*. Often presenting as tracheobronchitis, or the common cold, this upper respiratory infection usually included a sore throat, but it sometimes evolved into the more serious form, pneumonia.[6] This was not uncommon in winter camps or deployments during the Civil War. Additionally, the different forms of bacteria that caused pneumonia were easily transferred in Civil War hospitals to wounded soldiers and those already ill with other diseases, such as malaria, dysentery, measles, malaria, and typhoid.

Viruses, such as the human parainflueza viruses (HPIV), were also leading causes of pneumonia. Often associated with the common cold, symptoms of viral pneumonias include runny noses, fevers, and coughs.[7] In Civil War encampments, such viruses spread rapidly through the ranks; even touching items held by others was enough to contract the illness. The *Haemophilus influenzae* virus was the second most common form of pneumonia contracted during the war. This virus was often already present in soldiers and simply waited for an opportunity to present itself when soldiers' immune systems were compromised by the conditions of war.[8] Most Civil War soldiers could recover on their own, especially if their diets included vegetables and fruits that supported the immune system. Compromised immune systems, the practice of military personnel of all ranks self-diagnosing and treating their ailments, and inadequate medical care resulted in severe viral infections that devolved into croup and pneumonia.

Finally, fungi also facilitated the spread of pneumonia among the military ranks during the Civil War. *Pneumocystis* pneumonia was a serious form of the disease caused by the fungus *Pneumocystis jirovecii*. Only recently have medical researchers discovered that a fungus caused this form of pneumonia; originally the medical community believed it to be caused by protozoa. *Pneumocystis* pneumonia spread through the air and was often carried by healthy people who eventually contracted the disease when their immune systems became compromised.[9]

Prevalence of Secondary Pneumonia amid Ineffective Medical Care

These same agents still cause pneumonia in the 21st century. Today, pneumonia remains the sixth leading cause of death in the United States and the leading cause of death among infectious diseases. Prior to acquiring the knowledge of its etiology, and therefore before the discovery of effective methods to counter the disease with proper medical treatment, pneumonia became the third most common cause of death from disease. Most reported cases of disease during the Civil War were attributed directly or indirectly to unhealthy environments and poor hygiene.[10] Dysentery, the most common disease of the Civil War, was responsible for approximately a third of all deaths. Dysentery and related diarrhea diseases were indicative of the unsanitary conditions that accompanied military units as they moved from place to place. Typhoid, the second highest recorded fatal disease in the Civil War, was attributed to unsanitary conditions and contaminated food and water. Pneumonia cases also occurred due to poor hygiene and the overcrowding in camps and hospitals. These conditions remained common throughout the war in the North and the South. The elevated number of pneumonia cases and fatalities during the war were due to its role as a secondary infection.

People who had already experienced traumatic injuries, surgeries, or other illnesses were susceptible to the contraction of secondary diseases such as pneumonia. The effect of other diseases or injuries on one's immune system served to compromise the body's defenses. Pneumonia was more easily acquired due to the deteriorated health of an individual, regardless of whether the bacteria or virus was already present in the system of a patient or was transferred to a patient while recovering from wounds or illness. Occasionally, pneumonia further weakened the immune system of Civil War soldiers and allowed the bacterial infection to invade the bloodstream, causing sepsis or blood poisoning. Such incidents were rare but deadly. Secondary or tertiary diseases were often overlooked in 19th-century medical records, as they often recorded the disease associated with the initial onset of symptoms. The complexity of recording morbidity and mortality rates during a war was difficult in the best of times. Amid the chaos of the Civil War, record keeping was initially very poor. This improved gradually over the course of the war, and more so in the Union than in the Confederacy. Recording the occurrence of diverse diseases, when the etiology of a disease was unknown and shared common symptoms with other ailments, added to the difficulty and resulted in questionable data.

Additionally, pneumonia was referred to by several names in the 19th century: pleuro-pneumonia, lung fever, or inflammation of the lungs.[11] Mild cases of pneumonia often went undiagnosed as soldiers contracted what they considered common colds (catarrh) or influenza (epidemic catarrh). Despite these various factors that could easily account for unrecorded incidences of pneumonia, enough documentation existed to justify the various forms of pneumonia as the third leading cause of death in the Civil War.

The high disease death rate during the Civil War was partially because military personnel placed little faith in the medical care available. Enlisted men and officers alike tended to self-diagnose and treat infirmities or depend on comrades and family members to help identify illnesses and provide necessary homeopathic treatments. As the symptoms of more serious diseases such as pneumonia (including fever, cough, shortness of breath, sweating, chills, headache, muscle pains, fatigue, and chest pain with breathing) were common for anything from the common cold to seasonal influenza outbreaks, it is unsurprising that the diagnosis of pneumonia was often missed or made belatedly. For those with mild cases of pneumonia, the homeopathic treatments either worked, and soldiers returned to their duties without serious complications and no record of the disease reported; or the patient's condition worsened, and he was compelled to report to sick call or be carried to a medical practitioner for treatment.

Prior to the development of antibiotics, the treatment for diagnosed pneumonia varied by practitioner. The method of medical practice in the military at the outset of the war was called regular, or "allopathic."[12] This practice involved the use of high dosages of harsh chemicals to counter the "humors"[13] that presented themselves in the human body, the common understanding of diseases in the mid-19th century. However, some medical practitioners (often contracted civilian doctors) also utilized new scientific approaches to treat patients. At the start of the Civil War, the Medical Department did not recognize many of the new medical techniques as befitting the professional heritage of army medicine, and it discouraged the use of contracted physicians as a result.

Treatments for pneumonia at the war's onset were quite varied and included bleeding (with lancets or leeches), cupping, quinine, calomel (mercury contraction), application of poultices, blistering through the application of harsh compresses or rags dipped in scalding water, purgatives, strychnine, antimony, and digitalis.[14] Designed to stimulate blood flow as a means of eliminating congestion in the lungs, these allopathic treatments often contributed to the deteriorating health of patients, if not their death. Some, such as antimony, had side effects that included irritation of the lungs and lung diseases. The newer treatments employed by the end of the war included quarantine and the use of expectorants and pain medications (morphine and opium, if available).[15] Untreated, approximately one-third of patients diagnosed with pneumonia died.[16] The people most susceptible to pneumonia had recently experienced a cold or contracted influenza; smoked; had other respiratory illnesses (measles, mumps); or had a recent injury.[17] The survival rate of people with bacterial pneumonia was determined by the strength of the causal bacteria, the timing of the diagnosis, the treatments used (or not used), the age and health of the patient, and the presence of other conditions or diseases. The presence of other diseases, malnutrition, respiratory illnesses, and concurrent recovery from wounds were the most common means of acquiring the bacterial form of pneumonia in the Civil War.

Context and Conditions at the Start of the Civil War

The conditions within the Union and Confederacy at the start of the Civil War provide an important contextual understanding of the state of medicine. The Union was more urbanized and industrial, with large cities along the coastal regions, rivers, canals, and railways. It additionally had vast farmlands that were used to produce foods that made their way to the cities, and later to the war effort via boat and railroad cars. The constant influx of foreigners migrating to America occurred primarily in northern port cities and brought future citizens for the Union, who in turn helped produce supplies and even joined its armies. These migrants also brought wave after wave of diseases that exposed the urban societies of the north to a wide variety of viruses and bacteria. The scattered rural regions, less exposed, boasted healthier environments, but they also reduced the possibility of exposure and immunity to diseases. Though unaware of this demographic dynamic, a Pennsylvania officer noted that the rough, backwoodsmen of one rural company fell sick at a higher rate after recruitment, with more severe cases of illness. Meanwhile, those living in immediately adjacent tents, but from cities, had only three light cases of illness.[18]

Unlike the Union, the Confederacy was primarily agricultural, though it had some large cities and even some industry. With less favorable port facilities and a reliance on slave labor, the South experienced far fewer migrants from Europe and elsewhere, thereby maintaining its more rural environment and isolation from repeated epidemics. Even though the isolation from waves of foreign migrants protected the region from repeated epidemics, it also prevented the ability for urban populations of the South to build up strong immunities to diseases, unlike the populations from the urban North that experienced endemic diseases. Additionally, the warmer climate, humid conditions, and low-lying terrain of the southern coastal plains made the spread of some epidemic diseases, such as measles, unlikely, while it provided the perfect environment for fostering the spread of such illnesses as malaria and yellow fever. The heavy rainfall and poor drainage, coupled with the mobilization of large armies throughout the war, resulted in the contamination of waters and the spread of diseases such as typhoid, dysentery, cholera and others.

The diseases found in Civil War America were not new to medical studies. New awareness of the importance of hygiene and sanitary systems gradually became known and were adopted by cities and some practitioners of medicine. Recent wars with Mexico and in the Crimea demonstrated the impact of disease on militaries and prompted the reform of medical practices. However, resistance within the Medical Department and its bureaucratic structure prevented rapid changes in time to have a positive impact at the start of the Civil War. Consequently, at the war's outset, a total of only 96 medical officers served in the Union military.[19] No dedicated ambulances were utilized; the transfer of wounded from the field of combat was often conducted by military musicians. Medical supplies, when available, were distributed through the Quartermaster Corps. In addition to a rigid infrastructure, the recruiting and conscription efforts unintentionally contributed to the spread of disease in the armies of the North and South.

At the outset of the war, volunteers and conscripts manned the Union Army, which was composed of a mixture of white Northern American farmers, city dwellers, and recent immigrants from Europe. Free African Americans from the North and escaped slaves from the South were belatedly formed into units that served the Union. The Confederacy was composed of mostly white Americans from farms and cities, with some immigrants (i.e., Irish units) and some African American slaves who served their white masters. This mixture of urban and rural and foreign and native recruits provided the necessary dynamics for the introduction of viruses and bacterial diseases, from urban areas where such diseases were endemic to susceptible rural populations that, though healthy, had no immunity to the diseases.

Health Issues for Union and Confederate Soldiers and African Americans during the Civil War

In the first year of the war, the common epidemic that rippled through the ranks of the Union and Confederate forces was measles. The hardest hit units were those from more rural locations. Outbreaks occurred within months of a unit's organization and reoccurred with each new admission of recruits. Measles, a respiratory virus, further undermined the health of new and old recruits, impaired their natural respiratory tract defenses, and resulted in frequent secondary infections of pneumonia. The resulting combination of measles and pneumonia cases was reported as high as 45 percent in some units, affecting the ability to conduct effective campaigns.[20]

In late 1861 and through much of 1862, typhoid appeared and spread rapidly in the close confines of military life and among soldiers who increasingly suffered from malnutrition and lived in unsanitary conditions on a daily basis. The increase in typhoid epidemics corresponded directly with the increased recruitment of military forces. Further complicating this disease, spread by feces-contaminated water and food, was the environment. Although typhoid typically emerged in the summer, the extreme rainfall of the spring of 1862 washed the human waste of large armies from poorly dug latrines into the streams and rivers that were used for drinking water and washing. The dry, nonproductive cough of typhoid along with accompanying muscle- and headaches closely approximated influenza and was occasionally self-treated or misdiagnosed. Those not treated became delirious and fell into trancelike states. It was in this later stage that secondary infections such as pneumonia occurred, as the natural cough-reflex defenses of the respiratory system that kept bacterial matter from accessing the lower respiratory tract were compromised. The resulting high death toll was typically attributed to the initial infection of typhoid, especially without the understanding of pneumonia's etiology or the ability to identify the bacterial agents present. Similar to measles, regiments experiencing typhoid and pneumonia complications reported a 23–40 percent reduction of effective forces, which affected military campaigns during the periods of high typhoid epidemics.[21]

By 1864, the rate of contagious illnesses had declined as rural soldiers from the North and the South developed immunities to diseases, though the rates of fatalities for reported disease cases remained constant.[22] The constant mortality rates of reported illness cases were especially true in the South as the tide of war turned in the Union's favor. Increasing numbers of Confederate wounded placed pressure on medical personnel to provide necessary care with rapidly diminishing resources.[23] Although the number of epidemics initially declined in the North and then in the South, these same epidemics increased among the new African American Union recruits. The reason for this belated increase was because African Americans were not initially accepted as recruits; therefore, their exposure to new diseases and military camp conditions occurred later in the war.

African Americans did not join the Union in large numbers until 1863. Approximately 180,000 served as soldiers in the Civil War, with one-fifth dying. While death from disease outstripped death from combat by a 2-to-1 ratio for white Northerners and Southerners, 10 African Americans died from disease to every 1 killed in combat—5 times the rate of white soldiers. As the number of African Americans participating in the war rose, so did epidemics within their units. It was not surprising that measles and then typhoid swept through African American military camps in early 1864. Similarly, the increase in secondary pneumonia infections occurred in the same camps.

Epidemics and secondary diseases also devastated "contraband camps" of African American women and children who had fled slavery in the South and awaited the return of fathers, brothers, and sons who fought for the Union.[24] The morbidity and mortality figures for women and children were not captured in the traditional accounting of lives lost in the Civil War. Contributing factors to the susceptibility and mortality rates of pneumonia in African Americans included their diets and overall health prior to enrolling in the Union forces. The inequity of rationing (food and medical supplies), unhealthy environments, and heavier fatigue duties in relation to other personnel further contributed to morbidity and mortality rates.[25] In addition to inferior provisions, the initial lack of medical personnel assigned to African American units contributed to increased illness and fatalities.[26] Another factor affecting their susceptibility to epidemics and secondary infections was the presence of sickle cell disease. This disease, more common in African Americans, compromised the antibody function of the spleen, especially in children, and left them open to infectious diseases.[27]

Whether Union or Confederate, black, white, or ethnic immigrant, the presence of large armies polluted the environment and therefore affected the health of the armies and neighboring societies. The sanitation systems of the mid-19th century were incapable of accommodating the vast quantities of human sewage and debris from food preparation, much less the burial of bodies and body parts that accumulated from battle. Moving large armies with their accompanying baggage, food supplies, munitions, artillery, and medical corps along inadequate roads and bridges wore out equipment and exhausted the livestock and men. It also made it difficult to ensure that food and potable water were readily available. The resulting malnutrition, so often a hardship of warfare, undermined the health of armies and opened the men up to contagious infections that their systems would otherwise have fought off.

The Role of Nutrition and Hygiene in the Health of Armies

The method of pneumonia diffusion in the military was assisted by the health of the soldiers. The Union had vast resources capable of feeding the armies, but getting resources to the soldiers in a timely fashion was problematic. At times, the goods arrived too soon and rotted before they were distributed. The resulting quality of the food was inferior. Hardtack, a common item, was an extremely dry biscuit or cracker that had to be soaked in coffee or other hot liquid to make it edible. The hardtack distributed to soldiers was often riddled with weevils and maggots and covered in cobwebs. Vegetables were a necessary component of a healthy diet to ward off scurvy. However, the land surrounding military camps was quickly scoured of any edible plant life and was left unsuitable for gardening, even if the military units had remained in place for any length of time. The spoilage rate of vegetables resulted in the use of dehydration to preserve them. The process produced an inferior product referred to as *desiccated vegetables* that were inedible and had little remaining nutritional value.[28]

Meat, seldom fresh, was often rancid, spoiled, and even crawling with maggots. Nonetheless, it was still used in stews with whatever supplemental food was available. The alternative was salted beef or pork, which was often discolored yellow and inedible until soaked in freshwater.[29] The water selected for this soaking process was of questionable quality. Typically drawn from wells, creeks, and rivers, the water was quickly contaminated by human waste as latrines were positioned too close to the water supplies and not properly covered. Whether armies remained stationary and contaminated their own environment or moved great distances and outpaced their supplies, the result was an overall decline in the health of personnel. The combined results of insufficient diets and contaminated foods created constant illnesses such as chronic bronchitis and viral infections in soldiers—Union, Confederate, black, and white. The impaired immune defenses allowed the already present strains of bacterial and viral pneumonias to infect military personnel, volunteers, and the medical staff that served in the hospitals.[30]

The placement and layout of military camps also contributed to illness. As indicated, latrines were dug too close to wells, tents, and water sources, or not dug at all in the case of constantly moving forces. Additionally, large numbers of personnel were crowded together in unventilated tents, where they shared food, warmth, and, unwittingly, diseases. Common colds were normal, and people were unable to distinguish between a cold and the early stages of respiratory diseases such as measles, mumps, influenza, and pneumonia.[31] The viral and bacterial forms of pneumonia easily passed from person to person through shared utensils, coughing, and accidental contact. Though sick, many men nonetheless refused to report to sick call.

Realities of Civil War Medicine and Care

Some soldiers with infections refused to seek medical care out of a sense of duty to their comrades, others out of fear. The lives of these common soldiers were deplorable. However, the reported horrors of the temporary military hospitals, where allopathic remedies were distributed daily beside piles of discarded human limbs from post-battle amputations, were far worse. Nonetheless, some soldiers did report for sick call when ill, but they were sent back to their tents due to misdiagnoses, medical perceptions of malingering, or because their disease condition had not progressed enough to justify the military's definition of necessary hospitalization. The result was the contamination of other soldiers with the same bacterial or viral infections.

Once a soldier was admitted to a temporary or permanent hospital, whether for an injury or serious illness, his chances of contracting another infection such as pneumonia increased. This was partially due to inadequate medical services and ineffective remedies as well as the conditions in many medical facilities, especially at the start of the war. Traditional military doctors, many aged or with limited practice gained at small Western outposts, continued to practice allopathic medicine, distributing calomel, purgatives, and opium for a vast array of diseases. They also resisted the inclusion of contract and volunteer civilian doctors, viewing them as an improper fit in the military environment. Medical volunteers also took the form of female nurses, most well-intentioned but inexperienced in nursing outside of care for family members at home. Dorothea Dix, noted for her recruiting and organization of nurses for the war effort, sought individuals with "high moral character, no less than thirty years of age, plain looking, and unadorned." Lacking in Dix's requirements for recruits was any experience or nursing capabilities.[32]

Experience in medical volunteers and officers did not necessarily translate into effective care. One example was the commonly held perception during the Civil War that the flow of pus out of a newly amputated wound was evidence of proper healing. It was not unusual for doctors to report successful surgeries with signs of "healthy discharge," to be followed by surprised medical entries of declining health and the deaths of their patients (likely sepsis). Other examples of ineffective care included the focus of medical attention on a wound while overlooking the emergence of secondary infections such as pneumonia.

A famous example of an amputation that was followed by signs of "healthy discharge" that evolved into pneumonia and death is Lt. Gen. Thomas "Stonewall" Jackson. In Jackson's case, his fall from the litter he was being carried on bruised his chest area, and pneumonia soon followed. The damage to the lung area possibly initiated the onset of pneumonia. However, Jackson had already complained of a sore throat prior to being accidentally shot by his own troops, a sign he may have already been a carrier of a pneumonia bacteria or virus. Additionally, the series of transportations of Jackson were quite rough and accompanied by repeated applications of whiskey, morphine, and other opiates. When amputation was finally required, chloroform was used to reduce his discomfort. It is not improbable that he aspirated bacterial debris into his distal air passages while under the influence of the whiskey, morphine, other opiates, or chloroform at a time that his cough reflex would have been impaired. The end result, whether from a damaged lung, already present virus or bacterial infection, or aspiration due to the use of sedatives before and during surgery, was the development of a fatal case of pneumonia.[33] The other possibility still debated is that while he showed clear signs of pneumonia, he may have died from sepsis, either from the "healthy discharge" on his amputated limb or from complications of his pneumonia.

Reforms in Medicine during the War

Reforms were gradually made that began to foster improvements in the deplorable medical care and conditions over the course of the Civil War. The process of reform for the Union was reflected in the selection of leaders for the Medical Department. At the start of the war, an elderly Thomas Lawson held the position of army surgeon general. Born in 1789, Lawson joined the navy in 1809, though his education and medical training is unknown. He rose to the rank of surgeon general in 1836 and instituted some reforms, but mainly in the form of improved conditions for medical officers and oversight of medical examinations to ensure quality personnel based on traditional standards. By the time he left office in 1861, there were only 30 surgeons and 83 assistant surgeons; 24 of those resigned to join the Confederate Army, and 3 were dismissed for questionable loyalties.[34]

A slightly less aged Clement Alexander Finley replaced Lawson in the summer of 1861. Lincoln appointed Finley over the objections of Secretary of War Cameron and the recommendations of the newly installed U.S. Sanitary Commission. Finley in turn appointed Surgeon Charles Tripler as the medical director of the Army of the Potomac.[35] What ensued was a series of actions and reactions as the war stumbled along in the first two years.

The initial fighting at the Battle of 1st Manassas witnessed an "over-whelmed and inexperienced medical corps that had no medical battle plan, suffered from a significantly fractured organization, and had endured a paucity of resources."[36]

The efforts of Tripler to address the high disease rate in and around the nation's capital were met with little support from his superiors, provided minimal relief, and triggered a jealous reaction by Surgeon General Finley. In Tripler's efforts to erect needed hospitals to alleviate overcrowded conditions, he failed to clear the request through Finley first. The curtailing of needed reforms due to bureaucratic inefficiencies and petty jealousies continued and were further exacerbated by the division of authority between the secretary of war and the surgeon general over the delivery and control of medical supplies and medical innovations. By December 1861, the Army of the Potomac had settled into overcrowded winter quarters with poor sanitation, widespread disease, and inadequate and overcrowded hospital capacity. Not surprisingly, one-quarter of the Union soldiers were ill.[37]

Early 1862 saw some improvements as Sen. Henry Wilson introduced legislation calling for reforms in the Medical Department, the construction of pavilion-style military hospitals, and the creation of an ambulance service. There were also improvements in the command structure with the appointment of William A. Hammond as the new and innovative surgeon general. Additionally, fellow classmate Jonathan Letterman was appointed as the medical director, first over the Department of West Virginia under General William Rosecrans and later as the medical director for the Army of the Potomac. The combined efforts of these two reform-minded doctors, along with support for reforms from Sen. Wilson and the Sanitary Commission, and the support for military organization by, first, Gen. George McClellan and, later, Gen. Joseph Hooker enabled the steady implementation of medical reforms in the Union Army.[38]

Letterman came into the position of medical director at a desperate time for army medical services in the Union, and he immediately set forth three targeted reforms. With little experience outside of army outpost medicine, Letterman used support from his friend and superior, Hammond, as well as support from commanders such as Gen. McClellan to implement his three-pronged strategy for military medical reform: improvements to the evacuation of wounded and ill soldiers, a tiered care system composed of field triage to temporary field hospitals to distant but well-provisioned general hospitals, and an efficient system for delivering medical supplies.[39] McClellan issued Special Order 197 and General Orders 139 and 150 that targeted the reorganization of the medical department and initiated a campaign against disease.[40]

The first test of Letterman's new system came at the Battle of Antietam in September 1862. With only days to prepare, Letterman managed to improve the delivery speed of medical supplies as well as the evacuation of wounded from the battlefield. Unfortunately, the lack of an efficient ambulance system prevented the transport of wounded to the well-provisioned general hospitals. Instead, temporary tent hospitals and existing structures like churches and barns were utilized. Letterman used the results to promote more collaboration with civilian agencies and for further legislation to support his ambulance-reform concepts.

Meanwhile, the erection of a series of well-ventilated pavilion hospitals with ample space for the growing number of injured and sick was developed, utilizing concepts employed in the Western campaign by Medical Director Bernard Irwin. The structure of these pavilion hospitals allowed for the segregation of patients to isolate known contagious infections from the wounded and ailing soldiers. Unfortunately, the bacterial and viral qualities of pneumonia were not known; therefore, those patients were not quarantined. Additionally, the new commander of the Army of the Potomac, Gen. Joe Hooker, supported Letterman's call for improved diets as a means of preventing illness and improving recovery time for the wounded. Commissary officers were not only tasked with delivering food, but also reporting on the efficient delivery and preparation of food for the Union forces. This combination of reform services and accountability set the stage for later integration of Letterman's system within the military command structure following the war.[41]

The Confederacy also advocated for reforms in its medical department and structure during the Civil War. Outside of the initial 24 surgeons and assistant surgeons that left the Union and joined the Confederacy at the outset of the war, no medical department existed for the Southern military. One of those who left the Union to join the Confederacy, David Camden DeLeon, was appointed the first surgeon general of the Confederacy in May 1861. Disorganized, poorly funded, and with full expectations of a quick war, the Confederate Medical Department began to realize the extent of its flawed nature following the South's victory at 1st Manassas, as uncared-for wounded continued to arrive at designated hospitals for a week following the battle. Many of these wounded, like their wounded Union opponents, were compelled to find their own way to the hospitals due to the lack of ambulances or any organized system of evacuating injured soldiers from the battlefield. With disease already filtering through the ranks, the wounded were quickly exposed to the secondary infections found in the hospitals, such as measles and the subsequent complications of pneumonia, further undermining their health and chances of survival. Measles was epidemic at this time and contributed twice as many soldiers who reported to the ineffective Confederate medical system in 1861; many of these also contracted pneumonia as a secondary infection. The lack of medical facilities resulted in the need for civilians to take ill and wounded soldiers into their homes, further spreading disease from the military ranks to rural communities in and around Manassas, Virginia.[42]

In an effort to combat the chaos of the Confederate Medical Department, Jefferson Davis replaced DeLeon with Samuel Preston Moore, an experienced surgeon from the former U.S. Army. Recognizing the chaos within the system, Moore set about efforts to reform it. Unfortunately, he tended to deflect blame from the Southern Medical Department to regimental commanders and transportation officials, and he called for new regulations to facilitate change. A Confederate congressional committee's investigation countered Moore's analysis, directing most blame to the "inadequacy of preparations by medical authorities." Similar in its recommendations to the civilian Sanitary Commission of the Union, this Southern governmental body criticized the method of hospitalization and inadequate staffing of medical officers, and it encouraged a relaxation of policies that had made the furlough of injured and sick soldiers improbable at the time.[43]

In the face of such recommendations that targeted his new command, Moore began to institute his own series of reforms and requests to support modifications in medical services. Using practices he had learned under the old U.S. Army, he implemented medical examining boards for all existing and future Confederate doctors. He sought additional funding targeted for building medical facilities, which were quickly used as "new hospitals sprang up all over the Confederacy."[44] Some of the new pavilion-style hospitals were larger and designed to facilitate the medical treatment of personnel from specific states, with the intention of enabling friends and relatives to locate the ill and wounded. Unfortunately, the implementation of this structure by the Southern Medical Department did not account for the highly infectious nature of such diseases as measles, much less bacterial and viral pneumonia.

The Peninsula Campaign of the spring of 1862 severely tested Moore's reforms, which proved inadequate in preparing for the vast numbers of ill and wounded. Similarly, the Vicksburg Campaign of 1863 further highlighted the inadequacy of the system.[45] The goals for reforming the Southern Medical Department were similar to those of Letterman and Hammond. However, while Letterman had the support of his superiors in the Medical Department and of specific military commanders, Moore's requests often fell on deaf ears.[46] Indeed, while Letterman's system was eventually embedded in the military structure, the perceptions and reception of Moore's system was lukewarm at best. One historian's description was damning, stating that "three great characteristics of the hospital support system of the Army of Tennessee were improvisation, the barter system, and reliance upon donated labor and material"[47] as a means of trying to accommodate necessary care in the face of diminishing Confederate resources. Nonetheless, Moore did increase funding for medical services and supported the construction or remodeling of hospitals throughout the war. The unprecedented numbers of ill and wounded soldiers, combined with the need to repeatedly relocate hospitals as the Confederate victories turned increasingly into defeats in 1864 and 1865, impeded Moore's efforts. Additionally, access to needed medical supplies and daily provisions declined, especially once Sherman began his march across the South and the Northern blockade of Southern coastlines became more effective. The decline in food supplies and constant movement of Confederate armies perpetuated the conditions experienced at the beginning of the war and increased the incidence of diseases and disease fatalities among Southern militaries.

Combined Impacts of Disease, Wounds, Conditions of War, and Secondary Pneumonia

Despite the improvements in the Medical Department structures, the realities of the Civil War continued to enable the spread of diseases such as pneumonia. Union and Confederate forces did improve their hospitals and medical treatments. In the North, the ability to fund reform measures that included a dedicated ambulance system greatly improved the evacuation of wounded from battlefields. Modifications in the Quartermaster Corps and accountability for the delivery of medical supplies improved the distribution time of needed goods, though problems with this delivery system returned in the next war fought by the United States. The organization of Northern pavilion-style hospitals into wards, which allowed for the isolation of contagious diseases, decreased the number of hospitalized soldiers contracting secondary illnesses. Unfortunately, the lack of medical knowledge regarding germ theory and a lack of knowledge about pneumonia's etiology resulted in the continued housing of pneumonia patients with those newly wounded or suffering from other ailments. Additionally, the winter camps with their overcrowded conditions and insufficient temporary housing continued to witness widespread outbreaks of colds, flus, and secondary infections of pneumonia.

The overall conditions and health of the Southern and Northern armies improved over the course of the war. The lessons learned from the Crimean and Mexican-American Wars helped formulate reforms that called for improved organization, hygiene, and nutrition. For the South, the limited resources in the last two years of the war and unstable economy of the fledgling nation proved unable to sustain the reforms proposed by Surgeon General Samuel Moore on a consistent basis, despite civilian support for ill and wounded soldiers. For the North, the continued financial support by the federal government, combined with numerous civilian organizations such as the U.S. Sanitary Commission, enabled the innovative and organizational reforms proposed by Medical Director Letterman and Surgeon General Hammond, even though Hammond was removed from office in late 1864. The influx of African American contraband camps and volunteer soldiers in the last two years of the war brought about a return of epidemics in the North at an unprecedented level, including reported cases of secondary infections of pneumonia. But support internally and externally for Letterman's three-tiered reforms ensured cleaner camps, improved nutrition, the faster evacuation of wounded soldiers, and even the reduction of secondary infections through initial attempts at quarantine.

Both sides witnessed improvements in medical treatments over the course of the war. The harsh treatments of the allopathic system gave way to more moderate remedies. However, the widespread use of morphine and opium for pain and chloroform and ether for anesthesia during surgery had an immediate impact on the development of secondary respiratory infections such as pneumonia, not to mention the long-term impacts on soldiers who carried their acquired addictions to these opiates from wartime into their postwar lives.

The attention of many Civil War historians and enthusiasts to the political origins and military strategies of the war often reduces the treatment of the human cost to a series of charts and numbers and as a necessary consequence of the conflict. The reality of the Medical Corps' treatment of 6 million cases of illnesses, when only 425,000 of those cases were combat-related injuries, brings that view into question.[48] It is important to note that the use of numbers regarding reported cases of illness, though helpful and informative, risks the oversight of how some less understood diseases, especially those associated with secondary infections, had a dramatic impact on the lives and deaths of so many Civil War soldiers, volunteers, and civilians.

NOTES

1. Louis Cruveilhier, quoted in David M. Morens, Jeffery K. Taubenberger, and Anthony S. Fauci, "Predominant Role of Bacterial Pneumonia as a Cause of Death in Pandemic Influenza: Implications for Pandemic Influenza Preparedness," *Journal of Infectious Diseases* 198, no. 7 (October 1, 2008): 962, accessed August 31, 2017, https://academic.oup.com/jid/article/198/7/962/2192118/Predominant-Role-of -Bacterial-Pneumonia-as-a-Cause.

2. Barbara Lee Maling, "Black Southern Nursing Care Providers in Virginia during the American Civil War, 1861–1865" (PhD diss., University of Virginia, December 2009), 105. The order of deadly diseases listed reflects the impact on Caucasian Americans. Among African American participants, dysentery still ranked the most fatal (20 percent mortality), with pneumonia second (14 percent mortality) and typhoid a close third (13 percent mortality). Chulhee Lee, "Socioeconomic Difference in the Health of Black Union Soldiers during the American Civil War," *Social Science History* 33, no. 4 (Winter 2009): 434, accessed August 27, 2017, http://www.jstor.org/stable/40587324.

3. Sheila Grossman and Carol Mattson Porth, *Porth's Pathophysiology: Concepts of Altered Health States*, 9th ed. (Philadelphia: Wolters Kluwer Health, Lippincott Williams & Wilkins, 2014), 934.

4. Centers for Disease Control and Prevention, "Pneumococcal Disease," accessed August 27, 2017, https://www.cdc.gov/pneumococcal/index.html.

5. Michael R. Gilchrist, "Disease and Infection in the American Civil War," *American Biology Teacher* 60, no. 4 (April 1998): 261, accessed August 27, 2017, http://www.jstor .org/stable/4450468.

6. Centers for Disease Control and Prevention, "*Mycoplasma pneumoniae* Infection," accessed August 27, 2017, https://www.cdc.gov/pneumonia/atypical/mycoplasma /index.html.

7. Centers for Disease Control and Prevention, "Human Parainfluenza Viruses (HPIVs)," accessed August 27, 2017, https://www.cdc.gov/parainfluenza/index.html.

8. "Bacterial Pneumonia: Symptoms, Treatment, and Prevention," *Healthline Newsletter*, accessed August 27, 2017, http://www.healthline.com/health/bacterial-pneumonia #overview1.

9. Centers for Disease Control and Prevention, "Fungal Diseases: *Pneumocystis* pneumonia," accessed August 27, 2017, https://www.cdc.gov/fungal/diseases/pneumocystis -pneumonia/index.html.

10. Richard H. Shryock, "A Medical Perspective on the Civil War," *American Quarterly* 14, no. 2, Pt. 1 (Summer 1962): 165.

11. Robert C. Myers, "Mortality in the Twelfth Michigan Volunteer Infantry, 1861–1866," *Michigan Historical Review* 20, no. 1 (Spring 1994): 32, accessed August 27, 2017, http://www.jstor.org/stable/20173432.

12. Dale C. Smith, "Military Medical History: The American Civil War," *OAH Magazine of History* 19, no. 5, Medicine and History (September 2005): 17, accessed August 27, 2017, http://www.jstor.org/stable/25161973?seq=1&cid=pdf-reference#references_tab _contents.

13. The teachings of Hippocrates and Galen held that the four humors (black bile, yellow bile, blood, and phlegm), when imbalanced in the human body, were the cause of illness. The cure for such imbalances was to cleanse the body through rigorous regimens of purging, bleeding, blistering, and other counters to the particular humoral imbalances. John Duffy, "Medical Practice in the Ante Bellum South," *Journal of Southern History* 25, no. 1 (February 1959): 54, accessed September 3, 2017, http://www.jstor.org/stable/2954479.

14. A. W. Barclay, "Treatment of Pneumonia," *British Medical Journal* (November 11, 1865): 509–510, accessed August 27, 2017, http://www.jstor.org/stable/25205119; W. J. J. Arnold, "The Treatment of Pneumonia," *British Medical Journal* (July 12, 1913): 102, accessed August 27, 2017, http://www.jstor.org/stable/25302225; "The Treatment of Pneumonia," *Scientific American* 55, no. 8 (August 21, 1886): 119, accessed August 27, 2017, http://www.jstor.org/stable/26093152; and H. H. Cunningham, *Doctors in Gray: The Confederate Medical Service* (Baton Rouge: Louisiana State University Press, 1986), 203.

15. Rachel M. Kellum, "Surgeons of the Severed Limb: Confederate Military Medicine in Arkansas, 1863–1865" (master's thesis, Jackson College, 2014), 99.

16. It is impossible to determine the number of total patients who died from untreated pneumonia, as many were misdiagnosed or refused to go to sick calls to be diagnosed and treated.

17. Sepsis Alliance, "Sepsis and Pneumonia," accessed August 27, 2017, http://www.sepsis.org/sepsis-and-pneumonia.

18. Bell Irvin Wiley, *The Life of Billy Yank: A Common Soldier of the Union* (Baton Rouge: Louisiana State University Press, 1987), 133.

19. George Worthington Adams, *Doctors in Blue: The Medical History of the Union Army in the Civil War* (Baton Rouge: Louisiana State University Press, 1996), 4.

20. Wiley, *The Life of Billy Yank*, 133; and Grossman and Porth, *Porth's Pathophysiology*, 938.

21. Wiley, *The Life of Billy Yank*, 134–135; and Grossman and Porth, *Porth's Pathophysiology*, 938.

22. Smith, "Military Medical History," 18.

23. Frank Reed Freemon, "Medical Care during the American Civil War" (PhD diss., University of Illinois at Urbana-Champaign, 1992), 96–109.

24. Drew Gilpin Faust, *This Republic of Suffering: Death and the American Civil War* (New York: Vintage Books, 2008), 48, 138; and Lee, "Socioeconomic Difference," 434.

25. Lee, "Socioeconomic Difference."

26. Andrew K. Black, "In the Service of the United States: Comparative Mortality among African-American and White Troops in the Union Army," *Journal of Negro History* 79, no. 4 (Autumn 1994): 323.

27. Wiley, *The Life of Billy Yank*, 133; and Grossman and Porth, *Porth's Pathophysiology* 937.

28. David Madden, ed., *Beyond the Battlefield: The Ordinary Life and Extraordinary Times of the Civil War Soldier* (New York: Simon and Schuster, 2000), 136–137.

29. Madden, *Beyond the Battlefield*, 134–135, 138.

30. Grossman and Porth, *Porth's Pathophysiology* 936.

31. Madden, *Beyond the Battlefield*, 237.

32. Dorothy Denneen Volo and James M. Volo, *Daily Life in Civil War America* (Westport, CT: Greenwood Press, 1998), 167.

33. Marvin P. Rozear and Joseph C. Greenfield Jr., "'Let Us Cross over the River': The Final Illness of Stonewall Jackson," *Virginia Magazine of History and Biography* 103, no. 1 (January 1995): 31–33.

34. U.S. Army Medical Department, Office of Medical History, "Thomas Lawson," accessed August 27, 2017, http://history.amedd.army.mil/surgeongenerals/T_Lawson.html.

35. Scott McGaugh, *Surgeon in Blue: Jonathan Letterman, the Civil War Doctor Who Pioneered Battlefield Care* (New York: Arcade Publishing, 2013), 51, 56.

36. McGaugh, *Surgeon in Blue*, 47.

37. McGaugh, *Surgeon in Blue*, 57–61.

38. U.S. Army Medical Department, Office of Medical History, "William A. Hammond," accessed August 27, 2017, http://history.amedd.army.mil/surgeongenerals/W _Hammond.html; and McGaugh, *Surgeon in Blue*, 62–68, 73.

39. Freemon, "Medical Care," 60–62.

40. McGaugh, *Surgeon in Blue*, 80.

41. Adams, *Doctors in Blue*, 198; and McGaugh, *Surgeon in Blue*, 154–155, 157.

42. Freemon, "Medical Care," 83–85.

43. Freemon, "Medical Care," 87–88; and Wiley, *The Life of Billy Yank*, 261–263.

44. Freemon, "Medical Care," 89.

45. Wiley, *The Life of Billy Yank*, 261–264; and Freemon, "Medical Care," 91–93.

46. Freemon, "Medical Care," 178.

47. Freemon, "Medical Care," 110.

48. Michael A. Flannery, "Civil War Medicine: Approaches for Teaching," *OAH Magazine of History* 19, no. 5, *Medicine and History* (September 2005): 41, accessed August 27, 2017, http://www.jstor.org/stable/25161979.

Epilogue

Epidemics and Wars in the Context of Historical Inquiry

Rebecca M. Seaman

> But however secure and well-regulated civilized life may become, bacteria, Protozoa, viruses, infected fleas, lice, ticks, mosquitoes, and bedbugs will always lurk in the shadows ready to pounce when neglect, poverty, famine, or war lets down the defenses.[1]
>
> —Hans Zinsser

Disease epidemiology is the study of how populations, rather than individuals, are affected by contagious illnesses. The field is inherently interdisciplinary. It requires epidemiologists to have an understanding of everything from statistics to geography to produce theories about different diseases. By studying a particular disease or population, public health policies can be used to resolve outbreaks or keep them from occurring. As such, epidemiology is more often an applied process than a purely academic one.[2] As public health is often focused on preventing outbreaks of illnesses, epidemiologists are particularly concerned with disease diffusion. Diffusion is the process whereby something moves in space from one place to another. This can be applied not only to a disease, but also cultural ideas, technology, or even people. Several models of diffusion have been developed. Although the spread of infectious disease could resemble many of them, the most effective models when studying disease diffusion in the context of war are contagious diffusion, hierarchical diffusion, and transference diffusion.

Using the first model, three things are needed for the successful diffusion of a disease. There must be a source of infection, a population that is vulnerable to that infection, and direct contact between populations that enables spread.[3] Without these three things, it is impossible for an epidemic to occur. However, to accommodate the processes of hierarchical and transference diffusion, one must also consider the modes of transportation, routes of human migration and travel, and numerous other variables associated with particular diseases and transport vehicles. Accounting for these three models of disease diffusion during periods of war brings the issues involved into sharper focus. It also helps historians and medical personnel track initial contact and trace the flow of contacts and disease regionally and even globally.

One of the many ways to create the necessary contact that spreads disease is through warfare. As civilizations clash over territory and resources, they exchange technology, material culture, customs, and language. They also exchange bacteria, viruses, and parasites. This diffusion is especially dramatic when one party is left more vulnerable to infection. This can happen because of existing stressors, such as famine, or simply because the population has no existing immunity.[4] Disease exchange during war can also be intentional—a form of biological warfare. Most attempts of intentional contamination discussed in this volume were either unsuccessful or the methods of spreading the disease were not fully understood by the parties involved, thereby diminishing the intended results. It is the ability of epidemics to influence events that has drawn historians to incorporate disease in their studies, including how diseases relate to warfare.

Military structures, and specifically periods of war, create conditions that are all too accommodating for the emergence and spread of contagious diseases. Among the common conditions are crowding, overpopulation for facilities and the ecology, insufficient drainage and sewage, and insufficient food and shelter. Mobilization of forces is a specific aspect that creates conditions for epidemics. As populations from varied regions and backgrounds coalesce in crowded camps, far more is shared than just training and cultural norms. The indiscriminate mixing of populations has rarely taken into account the epidemiological backgrounds of the people clustered together in barracks, tents, trains, and ships.[5] While the health of troops has been a concern of good military leaders over the centuries, the ability to affect healthy conditions has not consistently existed. This has especially been true of physical and mental health, as fatigue, trauma, and stress blend with inadequate diets to undermine the resistance of even healthy individuals to diseases they become exposed to on a regular basis.

Disease history is a relatively new and, some would argue, underestimated field. In *Rats, Lice and History*, the physician Hans Zinsser wrote, "We are dealing with a phase of man's history on earth which has received too little attention from poets, artists, and historians. Swords and lances, arrows, machine guns, and even high explosives have had far less power over the fates of the nations than the typhus louse, the plague flea, and the yellow-fever mosquito."[6] Different observations have been made about how warfare could trigger or increase the impact of epidemics. For example, military campaigns were especially effective in causing outbreaks in rural areas, where the population was too low-density to support any infectious disease becoming endemic without in influx of armed forces on their way to battle. It is these outbreaks that caught the attention of chroniclers in urban areas, even if the disease never caused many deaths in the cities.[7] Epidemics have also sometimes demonstrated an apparent cycle of war, famine, and pestilence; wars leave populations malnourished, which in turn weakens the immune system and opens the way for an increase in disease-related deaths.[8]

It would be comparatively easy to demonstrate that warfare has historically encouraged the dissemination of disease, with certain diseases leading the way in terms of prevalence on battlefields: dysentery, typhus, malaria, typhoid fever, and problems from secondary infections have been the worst offenders. It is also a sober reminder that until the 20th century, humanity had lost more military personnel to such diseases than to actual combat. Yet, while diseases influence war, they do not necessarily determine war, and such virulent diseases as these, based on the proximity of opposed forces, may well affect multiple camps more or less simultaneously. As a result, studying how diseases historically affected warfare may prove as complex as making a "retrospective diagnosis" of any particular disease in the first place.

The historian's objective is not necessarily to conduct a diagnosis of patients from 200 or even 2,000 years ago. Our curiosity will always ask, what was this plague? That is an important question for the medical community and the continued growth and development of medicine. However, an equally important task is to assess the impact of epidemics in a 360-degree worldview, from the most basic questions to the more nuanced. Which population was affected? What were the symptoms? How did the society react? How did it impact war efforts or how did the war impact the sickness? Did the epidemic cause a fundamental change to the society in terms of its approach to medicine? An increasingly important question for military historians and leaders to ask includes, what lessons can be learned from the conflict and associated epidemic? Regardless of whether we can make a confirmed diagnosis of what a particular epidemic was, historians can and should still measure the impact epidemics have on societies and, in the case of this book, their overall relationships with their contemporaneous wars.

Within this volume, specific epidemics and wars were selected to highlight differing aspects regarding the interrelation between the two as well as to bring to light information not commonly known to readers unless they are military or medical historians. The first three chapters in part I deal directly with the problem of studying diseases from the past, or the difficulties associated with retrospective diagnosis. Because of the need to find epidemics and wars that fit this purpose and yet had extensive resources available, the Plague of Athens, the Antonine Plague of Rome, and the sweating sickness of England were targeted. The intention was not to provide a new diagnosis, but to reveal to readers why the diagnoses of these epidemics remain a mystery. This section also served to introduce the basic concepts of studying epidemics in the context of wars.

Part II of the volume targets bacterial epidemics that have impacted wars across the centuries. Decisions about which wars to target were sometimes made to intentionally highlight a particular epidemic that has been well studied in the context of another well-known war. Additionally, due to the reality of virulent contagious diseases to spread into pandemics that affected many societies simultaneously, the chapters on cholera and the plague pull together information from around the world or continents, thereby including societies involved in various wars or not involved in wars at all. Finally, the chapter on diphtheria tackles the task of showing how diseases thought to be understood and in check nonetheless return as epidemics, especially in shatter zones and underdeveloped regions. This concept is an important lesson that all societies need to keep in mind, as progress tends to breed overconfidence regarding the reemergence of contagious diseases.

Part III targets viral diseases that plagued periods of war. Smallpox, one of the oldest known diseases to impact humans in periods of peace and war, is broken into two chapters, demonstrating the eventual outcomes of the disease on victors and vanquished in two different eras of history. Some of the epidemics in these chapters capture the impact of diseases during wars already studied in other works, but they typically bring in the lessons learned from past wars and epidemics and how some were built upon and others temporarily disregarded due to the urgencies of warfare. The chapter on measles in World War I targets the impact of mobilization processes on the health of military personnel, especially in nations with conscripted urban and rural populations. Likewise, the chapter on HIV/AIDS in the African wars demonstrates how the movements of nonmilitary refugees during periods of war impacted the spread of disease regionally and even globally. The final chapter in this section, covering mumps following the Bosnian Wars, takes a different approach and shows how the costs and decisions associated with periods of war sometimes impact the outbreak of epidemics in later generations.

Not all diseases are easily grouped by categories of bacterial or viral origins. Part IV provides the opportunity to highlight examples of protozoan epidemics (malaria) as well as epidemics common during wars throughout the ages but that spread through bacteria, viruses, protozoa, fungi, arthropods, and even inhalation of fumes (malaria, pneumonia, and dysentery). The chapter on malaria provides another opportunity to examine a disease thought well under control that managed to reemerge to impact not only soldiers fighting in a later war but also to spread back to their families and communities upon their return home. Dysentery, one of the most common diseases throughout history, is included to highlight how and why this disease continues to plague militaries, though thankfully the impact on its victims has been significantly reduced with modern medicine. The chapter on pneumonia in the Civil War demonstrates how disease often took different forms in the confines of military hospitals. The original reasons for admission to camp hospitals were often recorded, and secondary infections, especially varying forms of pneumonia, that undermined the already fragile health of wounded and ill soldiers were intermittently recorded in the medical case histories.

Throughout the book, efforts were made to connect the lessons of the past with new struggles as each epidemic and period of war was examined. Additionally, failures to employ lessons from the past were also examined where appropriate, including reasons for such decisions. Finally, the prevailing perceptions of disease were provided to give context to the era studied. The contributing authors and editor of this volume may not be able to answer all questions pertaining to the historical examination of wars and epidemics for individual readers. However, their intent was to spur a curiosity in the minds of their readers and to provide guidance and structure for others to continue seeking answers to these and other relevant questions regarding the study of epidemics and wars.

NOTES

1. Hans Zinsser, *Rats, Lice and History* (London: Routledge, 1935), 13–14.
2. Carol Hand, *Epidemiology: The Fight against Ebola and Other Diseases* (Minneapolis: Abdo Publishing, 2015), 19–20.
3. Kathleen Hornsby, "Spatial Diffusion: Conceptualizations and Formalizations," National Center for Geographic Information and Analysis and Department of Spatial Information Science and Engineering (Orono, ME: University of Maine), 1–5.
4. Frederick F. Cartwright and Michael D. Biddiss, *Disease and History* (New York: Dorset Press, 1972), 1–4.
5. Matthew Smallman-Raynor and Andrew D. Cliff, "Epidemic Diffusion Processes in a System of U.S. Military Camps: Transfer Diffusion and the Spread of Typhoid Fever in the Spanish-American War, 1898," *Annals of the Association of American Geographers* 91, no. 1 (March 2001): 72, accessed July 30, 2017, http://www.jstor.org/stable/3651192.
6. Zinsser, 9.
7. William H. McNeill, *Plagues and Peoples* (New York: Anchor Books, 1998), 98.
8. Cartwright, *Disease and History*, 3.

Bibliography

Ackeren, Marcel van. *A Companion to Marcus Aurelius.* Oxford, UK: John Wiley & Sons, 2012.

Adams, George Worthington. *Doctors in Blue: The Medical History of the Union Army in the Civil War.* New York: Henry Schuman. Reprint. Baton Rouge: Louisiana Paperback Edition, 1996.

Aginam, Obijiofor. "Rape and HIV as Weapons of War." United Nations University (June 27, 2012). Accessed September 2, 2017. https://unu.edu/publications/articles/rape-and-hiv-as-weapons-of-war.html.

Agnew, Jeremy. *Alcohol and Opium in the Old West: Use, Abuse and Influence.* Jefferson, NC, and London: McFarland & Company, Inc., Publishers, 2014.

Akiner, Shirin, and Catherine Barnes. "The Tajik Civil War: Causes and Dynamics." From "Tajikistan: Disintegration or Reconciliation?" Royal Institute of International Affairs, London (Spring 2001): 16–22. Conciliation Resources. Accessed September 2, 2017. http://www.c-r.org/accord-article/tajik-civil-war-causes-and-dynamics.

Alkire, Sabina. "A Conceptual Framework for Human Security, Working Paper 2." Centre for Research on Inequality, Human Security, and Ethnicity, CRISE (2003): 3–5.

American Association for the Advancement of Science. "Medical Inspection of Camp Wheeler." *Science* 46, no. 1197 (1917): 558–559. Accessed September 2, 2017. http://science.sciencemag.org/content/46/1197/558.

Anderson, Jeffrey. "When We Have a Few More Epidemics the City Officials Will Awake: Philadelphia and the Influenza Epidemic of 1918–1919." *Maryland Historian* 27, no. 1-2 (1996): 1–26.

Andrews, Justin M. "North Africa, Italy, and the Islands of the Mediterranean." In *Preventive Medicine in World War II.* Vol. 6, *Communicable Diseases, Malaria,* edited by John Boyd Coates. Washington, D.C.: Office of the Surgeon General, U.S. Army Medical Department, 1963: 249–302. Accessed September 7, 2017. http://history.amedd.army.mil/booksdocs/wwii/Malaria/chapterV.htm.

"Anopheles Mosquitoes." Centers for Disease and Prevention. Accessed September 2, 2017. https://www.cdc.gov/malaria/about/biology/mosquitoes.

Aristides, P. Aelius. *The Complete Works.* Volume 2, *Orations XVII–LIII.* Translated by Charles A. Behr. Leiden: E. J. Brill, 1981.

Armytage, W. H. G. "William Crawford Gorgas, 1854–1920." *British Medical Journal* 2, no. 4894 (October 1954): 985–986.

Arnold, W. J. J. "The Treatment of Pneumonia." *British Medical Journal* (July 12, 1913): 102. Accessed August 27, 2017. http://www.jstor.org/stable/25302225.

ar-Razi, Abu Becr Mohammed ibn Zacariya. *A Treatise on the Smallpox and Measles.* Translated by William Alexander Greenhill, MD. London: C. and J. Adlard, 1848.

Arrow, Kenneth J., Claire B. Panosian, and Hellen Gelband, eds. *Saving Lives, Buying Time: Economics of Malaria Drugs in an Age.* Washington, D.C.: National Academies Press, 2004.

Ashburn, P. M. *The Ranks of Death: A Medical History of the Conquest of America.* New York: Coward-McCann, 1947.

Aurelius, Marcus. *Meditations.* Translated by Meric Casaubon. Auckland, NZ: The Floating Press, 2011.

Autrand, Françoise. "The Battle of Crecy: A Hard Blow for the Monarchy of France." In *The Battle of Crécy, 1346,* edited by Andrew Ayton and Philip Preston. Rochester, NY: Boydell & Brewer, Ltd., 2005: 273–286.

Auyang, Sunny Y. "Reality and Politics in the War on Infectious Diseases." Accessed, September 16, 2017. http://www.creatingtechnology.org/biomed/germs.pdf.

Ayers, Leonard P., Col. "Health and Casualties." In *The War with Germany, A Statistical Summary.* Washington, D.C.: Government Printing Office, 1919: 119–130.

Ayton, Andrew. *Knights and Warhorses: Military Service and the English Aristocracy under Edward III.* Rochester, NY: The Boydell Press, 1994.

Ayton, Andrew. "The English Army at Crécy." In *The Battle of Crécy, 1346,* edited by Andrew Ayton and Philip Preston. Rochester, NY: Boydell & Brewer, Ltd., 2005: 159–252.

Babkin, Igor V., and Irina N. Babkina. "The Origin of the Variola Virus." *Viruses* 7 (2015): 1100–1112.

"Bacterial Pneumonia: Symptoms, Treatment, and Prevention." *Healthline Newsletter.* Accessed August 27, 2017. http://www.healthline.com/health/bacterial-pneumonia#overview1.

Balić, Emily Greble. "When Croatia Needed Serbs: Nationalism and Genocide in Sarajevo 1941–1942." *Slavic Review* 68, no. 1 (Spring 2009): 116–137. Accessed August 12, 2017. http://www.jstor.org/stable/20453271.

Barclay, A. W. "Treatment of Pneumonia." *British Medical Journal* (November 11, 1865): 509–510. Accessed August 27, 2017. http://www.jstor.org/stable/25205119.

Barnes, Ethne. *Diseases and Human Evolution.* Albuquerque: University of New Mexico Press, 2007.

Baron, S., ed. *Medical Microbiology.* 4th edition. Galveston: University of Texas Medical Branch at Galveston, 1996. Accessed August 25, 2017. https://www.ncbi.nlm.nih.gov/books/NBK8461.

Barrett, O'Neill, Jr. "Malaria: Epidemiology." In *Internal Medicine in Vietnam.* Edited by Andre Ognibene and O'Neill Barrett Jr. Vol. 2, *General Medicine and Infectious Disease.* Washington, D.C.: Office of the Surgeon General & Center for Military History, 1982: 279–291.

Barry, John M. *The Great Influenza: The Story of the Deadliest Pandemic in History.* New York: Penguin Books, 2004.

Baxby, Derrick. *Jenner's Smallpox Vaccine: The Riddle of Vaccinia Virus and Its Origin.* London: Heinemann Educational Books Ltd, 1981.

Bayne-Jones, Stanhope, ed. "The American Civil War (15 April 1861–30 June 1865)—Beginnings of Bacteriological Era and Scientific Preventive Medicine (1861–1898)." In *The Evolution of Preventive Medicine in the United States Army, 1607–1939.* Washington, D.C.: U.S. Government Printing Office, 1968: 97–121. Accessed September 7, 2017. http://history.amedd.army.mil/booksdocs/misc/evprev/ch6.htm.

Beadle, Christine, and Stephen L. Hoffman. "History of Malaria in the United States Naval Forces at War: World War I through the Vietnam Conflict." *Clinical Infectious Diseases* 16, no. 2 (February 1993): 320–329.

Becker, Ann M. "Smallpox in Washington's Army: Strategic Implications of the Disease during the American Revolutionary War." *Journal of Military History* 68 (2004): 381–430.

Bell, Andrew McIlwaine. *Mosquito Soldiers: Malaria, Yellow Fever, and the Course of the American Civil War.* Baton Rouge: Louisiana State University Press, 2010.

Beltran, Gonzalo Aguirre. *Medicina y magia: El proceso de aculturacion en la estructura colonial*. Mexico: Instituto Nacional Indigenista, 1963.

Benedictow, Ole J. *The Black Death 1346–1353: A Complete History*. Woodbridge, Suffolk: Boydell Press, 2004.

Berger, Darlene. "A Brief History of Medical Diagnosis and the Birth of the Clinical Laboratory: Part I, Ancient Times through the 19th Century." (July 1999): 1–8. Accessed April 8, 2017. http://www.academia.dk/Blog/wp-content/uploads/KlinLab-Hist/Lab History1.pdf.

Berner, Brad K., ed. *The Spanish-American War: A Documentary History with Commentaries*. Madison, NJ: Fairleigh Dickinson University Press, 2014.

Beveridge, William Henry. *Prices and Wages, from the Twelfth to the Nineteenth Century*. Vol. 1. London: Longmans Green & Co., 1939.

Beyer, Henry G., MD. "The Dissemination of Disease by the Fly." *New York Medical Journal* 91, no. 14 (April 2, 1910): 677–685.

Beyrer, Chris, Stefan D. Baral, Frits van Griensven, Steven M. Goodreau, Suwat Chariyalertsak, Andrea L. Wirtz, and Ron Brookmeyer. "Global Epidemiology of HIV Infection in Men Who Have Sex with Men," *The Lancet* 380, no. 9839 (2012): 367–377.

Bianchine, Peter J., MD, and Thomas A. Russo, MD. "The Role of Epidemic Infectious Disease in the Discovery of America." In *Columbus and the New World: Medical Implications*, edited by Guy A. Settipane, MD. Providence, RI: OceanSide Publications, Inc., 1995: 11–18.

Bickel, M. H. "The American Malaria Program (1941–1946) and Its Sequelae for Biomedical Research after World War II." *Gesnerus* 56, no. 1-2 (1999): 107–119.

Billings, J. S. "Memoir of Joseph Janvier Woodward, 1833–1884." In *Biographical Memoirs*. Vol. 2, 205–307. Washington, D.C.: National Academy of Sciences, 1886. Accessed September 7, 2017. http://www.nasonline.org/publications/biographical-memoirs/memoir -pdfs/woodward-joseph-j.pdf.

Biotechin.Asia. "Scientists Illustrate How Host Cell Responds to Zika Virus Infection." Accessed September 2, 2017. https://biotechin.asia/2017/05/09/scientists-illustrate-how-host-cell-responds-to-zika-virus-infection.

Birley, Anthony. *Marcus Aurelius: A Biography*. New Haven, CT: Yale University Press, 1987.

Black, Andrew K. "In the Service of the United States: Comparative Mortality among African -American and White Troops in the Union Army." *Journal of Negro History* 79, no. 4 (Autumn 1994), 317–333.

Black, Mary E. "Abdullah Nakas, Bosnia and Hercegovina's Most Famous War Surgeon." *British Medical Journal* 332, no. 7545 (April 8, 2006): 856. Accessed August 14, 2017. http://www.jstor.org/stable/25456613.

Bland, Edward F., MD. "Heart Disease." In *Infectious Diseases and General Medicine*, 419–455. Internal Medicine in World War II Series. Washington, D.C.: Office of Medical History, U.S. Army Medical Department):. Accessed September 2, 2017. http://history.amedd .army.mil/booksdocs/wwii/internalmedicinevolIII/chapter16.htm.

Blondo, Richard A. "A View of Point Lookout Prison Camp for Confederates." *OAH Magazine of History* 8, no. 1, *The Civil War* (Fall 1993): 30–34. Accessed September 7, 2017. http://www.jstor.org/stable/25162923?seq=1#page_scan_tab_contents.

Boak, Arthur E. R. *Manpower Shortage and the Fall of the Roman Empire in the West*. Ann Arbor: University of Michigan Press, 1955.

Boccaccio, Giovanni. *Decameron*. Quoted in *The Black Death*, edited and translated by Rosemary Horrox. Manchester and New York: Manchester University Press, 1994.

Boorde, Andrew. *The Fyrst Boke of the Introduction of Knowledge: A Compendious Regyment, or, a Dyetary of Helth Made in Mountpyllier. Barnes in the Defence of the Berde.* 1542, 1870, 1952. London: Adamant Media, 2001.

Bos, Kirsten I., Verena J. Schuenemann, G. Brian Golding, Hernán A. Burbano, Nicholas Waglechner, Brian K. Coombes, Joseph B. McPhee, Sharon N. DeWitte, Mattias Meyer, Sarah Schmedes, James Wood, David J. D. Earn, D. Ann Herring, Peter Bauer, Hendrik N. Poinar, and Johannes Krause. "A Draft of *Yersinia pestis* from Victims of the Black Death." *Nature* 478, no. 7370 (October 27, 2011): 506–510.

Boslough, Sarah, ed. *Encyclopedia of Epidemiology.* Thousand Oaks, CA: Sage Publications, 2008.

Bougarel, Xavier. "Review Essay." *Southeast European and Black Sea Studies* 15, no. 4 (2015): 683–688.

Bowersock, G. W. "The Personality of Thucydides." *The Antioch Review* 25, no. 1, Special Greek Issue (Spring 1965): 135–146.

Boyd, Charles G. "Making Peace with the Guilty: The Truth about Bosnia." *Foreign Affairs* 74, no. 5 (September–October 1995): 22–38. Accessed August 12, 2017. http://www.jstor.org/stable/20047298.

Bradford, James C., ed. *Crucible of Empire, The Spanish-American War and Its Aftermath.* Annapolis, MD: Naval War College, 1993.

Bradbury, Jim. *The Medieval Archer.* New York: St. Martin's Press, 1985.

Bresalier, Michael. "Fighting Flu: Military Pathology, Vaccines, and the Conflicted Identity of the 1918–19 Pandemic in Britain." *Journal of the History of Medicine and Allied Science* 68, no. 1 (2013): 15–28.

Brown, R. A., and H. M. Colvin. "The King's Works 1272–1485." In *The History of the King's Works.* Vol. 1. Edited by H. M. Colvin. London: Her Majesty's Stationary Office, 1963.

Bryant, J. E., E. C. Holmes, and A. D. T. Barrett. "Out of Africa: A Molecular Perspective on the Introduction of Yellow Fever Virus into the Americas." *PLoS Pathogens* 3, no. 5, e75 (May 2007). Accessed September 2, 2017. http://dx.doi.org/10.1371/journal.ppat.0030075.

Bugl, Paul. "History of Epidemics and Plagues." Hartford.edu. Accessed September 2, 2017. http://uhavax.hartford.edu/bugl/histepi.htm#plague.

Butler, Hilary. "Diphtheria." Whale.to. Accessed September 2, 2017. http://www.whale.to/m/butler.html.

Buve, Anne, Kizito Bishikwabo-Nsarhaza, and Gladys Mutangadura. "The Spread and Effect of HIV-1 Infection in Sub-Saharan Africa." *The Lancet* 359 (2002): 2011–2017.

Byerly, Carol R. "The Politics of Disease and War: Infectious Disease in the United States Army during World War I." PhD diss., University of Colorado, 2001.

Byerly, Carol R. "The U.S. Military and the Influenza Pandemic of 1918–1919." *Public Health Reports (1974–)* 125, Supplement 3, "The 1918–1919 Influenza Pandemic in the United States." (April 2010): 82–91. Accessed September 2, 2017. http://www.jstor.org/stable/41435302.

Byrne, Aisling, and Victoria Flood. "The Romance of the Stanleys: Regional and National Imaginings in the Percy Folio." *Viator* 46, no. 1 (2015): 327–351.

Byrne, Joseph P. *The Black Death.* Westport, CT: Greenwood Press, 2004.

Caius, John. *The Sweating Sickness: A Boke or Counseill Against the Disease Commonly Called the Sweate or Sweatyng Sicknesse.* Reprint. Memphis, TN: General Books, 2010. First published in 1552.

Calderaro, Adriana, Giovanna Piccolo, Chiara Gorrini, Sabina Rossi, Sara Montecchini, Maria Loretana Dell'Anna, Flora De Conto, Maria Cristina Medici, Carlo Chezzi, and Maria Cristina Arcangeletti. "Accurate Identification of the Six Human *Plasmodium* Spp. Causing Imported Malaria, including *Plasmodium ovale wallikeri* and *Plasmodium knowlesi*." *Malaria Journal* 12, no. 321 (2013). Accessed September 2, 2017. https://malariajournal.biomedcentral.com/articles/10.1186/1475-2875-12-321.

Calloway, Colin. *The Indian History of an American Institution: Native Americans and Dartmouth.* Dartmouth, MA: Dartmouth College Press, 2010.

Campbell, Bruce M. S. "Physical Shocks, Biological Hazards, and Human Impacts: The Crisis of the Fourteenth Century Revisited." In *Economic and Biological Interactions in Pre-Industrial Europe from the 13th to the 18th Centuries.* Edited by S. Cavaciocchi. Florence, Italy: Firenze University Press, 2010.

Canfield, C. J. "Malaria in U.S. Military Personnel 1965–1971." *Proceedings of the Helminthological Society of Washington* 39 (Special Issue, Basic Research in Malaria, 1972): 15–18.

Capps, Joseph A. "A New Adaptation of the Face Mask in Control of Contagious Disease." *JAMA* 70, no. 13 (1918): 910–911.

Carlson, James R., and Peter W. Hammond. "The English Sweating Sickness (1485–c. 1551): A New Perspective on Disease Etiology." *Journal of the History of Medicine and Allied Sciences* 54, no. 1 (1999): 23–54.

Cartwright, Frederick F., and Michael D. Biddiss. *Disease and History.* New York: Barnes & Noble, 1991.

Casadesus, Josep, and David Low. "Epigenetic Gene Regulation in the Bacterial World." *Microbiology and Molecular Biology Reviews* (September 2006): 830–856.

Cash, Philip. "1775: Smallpox Epidemic in the American Revolution." *Disasters, Accidents, and Crises in American History: A Reference Guide to the Nation's Most Catastrophic Events.* Edited by Ballard C. Campbell. New York: Facts on File, 2008.

Castiglioni, Arturo. *A History of Medicine.* Translated by E. B. Krumbhaar. New York: Jason Aronson, Inc., 1975.

Castillo, Bernal Diaz del. *The Conquest of New Spain.* Translated with introduction by John M. Cohen. London: Penguin Books, 1963.

Caulaincourt, Eilleaux (Countess) Armand Augustin Louis de. *Recollections of Caulaincourt, Duke of Vicenza.* London: Henry Colburn Publisher, 1838.

Cecil, Paul F., Sr., and Alvin L. Young. "Operation FLYSWATTER: A War within a War." *Environmental Science and Pollution Research* 15, no. 1 (2007): 3–7.

Centers for Disease Control and Prevention. "Fungal Diseases: *Pneumocystis* Pneumonia." Accessed August 27, 2017. https://www.cdc.gov/fungal/diseases/pneumocystis-pneumonia/index.html.

Centers for Disease Control and Prevention. "HIV among Gay and Bisexual Men." National Center for HIV/AIDS, Viral Hepatitis, STD, and TB Prevention. (September 2016). Accessed Sept 17, 2017. https://www.cdc.gov/hiv/pdf/group/msm/cdc-hiv-msm.pdf.

Centers for Disease Control and Prevention. "How the Flu Virus Can Change: 'Drift' and 'Shift.'" Accessed September 2, 2017. https://www.cdc.gov/flu/about/viruses/change.htm.

Centers for Disease Control and Prevention. "Human Parainfluenza Viruses (HPIVs)." Accessed August 27, 2017. https://www.cdc.gov/parainfluenza/index.html.

Centers for Disease Control and Prevention. "Induced Malaria—California." *Morbidity and Mortality Weekly Report* (March 27, 1971): 99–100.

Centers for Disease Control and Prevention. "*Mycoplasma pneumoniae* Infection." Accessed August 27, 2017. https://www.cdc.gov/pneumonia/atypical/mycoplasma/index.html.

Centers for Disease Control and Prevention. "Pneumococcal Disease." Accessed August 27, 2017. https://www.cdc.gov/pneumococcal/index.html.

Centers for Disease Control and Prevention. "*Pneumocystis* Pneumonia—Los Angeles." *Morbidity and Mortality Weekly Report* 30, no. 21 (1981): 1–3. Accessed September 18, 2017. https://www.cdc.gov/mmwr/preview/mmwrhtml/june_5.htm.

Centers for Disease Control and Prevention. "Transmission of Yellow Fever Virus." Accessed September 2, 2017. http://www.cdc.gov/yellowfever/transmission/index.html.

Centers for Disease Control and Prevention. "Types of Influenza Viruses." Accessed September 2, 2017. https://www.cdc.gov/flu/about/viruses/types.htm.

Centers for Disease Control and Prevention. "Yellow Fever: Symptoms and Treatment" (August 13, 2015). Accessed September 2, 2017. https://www.cdc.gov/yellowfever/symptoms/index.html.

Centers for Disease Control and Prevention and the World Health Organization. "History and Epidemiology of Global Smallpox Eradication." Atlanta: Stephen B. Thacker CDC Library Collection, Centers for Disease Control and Prevention, U.S. Department of Health and Human Services, 2014.

"A Century of Social Achievement: The Society of Medical Officers of Health." *The British Medical Journal* 1, no. 4975 (May 12, 1956): 1102–1104. Accessed September 16, 2017. http://www.jstor.org/stable/20335411.

Chain, Patrick S. G., Ping Hu, Stephanies A. Malfatti, Lyndsay Radnedge, Frank Larimer, Lisa M. Vergez, Patricia Worsham, May C. Chu, and Gary L. Andersen. "Complete Genome Sequence of *Yersinia pestis* Strains Antiqua and Nepal516: Evidence of Gene Reduction in an Emerging Pathogen." *Journal of Bacteriology* 188, no. 12 (June 2006): 4453–4463.

Chandler, David. *The Campaigns of Napoleon.* New York: The MacMillan Company, 1966.

Chin, William, Peter G. Contacos, G. Robert Coatney, and Harry R. Kimball. "A Naturally Acquired Quotidian-Type Malaria in Man Transferable to Monkeys." *Science* 149, no. 3686 (August 1965): 865. doi:10.1126/science.149.3686.865.

Chitnis, Amit, Diana Rawls, and Jim Moore. "Origin of HIV Type 1 in Colonial French Equatorial Africa?" *AIDS Research and Human Retroviruses* 16, no. 1 (2004): 5–8.

Churchill, Winston. "Parliamentary Debate" (March 21, 1902). Quoted in *Churchill by Himself: The Definitive Collection of Quotations*, edited by Richard Lanworth. New York, PublicAffairs, 2008: 469.

Cirillo, Vincent J. *Bullets and Bacilli: The Spanish-American War and Military Medicine.* New Brunswick, NJ: Rutgers University Press, 2004.

Cirillo, Vincent J. "Two Faces of Death: Fatalities from Disease and Combat in America's Principal Wars, 1775 to Present." *Perspectives in Biology and Medicine* 51, no. 1 (2008): 121–133.

Clancy, Jacqueline. "Hell's Angel: Eleanor Kinzie Gordon's Wartime Summer of 1898." *Tequesta* 63 (2003): 37–61.

Clausewitz, Carl von. *On War.* Edited by Michael Howard and Peter Paret. New York: Oxford University Press, 2006.

Clendening, Logan. "Reinfection with Streptococcus Hemolyticus in Lobar Pneumonia, Measles and Scarlet Fever and Its Prevents." *American Journal of the Medical Sciences* 156 (1918): 575–586.

Coates, John Boyd, ed. *Preventive Medicine in World War II.* Vol. 6, *Communicable Diseases, Malaria.* Washington, D.C.: Office of the Surgeon General, U.S. Army Medical Department, 1963.

Cobo, Father Bernabe. *History of the Inca Empire*. Translated and edited by Roland Hamilton. Austin: University of Texas Press, 1979.

Coffman, Sherrilyn. "Margaret Utinsky: A Nurse Undertook Heroic Underground Activities in Support of American Prisoners in the Philippines during WWII." *American Journal of Nursing* 109, no. 5 (May 2009): 72–76. Accessed September 2, 2017. http://www.jstor.org/stable/40384988.

Cohn, Samuel K. "The Black Death and the Burning of Jews." *Past & Present* 196, no. 1 (August 2007): 3–36.

Cohn, Samuel K. "The Black Death: End of a Paradigm." *The American Historical Review* 107, no. 3 (2002): 703–738.

Cole, Rufus, and W. G. MacCallum, "Pneumonia at Base Hospital," *JAMA* 70, no. 16 (1918): 1146–1156. Accessed September 2, 2017. https://babel.hathitrust.org/cgi/pt?id=mdp.39015082605612;view=2up;seq=6.

Conlon, Joseph M. "The Historical Impact of Epidemic Typhus." Montana University. Accessed September 2, 2017. www.montana.edu/historybug/documents/TYPHUS-Conlon.pdf.

"The Control of Diphtheria." *British Medical Journal* 2, no. 2276 (August 13, 1904): 340–341. Accessed September 2, 2017. http://www.jstor.org/stable/20281717.

Cook, David Noble. *Born to Die: Disease and New World Conquest, 1492–1650*. Cambridge, UK: Cambridge University Press, 1998.

Cook, Sherburne F. *An Expanding World*. Vol. 26, *Biological Consequences of the European Expansion, 1450–1800*. Edited by Kenneth F. Kiple and Stephen V. Beck. Aldershot, UK: Variorum, Ashgate Publishing Limited, 1997.

Cook, Sherburne F., and Lesley Byrd Simpson. *The Population of Central Mexico in the Sixteenth Century*. Berkeley and Los Angeles: University of California Press, 1948.

Cortés, Hernán. *Letters from Mexico*. Translated and edited by Anthony Pagden, with an introduction by J. H. Elliott. New Haven, CT: Yale University Press, 1986.

Costa, Dora L., and Matthew E. Kahn. "Surviving Andersonville: The Benefits of Social Networks in POW Camps." *American Economic Review* 97, no. 4 (Sept. 2007): 1467–1487. Accessed September 7, 2017. http://www.jstor.org/stable/30034102.

Creighton, Charles. *A History of Epidemics in Britain*. Cambridge, UK: Cambridge University Press, 1894.

"Crimean War, Chapter 1: Loss of Life in Different Ways." *Advocate of Peace,* New Series I, no. 7 (July 1869): 106–107.

Crosby, Alfred W. *America's Forgotten Pandemic: The Influenza of 1918*. Cambridge, UK: Cambridge University Press, 2003.

Crosby, Alfred W. *The Columbian Exchange: Biological and Cultural Consequences of 1492*. Westport, CT: Greenwood Press, 1972.

Cruttwell, Charles Robert Mowbray Fraser. *A History of the Great War: 1914–1918*. 2nd ed. Chicago: Academy Chicago Publishers, 1991.

Cubbison, Douglas R. *The American Northern Theater Army in 1776: The Ruin and Reconstruction of the Continental Force*. Jefferson, NC: MacFarland and Co., 2010.

Cumming, James G., Charles B. Spruit, and Charles Lynch. "The Pneumonias: Streptococcus and Pneumonococcus Groups." *Journal of the American Medical Association [JAMA]* 70, no. 15 (1918): 1066.

Cunha, Burke A. "The Cause of the Plague of Athens: Plague, Typhoid, Typhus, Smallpox, or Measles?" *Infectious Disease Clinics North America* 18 (2004): 29–43. Accessed September 16, 2017. https://doi.org/10.1016/S0891-5520(03)00100-4.

Cunha, Cheston B., and Burke A. Cunha. "Great Plagues of the Past and Remaining Questions." In *Paleomicrobiology: Past Human Infections*, edited by Didier Raoult and Michel Drancourt, 1–20. Berlin: Springer-Verlag, 2008.

Cunningham, Andrew. "Identifying Disease in the Past: Cutting the Gordian Knot." *Asclepio* 54, no. 1 (2002): 13–34.

Cunningham, H. H. *Doctors in Gray: The Confederate Medical Service*. Baton Rouge: Louisiana State University Press, 1986.

Cunningham, Sean. *Henry VII*. London: Routledge, 2007

"Cutaneous Diphtheria." *British Medical Journal* 1, no. 4345 (April 15, 1944): 534–535. Accessed September 2, 2017. http://www.jstor.org/stable/20345103.

Cruveilhier, Louis. Quoted in David M. Morens, Jeffery K. Taubenberger, and Anthony S. Fauci. "Predominant Role of Bacterial Pneumonia as a Cause of Death in Pandemic Influenza: Implications for Pandemic Influenza Preparedness." *Journal of Infectious Diseases* 198, no. 7 (October 1, 2008): 962–970. Accessed August 31, 2017. https://academic.oup.com/jid/article/198/7/962/2192118/Predominant-Role-of-Bacterial-Pneumonia-as-a-Cause.

Davidson, James West, and Mark H. Lytle. "Contact." *After the Fact: The Art of Historical Detection*. 6th ed. New York: McGraw Hill, 2010.

Devakumar, Delan, Marion Clare Birch, David Osrin, and Jonathan C. K. Wells. "The Intergenerational Effects of War on the Health of Children." *BMC Medicine* 12, no. 1 (April 2014): 1–15. Accessed August 13, 2017. https://www.researchgate.net/publication/261325728_The_Intergenerational_Effects_of_War_on_the_Health_of_Children.

DeWitte, Sharon N., and Philip Slavin. "Between Famine and Death: England on the Eve of the Black Death—Evidence from Paleoepidemiology and Manorial Accounts." *Journal of Interdisciplinary History* 44, no. 1 (Summer 2013): 37–60.

DeWitte, Sharon N., and James W. Wood. "Selectivity of Black Death Mortality with Respect to Preexisting Health." *Proceedings of the National Academy of Sciences of the United States of America* 105, no. 5 (November 13, 2007): 1436–1441.

Dio, Cassius. *Roman History*. Vol. 9. Translated by Earnest Cary, PhD. London: William Heinemann LTD, 1927.

"Diphtheria Epidemic: New Independent States of the Former Soviet Union, 1990–1994." *Morbidity and Mortality Weekly Report*. CDC 44, no. 10 (March 17, 1995): 177–181.

"Diphtheria: Medical Research Council's Report." *British Medical Journal* 1, no. 3297 (March 8, 1924): 439–441. Accessed September 2, 2017. http://www.jstor.org/stable/20435984.

Directorate for Information, Operations, and Reports. *Department of Defense Selected Manpower Statistics, Fiscal Year 1983*. Washington, D.C.: Department of Defense, 1984.

Division of Vector-Borne Diseases. "Plague." Centers for Disease Control and Prevention. Accessed September 2, 2017. http://www.cdc.gov/plague.

Dixon, Bernard. "Ebola in Greece?" *British Medical Journal* 313, no. 7054 (August 17, 1996): 430.

Dixon, C. W. *Smallpox*. London: J&A Churchill, 1962.

Doder, Dusko. "Yugoslavia: New War, Old Hatreds." *Foreign Policy* 91 (Summer 1993): 3–23.

Dollar, Emily, and Lee A. Witters. "That Bourne from Whence No Traveler Returns." *Dartmouth Medicine* 39, no. 1 (Fall 2014): 36–41.

Donovan, Paula. "Rape and HIV/AIDS in Rwanda." *The Lancet Supplement* 360 (December 2002): s17–s18.

Dubois, Laurent. *Avengers in the New World: The Story of the Haitian Revolution*. Cambridge, UK: Belknap Press, 2004.

Dubois, Laurent. *Haiti: The Aftershocks of History.* New York: Picador, 2012.

Duffy, John. "Medical Practice in the Ante Bellum South." *Journal of Southern History* 25, no. 1 (February 1959): 53–72. Accessed September 3, 2017. http://www.jstor.org/stable /2954479.

Dunn, Carroll H. *Base Development in South Vietnam, 1965–1970.* Washington, D.C.: GPO, 1991.

Durack, David T., Robert J. Littman, R. Michael Benitez, and Philip A. Mackowiak. "Hellenic Holocaust: A Historical Clinico-Pathologic Conference." *American Journal of Medicine* 109 (2000): 391–397.

"Dysentery." *Gale Encyclopedia of Medicine.* 3rd edition (2006). Accessed September 7, 2017. http://www.encyclopedia.com/medicine/diseases-and-conditions/pathology/dysentery #1G23451600534.

Dzidic, Denis. "Bosnia Still Living with Consequences of War." Balkan Transitional Justice (April 2012). Accessed August 13, 2017. http://www.balkaninsight.com/en/article /bosnia-still-living-with-consequences-of-war.

Elbe, Stefan. "HIV/AIDS and the Changing Landscape of War in Africa." *International Security* 27, no. 2 (2002): 159–177.

"Entamoeba Histolytica." Stanford University. Accessed September 7, 2017. https://web .stanford.edu/group/parasites/ParaSites2006/Amoebiasis/Agents&History.html.

"The Epidemic of Influenza in England." *Science, New Series* 52, no.1336 (1920): 124

Epitome de Caesaribus. Translated by Thomas M. Banchich. Buffalo, NY: Canisius College, 2009.

Erskine, Edgar. *Victories of Army Medicine; Scientific Accomplishments of the Medical Department of the United States Army.* Philadelphia: J. B. Lippincott Co., 1943.

Espinosa, Mariola. "A Fever for Empire: U.S. Disease Eradication in Cuba as Colonial Public Health." In *Colonial Crucible,* edited by Alfred W. McCoy and Francisco A. Scarano, 288–296. Madison: University of Wisconsin Press, 2009.

Eutropius. *Abridgement of Roman History.* Translated by Rev. John Selby Watson, MA. London: Henry G. Bohn, 1853.

Evans, Richard J. "Epidemics and Revolutions: Cholera in Nineteenth-Century Europe." *Past & Present* no. 120 (August 1988): 123–146.

Farmer, David. "Prices and Wages, 1041–1350." *The Agrarian History of England and Wales.* Vol. 2, *1042–1350.* Edited by Joan Thirsk. Cambridge, UK: Cambridge University Press, 1988.

Farmer, David. "Prices and Wages, 1350–1500." In *The Agrarian History of England and Wales* Vol. 3, *1350–1500,* edited by Edward Miller. Cambridge, UK: Cambridge University Press, 1988.

Faust, Drew Gilpin. *This Republic of Suffering: Death and the American Civil War.* New York: Vintage Books, 2008.

Fenn, Elizabeth A. *Pox Americana: The Great Smallpox Epidemic of 1775–82.* New York: Hill and Wang New York, 2001.

Fenner, Frank, Donald A. Henderson, Isao Arita, Zdenek Jezek, and Ivan Ladnye. *Smallpox and Its Eradication.* Geneva: World Health Organization, 1988.

Flint, Austin, MD, ed. *A Report of the Diseases, etc., Among the Prisoners at Andersonville, GA.* Riverside, Cambridge: H.O. Houghton and Company.

Following the Twenty-Second. "Sickness & Disease: The Impact of Non-Combat Casualties on Fighting Strength in the AIF." Accessed September 2, 2017. https://anzac-22nd -battalion.com/sickness-disease-the-impact-of-non-combat-casualties-on-fighting -strength-in-the-aif.

Fox, Herbert. *Thucydides Histories: Book III.* Oxford: Clarendon Press, 1901.

Fracastoro, Girolamo (Fracastorius, Hieronymus). *De Contagione et Contagiosis Morbis et eorum Curatione*. Edited by William C. Wright. Reprint. New York: G. P. Putnam's Sons, 1930. First published in 1546.

Francis, Thomas, and Jonas Salk. "A Simplified Procedure for the Concentration and Purification of Influenza Virus." *Science, New Series* 96, no. 2500 (1942): 499–500.

Francis, Thomas, Jonas Salk, Harold Pearson, and Philip Brown. "Protective Effect of Vaccination against Induced Influenza A." *Journal of Clinical Investigation* 24, no. 4 (1945): 536–546.

Freemon, Frank Reed. "Medical Care during the American Civil War." PhD diss., University of Illinois at Urbana-Champaign, 1992.

Froland, A. "The Great Plague of Athens 430 BCE," *Danish Medicine History Journal* 38 (2010): 63–80.

Fukuda, Mark M. "Editorial: Malaria in the U.S. Armed Forces: A Persistent but Preventable Threat." *Medical Surveillance Monthly Report* 19, no.1 (January 2012): 12–13.

Furuse, Yuki, Akira Suzuki, and Hitoshi Oshitani. "Origin of Measles Virus: Divergence from Rinderpest Virus between the 11th and 12th Centuries." *Virology Journal* 7 (2010): 52–55.

Gagnon, Alain, Matthew S. Miller, Stacey A. Hallman, Robert Bourbeau, D. Ann Herring, David J. D. Earn, and Joaquin Madrenas. "Age-Specific Mortality during the 1918 Influenza Pandemic: Unraveling the Mystery of High Young Adult Mortality." *PLoS One* (2013): e69586.

Galazka, A. M., S. E. Robertson, and A. Kraigher. "Mumps and Mumps Vaccine: A Global Review." *Bulletin of the World Health Organization* 77, no. 1 (1999): 3–14.

Geggus, David. *The Haitian Revolution: A Documentary History*. Indianapolis: Hackett Publishing Company, 2014.

Gibson, James E. *Dr. Bodo Otto and the Medical Background of the American Revolution*. Springfield, IL: Charles C Thomas, 1937.

Gigas, Herman. "Hermanni Gygantis, ordinis fratrum minorum, Flores Temporum seu Chronicon Universale ad Orbe condito ad annum Christi MCCCXLIX." In *The Black Death*, edited and translated by Rosemary Horrox. Manchester, UK: Manchester University Press, 1984: 138–139.

Gilbert, William. "The Italian City-States of the Renaissance." Accessed September 2, 2017. http://vlib.iue.it/carrie/texts/carrie_books/gilbert/03.html.

Gilchrist, Michael R. "Disease & Infection in the American Civil War." *The American Biology Teacher* 60, no. 4 (April 1998): 258–262.

Giles-Vernick, Tamara, Ch. Didier Gondola, Guillaume Lachenal, and William H. Schneider. "Social History, Biology, and the Emergence of HIV in Colonial Africa." *Journal of African History* 54, no. 1 (2013): 11–30.

Gillgannon, Sister Mary McAuley. "The Sisters of Mercy as Crimean War Nurses." PhD diss., University of Notre Dame, 1962.

Gilliam, J. F. "The Plague under Marcus Aurelius." *American Journal of Philology* 82, no. 3 (July 1961): 225–251.

Ginn, Richard V. N. *The History of the U.S. Army Medical Service Corps*. Washington, D.C.: GPO, 1996.

Girard, Philippe R. *The Slaves Who Defeated Napoleon: Toussaint Louverture and the Haitian War for Independence, 1801–1804*. Tuscaloosa: University of Alabama Press, 2011.

Global Security.Org. "Tajikistan Civil War." Accessed September 2, 2017. http://www.globalsecurity.org/military/world/war/tajikistan.htm.

Gorgas, William Crawford. Papers. University of Alabama, Tuscaloosa, AL.

Gorgas, William Crawford. "A Record of Brilliant and Gallant Service of More Than Twenty Years." In Articles, *Commoner*, Lincoln, NE, March 4–11, 1910.

Gorgas, William Crawford. Hill, Lister. "William Crawford Gorgas—Speech of the Honorable Lister Hill of Alabama in the House of Representatives, March 28, 1928."

Gorgas, William Crawford. United States. Congress. Senate. Report on Senate Bill 2842, concerning Army promotion of Dr. W. C. Gorgas, February 6, 1903.

Gorgas, William Crawford. Boykin, Frank W. Commemorative Exercises of the Thirtieth Anniversary of the Death of Major General William Gorgas at His Grave, Arlington National Cemetery. Speech of Honorable Frank W. Boykin of Alabama, House of Representatives, August 3, 1950.

Gottfried, R. S. "Population, Plague, and the Sweating Sickness: Demographic Movements in Late Fifteenth-Century England." *Journal of British Studies* 17, no. 1 (Fall, 1977): 12–37.

Gransden, Antonia, ed. "A Fourteenth-Century Chronicle from the Grey Friars Lynn." *English Historical Review* 72 (1957): 270–278.

Grant, James, MD, DPH. "The Problems of Diphtheria." *British Medical Journal* 1, no. 4443 (March 2, 1946): 309–312. Accessed May 13, 2017. http://www.jstor.org/stable /20365647.

Gray, Sir Thomas. "Scalacronica 1271–1363." *The Publications of the Surtees Society*. Vol. 209. Edited and translated by Andy King. Rochester, NY: The Boydell Press, 2005.

Greenway, James C., Carl Boettiger, and Howard S. Colwell. "Pneumonia and Some of Its Complications at Camp Bowie." *Archives of Internal Medicine* 24, no. 1 (1919): 1–34.

Grenfell, Bernard P., and Arthur S. Hunt. *The Oxyrhynchus Papyri*. Part 1. London: Egypt Exploration Society, 1898, 39–44.

Griffith, David. "Local Knowledge, Multiple Livelihoods, and the Use of Natural and Social Resources in North Carolina." *Traditional Ecological Knowledge and Natural Resource Management*. Norman: University of Nebraska Press, 2006.

Grossman, Sheila C., and Carol Mattson Porth. *Porth's Pathophysiology: Concepts of Altered Health States*. 9th ed. Philadelphia: Wolters Kluwer Health, Lippincott Williams and Wilkins, 2014.

Guerrero, Isabel C., Bruce C. Weniger, and Myron G. Schultz. "Transfusion Malaria in the United States, 1972–1981." *Annals of Internal Medicine* 99 (1983): 221–226.

Hackett, F. J. Paul. *"A Very Remarkable Sickness": Epidemics in the Petit Nord, 1670–1846*. Winnipeg: University of Manitoba Press, 2002.

Haensch, Stephanie, Raffaella Bianucci, Michel Signoli, Minoarisoa Rajerison, Michael Schultz, Sacha Kacki, Marco Vermunt, Darlene A. Weston, Derek Hurst, Mark Achtman, Elisabeth Carniel, and Barbara Bramanti. "Distinct Clones of *Yersinia pestis* Caused the Black Death." *PLoS Pathogens* 6, no. 10 (October 2010). Accessed September 16, 2017. http://journals.plos.org/plospathogens/article?id=10.1371/journal .ppat.1001134.

Hahn, Beatrice H., George M. Shaw, Kevin M. De Cock, and Paul M. Sharp. "AIDS as a Zoonosis: Scientific and Public Health Implications." *Science* 28, no. 287 (2000): 607–614.

Hall, Edward. *The Union of the Two Noble and Illustre Femelies of Lancastre & Yorke, Beeying Long in Continual Discension for the Croune of this Noble Realme, with all the Actes done in bothe the Tymes of the Princes, bothe of the One Linage and of the Other, Beginnyng at the Tyme of Kyng Henry the Fowerth, the First Aucthor of this Deuision, and so Successiuely Proceadyng to the Reigne of the High and Prudent Prince Kyng Henry the Eight, the Vndubitate*

Flower and very Heire of both the Sayd Linages. Reprint. New York: AMS Press, 1965. First published in 1548, 1809.

Hamel, Debra. *The Battle of Arginusae: Victory at Sea and Its Tragic Aftermath in the Final Years of the Peloponnesian War.* Witness to Ancient History Series. Baltimore, MD: Johns Hopkins University Press, 2015.

Hammerlund, Erika, Matthew W. Lewis, Jon M. Hanifin, Motomi Mori, Caroline W. Koudelka, and Mark K. Slifka. "Antiviral Immunity Following Smallpox Virus Infection: A Case-Control Study." *Journal of Virology* 84, no. 24 (December 2010): 12754. Published online October 6, 2010. Accessed September 16, 2017. https:/ncbi.nlm.nih .gov/pmc/articles/PMC3004327.

Hammond, William A. *A Treatise on Hygiene with Special Reference to the Military Service.* Philadelphia: J. B. Lippincott & Co.

Hand, Carol. *Epidemiology: The Fight against Ebola and Other Diseases.* Minneapolis: Abdo Publishing, 2015.

Handlos, Line Neerup, Karen Fog Olwig, Ib Christian Bygbjerg, and Marie Norredam. "Return Migrants' Experience of Access to Care in Corrupt Healthcare Systems: The Bosnian Example." *International Journal of Environmental Research and Public Health* 13, no. 9 (September 2016): 1–12. Accessed August 13, 2017. www.mdpi.com/1660 -4601/13/9/924/pdf.

Hanna, Eriny. "The Route to Crisis: Cities, Trade, and Epidemics in the Roman Empire." *Vanderbilt Undergraduate Research Journal* 10 (Fall 2015): 1–10.

Hansen, Morgen. "Athenian Population Losses 431–403 B.C. and the Number of Athenian Citizens in 431 B.C." In *Three Studies in Athenian Demography.* Copenhagen, Denmark: Munkgaard Historisk-Filosopfiske Meddelelser, 1988: 14–28.

Hanson, Victor. *A War Like No Other: How the Spartans and Athenians Fought the Peloponnesian War.* New York: Random House, 2005.

Harleian Manuscripts. Harleian Collection. The British Museum, London.

Harper, Douglas. "Typhus." Dictionary.com, Online Etymology Dictionary. Accessed September 2, 2017. http://www.etymonline.com.

Harrison, Mark. *Contagion: How Commerce Has Spread Disease.* New Haven, CT, and London: Yale University Press, 2012.

Harrison, Mark. "Disease, Diplomacy and International Commerce: The Origins of International Sanitary Regulation in the Nineteenth Century." *Journal of Global History* 1 (2006): 197–217. Accessed September 16, 2017. https:/www.cambridge.org/core/terms.

Harriss, G. L. "Budgeting at the Medieval Exchequer." In *War, Government and Aristocracy in the British Isles, c. 1150–1500: Essays in Honour of Michael Prestwich,* edited by Chris Given-Wilson, Ann Kettle, and Len Scales. Rochester, NY: The Boydell Press, 2008: 179–196.

Haydon, F. S., ed. *Eulogium Historiarum sive Temporis.* Vol. 3. London: Rolls Series,1863.

Hays, Jeffrey. "Economy of Tajikistan." *Facts and Details* (April 2016). Accessed September 2, 2017. http://factsanddetails.com/central-asia/Tajikistan/sub8_6d/entry-4896.html.

Heaton, Matthew, and Toyin Falola. "Global Explanations versus Local Interpretations: The Historiography of the Influenza Pandemic of 1918–19 in Africa." *History of Africa* 33 (2006): 205–230.

Heizmann, Charles. "Military Sanitation in the 16th, 17th, and 18th Centuries." In *Journal of the Military Service Institution of the United States,* Vol. 14, No. 64, edited by William Huskin and James Bush. Governor's Island, NY: Military Service Institution, 1893: 709–738.

Henderson, Donald A. "Smallpox: Clinical and Epidemiologic Features." *Emerging Infectious Diseases* 5, no. 4 (July–August 1999): 537–539.

Hendricks, Kenneth E., Jr. *The Spanish-American War.* Westport, CT: Greenwood Press, 2003.

Henry, Fitzroy J. "The Epidemiologic Importance of Dysentery in Communities." *Reviews of Infectious Diseases* 13, no. 4 (April 1991): S238.

Herlihy, David. *The Black Death and the Transformation of the West.* Cambridge, MA: Harvard University Press, 1997.

Herodian. *History.* Vol. 1. Translated by C. R. Whittaker. Cambridge, MA: Harvard University Press, 1969.

Hewitt, H.J. *The Organization of War under Edward III.* Manchester, UK: Manchester University Press, 1966.

Heyman, Paul, Leopold Simons, and Christel Cochez. "Were the English Sweating Sickness and the Picardy Sweat Caused by Hantaviruses?" *Viruses* 6 (2014): 151–171.

Higden, Rudolf. "Polychronicon." *The Black Death.* Edited and translated by Rosemary Horrox. Manchester, UK: Manchester University Press, 1984.

Higgins, Brian Thomas. "Epidemic Proportions: Cholera in the British West Indies, 1850–1855." PhD diss., Bowling Green State University, 1993.

Hilley, Richard. *A Compendium of European Geography and History.* London: Spottiswoode and Co., 1870.

Hinnenbusch, B. J., A. E. Rudolph, P. Cherepanov, J. E. Dixon, T. G. Schwan, and A. Forsberg. "Role of Yersinia Murine Toxin in Survival of *Yersinia pestis* in the Midgut of the Flea Vector." *Science* 296, no. 5568 (April 2002): 733–735.

Hippocrates. "Epidemics I: First Constitution." In *Hippocrates.* Vol. 1. Translated by W. H. S. Jones, 147–149. London: William Heinemann, LTD, 1957.

Hirsch, August. *Handbook of Geographical and Historical Pathology.* Vol. 1, *Acute Infective Diseases.* Translated by Charles Creighton, MD. London: J. B. Adlard, Bartholomew Close, 1883.

Hodge, William Barwick. "On the Mortality Arising from Military Operations." *The Assurance Magazine, and Journal of the Institute of Actuaries* 7, no. 2 (July 1857): 80–90. Accessed June 26, 2017. http://www.jstor.org/stable/41134778.

Hoehling, A. A. *The Great Epidemic.* Boston: Little Brown and Company, 1961.

Holmes, Frederick F. "Anne Boleyn, the Sweating Sickness, and the Hantavirus: A Review of an Old Disease with a Modern Interpretation." *Journal of Medical Biography* 6, no. 1 (February 1998): 43–48.

Hopkins, Donald. *Princes and Peasants: Smallpox in History.* Chicago: University of Chicago Press, 1983.

Hornsby, Kathleen. "Spatial Diffusion: Conceptualizations and Formalizations." National Center for Geographic Information and Analysis and Department of Spatial Information Science and Engineering. Orono: University of Maine, 2003.

Horrox, Rosemary, trans. and ed. *The Black Death.* Manchester, UK: Manchester University Press, 1994.

Hovanec, Caroline. "The 1918 Influenza Pandemic in Literature and Memory." Master's thesis, Vanderbilt University, 2009.

Hukic, M., A. Hajdarpasic, J. Ravlija, Z. Ler, R. Baljic, A. Dedeic Ljubovic, A. Moro, I. Samlimović-Besic, A. Sausy, C. P. Muller, and J. M. Hübschen. "Mumps Outbreak in the Federation of Bosnia and Herzegovina with Large Cohorts of Susceptibles and Genetically Diverse Strains of Genotype G, Bosnia and Herzegovina, December 2010 to September 2012." *European Surveillance* 19, no 33 (2014). Accessed August 13, 2017. http://www.eurosurveillance.org/ViewArticle.aspx?ArticleId=20879.

Humphries, Mark Osborne. "Paths of Infection: The First World War and the Origins of the 1918 Influenza Pandemic." *War in History* 21, no. 1 (January 8, 2014): 55–81.

Hunt, Margaret. "Virology, Chapter Fourteen: Measles (Rubeola) and Mumps Viruses." *Microbiology and Immunology On-line.* University of South Carolina School of Medicine. Accessed August 7, 2017. http://microbiologybook.org/mhunt/mump-meas.htm.

Hunter, Paul R. "The English Sweating Sickness, with Particular Reference to the 1551 Outbreak in Chester." *Reviews of Infectious Diseases* 13, no. 2 (March–April, 1991): 303–306.

"Influenza, Pneumonia, and Common Respiratory Diseases." In *Annual Report of the Surgeon General for Fiscal Year 1919.* Vol. 1. Washington, D.C.: GPO, 1919: 740–786.

"Influenza—Prevalence in the United States." *Public Health Reports* 35, no. 6 (February 6, 1920): 269–275.

Institute of Medicine and Committee on Envisioning a Strategy to Prepare for the Long-Term Burden of HIV/AIDS: African Needs and U.S. Interests. *Preparing for the Future of HIV/AIDS in Africa: A Shared Responsibility.* Washington, D.C.: The National Academies Press, 2011.

Ixtlilxochitl, Fernando de Alva. *Horribles crueldades de los conquistadores de Mexico, y de los indios que los auxiliaron para subyugarlo a la corona de Castilla.* Suplemento a la historia del Padre Sahagun, redactado por Carlos Maria Bustamante. Mexico: Imprenta de Alejandro Valdes, 1829.

Jaffin, Jonathan H. "Medical Support for the American Expeditionary Forces in France during the First World War." Master's thesis, U.S. Army Command and General Staff College, 1991.

James, C. L. R. *The Black Jacobins: Toussaint L'Ouverture and the San Domingo Revolution.* Reprint. New York: Vantage Books, Random House, 1989. First published in 1963.

Johnson, N. P., and J. Mueller. "Updating the Accounts." *Bulletin of the History of Medicine* 76, no. 1 (Spring 2002): 105–115.

Jones, Lynne. "On a Front Line." *British Medical Journal* 310, no. 6986 (April 22, 1995): 1052–1054. Accessed August 14, 2017. http://www.jstor.org/stable/29727045.

Jones, Michael. *Bosworth, 1485: The Battle That Transformed England.* Reprint. New York: Pegasus Books, 2015. First published in 2002.

Jones, Ryan T., Sara M. Vetter, and Kenneth L. Gage. "Exposing Laboratory-Reared Fleas to Soil and Wild Flea Feces Increases Transmission of *Yersinia pestis.*" *American Journal of Tropical Medicine and Hygiene* 89, no. 4 (October 9, 2013): 784–787.

Jonsson, Colleen B., Luiz Tadeu Moraes Figueiredo, and Olli Vapalahti. "A Global Perspective on Hantavirus Ecology, Epidemiology, and Disease." *Clinical Microbiology Reviews* 23, no. 2 (2010): 412–441.

Kagan, Donald. *The Peace of Nicias and the Sicilian Expedition.* Ithaca, NY: Cornell University Press, 1981.

Kagan, Donald. *The Peloponnesian War.* New York: Penguin Books, 2003.

Kalonda-Kanyama, Isaac. "Civil War, Sexual Violence and HIV Infections: Evidence from the Democratic Republic of the Congo." *Journal of African Development* 12, no. 2 (2010): 47–60.

Kansas State Board of Health. "Ninth Biennial Report Being the Thirty-Third and Thirty-Fourth Annual Reports of the State Board of Health of the State of Kansas, June 30, 1916, to June 30, 1918." In *Influenza Encyclopedia: The American Influenza Epidemic of 1918–1919, a Digital Encyclopedia.* University of Michigan Center for the History of Medicine and Michigan Publishing: 5–30. Accessed September 2, 2017. http://quod.lib.umich.

edu/f/flu/7740flu.0013.477/17/--ninth-biennial-report-being-the-thirty-third-and-thirty?page=root;rgn=full+text;size=150;view=image;q1=Fort+Riley.

Kantele, Anu, and T. Sakari Jokiranta. "Review of Cases with the Emerging Fifth Human Malaria Parasite, *Plasmodium knowlesi*." *Clinical Infectious Diseases* 52, no. 11 (2011): 1356–1362. Accessed September 2, 2017. http://cid.oxfordjournals.org/content/52/11/1356.full.

Kazanjian, Powel. "Ebola in Antiquity?" *Clinical Infectious Diseases, Oxford Journals* 61, no. 6 (2015): 964–965. Accessed September 16, 2017. http://cid.oxfordjournals.org/content/61/6/963.

Kellum, Rachel M. "Surgeons of the Severed Limb: Confederate Military Medicine in Arkansas, 1863–1865." Master's thesis, Jackson College, 2014.

Kennan, George. *Campaigning in Cuba*. Reprint. Charleston: BiblioLife, 2009. First published in 1899.

Kharsany, Ayesha B. M., and Quarraisha A. Karim. "HIV Infection and AIDS in Sub-Saharan Africa: Current Status, Challenges, and Opportunities." *Open AIDS Journal* 10 (2016): 34–48.

Kiel, F. W. "Some Medical Aspects of the History of Fort Sam Houston." *Military Medicine* 129 (November 1964): 1044–1051. Accessed September 2, 2017. http://www.dtic.mil/dtic/tr/fulltext/u2/454027.pdf.

Kinra, Sanjay, Mary E. Black, Sanja Mandic, and Nora Selimovic. "Impact of the Bosnian Conflict on the Health of Women and Children." *Bulletin of the World Health Organization* 80, no. 1 (2002): 75–76. Accessed August 14, 2017. http://www.who.int/bulletin/archives/80(1)75.pdf.

Kirimli, Hakan. "Emigrations from the Crimea to the Ottoman Empire during the Crimean War." *Middle Eastern Studies* 44, no. 5 (2008): 751–773. Accessed July 22, 2017. http://dx.doi.org/10.1080/00263200802315778.

Knight, Joe. "Napoleon Wasn't Defeated by the Russians." *Health and Science: Pandemics* (December 11, 2012). Accessed September 17, 2017. http://www.slate.com/articles/health_and_science/pandemics/2012/12/napoleon_march_to_russia_in_1812_typhus_spread_by_lice_was_more_powerful.html.

Knighton, Henry. *Knighton's Chronicle*. Edited and Translated by G. H. Martin. Oxford: Clarendon Press, 1995.

Kotwal, Russ S., Robert B. Wenzel, Raymond A. Sterling, William D. Porter, Nikki N. Jordan, and Bruno P. Petruccelli. "An Outbreak of Malaria in US Army Rangers Returning from Afghanistan." *JAMA* 293, no. 2 (January 12, 2005): 212–216.

Kozelsky, Mara. "Casualties of Conflict: Crimean Tatars during the Crimean War." *Slavic Review* 67, no. 4 (Winter 2008): 866–891

Kreidberg, Marvin A., and Merton G. Henry. *History of Military Mobilization in the United States Army 1775–1945*. Department of the Army pamphlet, no. 20-212. Washington, D.C.: Department of the Army, 1955.

Lambert, Craig L. *Shipping the Medieval Military: English Maritime Logistics in the Fourteenth Century*. Rochester, NY: The Boydell Press, 2011.

Lambert, Craig L. "Taking the War to Scotland and France: The Supply and Transportation of English Armies by Sea, 1320–60." PhD diss., University of Hull, 2009.

Landa, Friar Diego de. *Yucatan before and after Conquest*. Translated with notes by William Gates. New York: Dover Publications, Inc., 1978.

Langford, Christopher. "Did the 1918–19 Influenza Pandemic Originate in China?" *Population and Development Review* 31, no. 3 (September 2005): 473–505.

Ledford, Heidi. "Tissue Sample Suggests HIV Has Been Infecting Humans for a Century." *Nature* (October 1, 2008). Accessed September 2, 2017. http://www.nature.com /news/2008/081001/full/news.2008.1143.html.

Lee, Chulhee. "Socioeconomic Difference in the Health of Black Union Soldiers during the American Civil War." *Social Science History* 33, no. 4 (Winter 2009): 427–457. Accessed August 27, 2017. http://www.jstor.org/stable/40587324.

Lee, Josh, Pvt. "The Flu." Quoted in Peter C. Wever and Leo van Bergen, "Death from 1918 Pandemic Influenza during the First Word War: A Perspective from Personal and Anecdotal Evidence." *Influenza and Other Respiratory Viruses* 8, no. 5 (September 2014): 538–546.

Lee, Kelley, and Richard Dodgson. "Globalization and Cholera: Implications for Global Governance." *Global Governance* 6, no. 2 (April–June 2000): 213–236. Accessed September 16, 2017. http://www.jstor.org/stable/27800260.

Lemarchand, Rene. *The Dynamics of Violence in Central Africa*. State College: University of Pennsylvania Press, 2009.

"LePrince, Malaria Fighter." *Public Health Reports* 71, no. 8 (August 1956): 756–758.

Leroy-Dupré, Louis Alexandre Hippolyte. Memoir of Baron Larrey: Surgeon-in-Chief of the Grande Armée, from the French. London: Henry Henshaw, 1861.

Letterman, Jonathan, MD. *Medical Recollections of the Army of the Potomac*. New York: D. Appleton & Company, 1866. Accessed September 7, 2017. http://history.amedd. army.mil/booksdocs/civil/lettermanmemoirs/medical_recollections.html#Letter_from _Letterman_to_Hooker_on_Layout_of_Unhealthy_Huts_by_Soldiers_on.

"Letters from the Crimea." *British Medical Journal* 2, no. 4896 (November 6, 1954): 1103. Accessed September 16, 2017. http://www.jstor.org/stable/20361410.

Levy, Robert L., and H. L. Alexander. "The Predisposition of Streptococcus Carriers to the Complications of Measles: Results of Separation of Carriers from Non-Carriers at a Base Hospital." *JAMA* 70, no. 20 (1919): 1827–1830.

Liebow, Averill A., MD, and John H. Bumstead, MD. "Cutaneous and Other Aspects of Diphtheria." In *Internal Medicine in World War II*. Vol. 2, *Infectious Diseases*, edited by John Boyd Coates Jr., MC, and W. Paul Havens Jr., MD., 275–327. Washington, D.C.: Office of the Surgeon General, U.S. Army Medical Department, 1963). Accessed September 16, 2017. http://history.amedd.army.mil/booksdocs/wwii/infectiousdisvolii /chapter10.htm.

Lieven, Dominic. *The True Story of the Campaigns of War and Peace: Russia against Napoleon*. New York: Penguin Group, 2010.

Littman, Robert J. "The Plague of Athens: Epidemiology and Paleopathology." *Mount Sinai Journal of Medicine* 76 (2009): 456–467.

Littman, Robert J., and M. L. Littman. "Galen and the Antonine Plague." *American Journal of Philology* 94, no. 3 (1973): 243–255.

Littman, Robert J., and M. L. Littman. "The Athenian Plague: Smallpox." *Transactions and Proceedings of the American Philological Association* 100 (1969): 261–275.

Lolaeva, Svetlana. "Tajikistan in Ruins: The Descent into Chaos of a Central Asian Republic." George Washington University. Accessed September 2, 2017. https://www2.gwu.edu /~ieresgwu/assets/docs/demokratizatsiya%20archive/01-4_Lolaeva.PDF.

Longrigg, James. "The Great Plague of Athens." *History of Science* 18 (1980): 209. SAO/NASA Astrophysics Data System. Accessed August 31, 2017. http://articles.adsabs.harvard .edu/cgi-bin/nph-iarticle_query?bibcode=1980HiSc..18..209L&db_key=AST&page _ind=0&data_type=GIF&type=SCREEN_VIEW&classic=YES.

Love, A. G., and Charles B. Davenport. "Immunity of City-Bred Recruits." *Archives of Internal Medicine* 24, no. 2 (1919), 129–153.

Luby, James P., Myron G. Schultz, Taras Nowosiwsky, and Robert L. Kaiser. "Introduced Malaria at Fort Benning, GA: 1964–1965." *American Journal of Tropical Medicine and Hygiene* 16 (1967): 146–153.

Lucchi, N. W., M. Poorak, J. Oberstaller, J. DeBarry, G. Srinivasamoorthy, I. Goldman, M. Xayavong, A. J. da Silva, D. S. Peterson, J. W. Barnwell, J. Kissinger, and V. Udhayakumar. "A New Single-Step PCR Assay for the Detection of the Zoonotic Malaria Parasite *Plasmodium knowlesi*." *PLoS One* 7, no. 2 (2012): e31848. Epub February 20, 2012. Accessed by September 2, 2017. http://www.ncbi.nlm.nih.gov/pubmed/22363751.

Lucian of Samosata. "The Way to Write History." *The Works of Lucian of Samosata*. Vol. 2. Translated by H. W. Fowler and F. G. Fowler. Oxford: Clarendon Press, 1905.

Lund, Mary Ann. "Richard's Back: Death, Scoliosis, and Myth Making." *Medical Humanities* 41, no. 2 (December 2015): 89–94.

Madden, David, ed. *Beyond the Battlefield: The Ordinary Life and Extraordinary Times of the Civil War Soldier.* New York: Simon and Schuster, 2000.

Maling, Barbara Lee. "Black Southern Nursing Care Providers in Virginia during the American Civil War, 1861–1865." PhD diss., University of Virginia, December 2009.

Manley, Jennifer. "Measles and Ancient Plagues: A Note on New Scientific Evidence." *Classical World* 107, no. 3 (Spring 2014): 393–397.

Marcellinus, Ammianus. *The Roman History of Ammianus Marcellinus during the Reigns of the Emperors Constantius, Julian, Jovianus, Valentinian, and Valens.* Translated by C. D. Yonge, MA. London: George Bell & Sons, 1902.

Marr, John S., MD, and John T. Cathey, MS. "The 1802 Saint-Domingue Yellow Fever Epidemic and the Louisiana Purchase." *Journal of Public Health Management and Practice* 19, no. 1 (January 2013): 77–82. Accessed September 2, 2017. https://www.researchgate.net/publication/233738388_The_1802_Saint-Domingue_Yellow_Fever_Epidemic_and_the_Louisiana_Purchase.

Marroquin, Horacio Figueroa. *Enfermedades de los Conquistadores.* San Salvador, Guatemala: Ministerio de Cultura, 1957.

May, Jacques M. "Map of the World Distribution of Cholera." *Geographical Review* 41, no. 2 (April 1951): 272–273. Accessed May 14, 2017. http://www.jstor.org/stable/211023.

Mayo Clinic Staff. "Symptoms." *Diseases and Conditions: Measles.* Accessed September 2, 2017. http://www.mayoclinic.org/diseases-conditions/measles/basics/symptoms/CON-20019675.

McCaa, Robert. "Spanish and Nahuatl Views on Smallpox and Demographic Catastrophe in the Conquest of Mexico." *Journal of Interdisciplinary History* 25, no. 3 (Winter 1995): 397–431. Accessed September 2, 2017. http://users.pop.umn.edu/~rmccaa/vircatas/vir6.htm.

McCartney, Paul T. *Power and Progress: American National Identity, the War of 1898, and the Rise of American Imperialism.* Baton Rouge: Louisiana State University Press, 2006.

McGaugh, Scott. *Surgeon in Blue: Jonathan Letterman, the Civil War Doctor Who Pioneered Battlefield Care.* New York: Arcade Publishing, 2013.

McGuinness, Aims C., MD. "Diseases Caused by Bacteria: Diphtheria." *Preventive Medicine in WWII.* Vol. 4, *Communicable Diseases, Transmitted Chiefly through Respiratory and Alimentary Tracts*, edited by John Boyd Coates Jr., MC, Ebbe Curtis Hoff, PhD, MD, and Phebe M. Hoff, MA. Washington, D.C.: Office of the Surgeon General, U.S. Army

Medical Department, 1958): 167–189. Accessed September 2, 2017. http://history
.amedd.army.mil/booksdocs/wwii/PM4/CH10.Diphtheria.htm.

McLynn, Frank. *Marcus Aurelius: A Life*. Cambridge, MA: De Capo Press, 2009.

McNeill, J. R. *Mosquito Empires: Ecology and War in the Greater Caribbean, 1620–1914*. New York: Cambridge University Press, 2010.

McNeill, William H. *Plagues and Peoples*. New York: Doubleday Press, 1977.

McQuiston, Jennifer. "Infectious Diseases Related to Travel." Centers for Disease Control and Prevention. Accessed September 2, 2017. https://wwwnc.cdc.gov/travel/yellow book/2016/infectious-diseases-related-to-travel/rickettsial-spotted-typhus -fevers-related-infections-anaplasmosis-ehrlichiosis.

McSweegan, Edward. "Anthrax and the Etiology of the English Sweating Sickness." *Medical Hypotheses* 62, no. 1 (2004): 155–157.

Meshnick, Steven R., and Mary J. Dobson. "The History of Antimalarial Drugs." In *Antimalarial Chemotherapy: Mechanisms of Action, Resistance, and New Directions in Drug Discovery*, edited by Philip J. Rosenthal, 15–25. Totowa, NJ: Humana Press Inc., 2001.

Metersky, Mark L., Robert G. Masterton, Hartmut Lode, Thomas M. File Jr., and Timothy Babinchak. "Epidemiology, Microbiology, and Treatment Considerations for Bacterial Pneumonia Complicating Influenza." *International Journal of Infectious Diseases* 16, no. 5 (May 2012): e321–331.

Michie, Henry C., and George E. Lull. "Measles." *Communicable and Other Diseases*. Vol. 9, *The Medical Department of the United States Army in the World War*. Washington, D.C.: U.S. Government Printing Office, 1928.

Mintz, S. "Lord Dunmore's Proclamation." *Digital History*. Accessed September 2, 2017. http:// www.umbc.edu/che/tahlessons/pdf/Fighting_for_Whose_Freedom_Black_Soldiers _in_the_American_Revolution_RS_4.pdf.

Mitrofan, Dragos. "The Antonine Plague in Dacia and Moesia Inferior." *Journal of Ancient History and Archeology*, no. 1.2 (2014): 9–13.

Mock, Nancy M., Sambe Duale, Lisanne F. Brown, Ellen Mathys, Heather C. O'Maonaigh, Nina K. L. Abul-Husn, and Sterling Elliot. "Conflict and HIV: A Framework for Risk Assessment to Prevent HIV in Conflict-Affected Settings in Africa." *Emerging Themes in Epidemiology* 1, no. 6 (2004). Accessed September 18, 2017. https://www.ncbi.nlm .nih.gov/pmc/articles/PMC544944.

Mollaret, H. H. "The Discovery by Paul-Louis Simond of the Role of the Flea in the Transmission of the Plague." *Bulletin de la Société de pathologie exotique* 92, no. 5, pt. 2 (December 1999): 383–387.

Montellano, Bernard R. Ortiz de. *Aztec Medicine, Health, and Nutrition*. New Brunswick, NJ: Rutgers University Press, 1990.

Moore, Samuel T. *America and the World War*. New York: Greenberg Publisher, Inc., 1937.

Morens, David M., and Robert J. Littman. "Epidemiology of the Plague of Athens." *Transactions of the American Philological Association* 122 (1992): 271–304.

Morens, David M., and Jeffery K. Taubenberger. "A Forgotten Epidemic That Changed Medicine: Measles in the U.S. Army, 1917–18." *The Lancet: Infectious Diseases* 15, no. 7 (2015): 852–861.

Morgan, James. "Black Death Skeletons Unearthed by Crossrail Project." *BBC News: Science & Environment* (March 30, 2014). Accessed December 12, 2017. http://www .bbc.com/news/science-environment-26770334.

Mortimer, P. P. "Historical Review: The Diphtheria Vaccine Debacle of 1940 That Ushered in Comprehensive Childhood Immunization in the United Kingdom." *Epidemiology and Infection* 139, no. 4 (April 2011): 487–497. Accessed September 2, 2017. www .jstor.org/stable/27975617.

Moss William J., and Diane E Griffin. "Measles." *The Lancet* 379, no. 9811 (2012): 153–164.

Muir, Rory. *Tactics and the Experience of Battle in the Age of Napoleon.* New Haven, CT: Yale University Press, 1998.

Mukharji, Projit Bihari. "The 'Cholera Cloud' in the Nineteenth Century 'British World': History of an Object-without-an-Essence." *Bulletin of the History of Medicine* 86, no. 3 (Fall 2012): 303–332. Accessed September 16, 2017. doi:https://doi.org/10.1353 /bhm.2012.0050.

Munro, John H. A. *Wool, Cloth, and Gold: The Struggle for Bullion in Anglo-Burgundian Trade, 1340–1478.* Toronto: University of Toronto Press, 1972.

Murphy, Jim. *An American Plague: The True and Terrifying Story of the Yellow Fever Epidemic of 1793.* New York: Clarion Books, 2003.

Murphy, Neil. *The Captivity of John II, 1356–60: The Royal Image in Later Medieval England and France.* New York: Palgrave MacMillan, 2016.

Murthy, R. Srinivasa, and Rashmi Lakshminarayana. "Mental Health Consequences of War: A Brief Review of Research Findings." *World Psychology* 5, no. 1 (February 2006): 25–30.

Mussis, Gabriele de'. "Historia de Morbo." In *The Black Death*, edited and translated by Rosemary Horrox. Manchester, UK: Manchester University Press, 1984.

Myers, Robert C. "Mortality in the Twelfth Michigan Volunteer Infantry, 1861–1866." *Michigan Historical Review* 20, no. 1 (Spring 1994): 29–47. Accessed August 27. 2017. http:// www.jstor.org/stable/20173432.

Nasir, Arshan, and Gustavo Caetano-Anollés. "A Phylogenomic Data-Driven Exploration of Viral Origins and Evolution." *Science Advances* 1, no. 8 (September 25, 2015): 1–24. Accessed on September 2, 2017. http://advances.sciencemag.org/content/1/8 /e1500527/tab-pdf.

National Archives. Kew, Richmond, Surrey. E101/25/11, E101/393/11.

Navarro, Julian A. "Influenza in 1918: An Epidemic in Images." *Public Health Reports (1974–)* 125 (April 2010): 9–14. Accessed September 2, 2017. http://www.jstor.org /stable/41435295.

Neel, Spurgeon. *Medical Support of the U.S. Army in Vietnam 1965–1970.* Washington, D.C.: GPO, 1973.

Nelson, Kenrad E., and Carolyn Masters Williams. *Infectious Disease Epidemiology: Theory and Practice.* Sudbury, MA: Jones and Bartlett Pub., 2005.

"News." *Journal of Infectious Diseases* 133, no. 1 (January 1976): 95.

Newton, Anna E., Janell A. Routh, and Barbara E. Mahon. "Typhoid & Paratyphoid Fever." Centers for Disease and Prevention. Accessed September 2, 2017. http:// wwwnc.cdc.gov/travel/yellowbook/2016/infectious-diseases-related-to-travel/typhoid -paratyphoid-fever.

Nicholas, David. *Medieval Flanders.* London: Longman, 1992.

Nicholas, David. *Town and Countryside: Social, Economic, and Political Tensions in Fourteenth-Century Flanders.* Brugge: De Tempel, 1971.

Niebuhr, Cheston B. *Nieburh's Lectures on Roman History.* London: Chatto & Windus, Piccadilly, 1875.

Nightingale, Florence. "Little Chats with Big People." *The Scrap Book* 5, no. 1 (January 1908): 42–45.

"Night Soil." The Phrase Finder. Accessed July 31, 2017. http://www.phrases.org.uk/meanings /256350.html.

Nourzhanov, Kirill, and Christian Bleuer. *Tajikistan: A Political and Social History.* Canberra: Australian National University Press, 2013.

Nowrojee, Binaifer. *Shattered Lives: Sexual Violence during the Rwandan Genocide and Its Aftermath.* New York: Human Rights Watch, 1996.

Oaks, Stanley C., Jr., Violaine S. Mitchell, Greg W. Pearson, and Charles C. J. Carpenter, eds. *Malaria: Obstacles and Opportunities.* Washington, D.C.: National Academies, 1991.

Obradovic, Zarema, Snjezana Balta, Amina Obradovic, and Salih Mesic. "The Impact of War on Vaccine Preventable Diseases." *Mater Sociomed* 26, no. 6 (December 2014): 382–84. Accessed August 14, 2017. https://www.ncbi.nlm.nih.gov/pmc/articles/PMC4314173/pdf/MSM-26-382.pdf.

Ognibene, Andre J., ed. *Internal Medicine in Vietnam* Vol. 2. Washington, D.C.: Center for Military History, 1982.

Ognibene, Andre J., and O'Neil Barrett. "Clinical Disorders: Malaria." In *Internal Medicine in Vietnam*, edited by Andre J. Ognibene. Vol. 2, *General Medicine and Infectious Disease.* Washington, D.C.: Center for Military History, 1982.

Ognibene, Andre J., and Nicholas F. Conte. "Malaria: Chemotherapy." In *Internal Medicine in Vietnam*, edited by Andre J. Ognibene. Vol. 2, *General Medicine and Infectious Disease.* Washington, D.C.: Center for Military History, 1982.

Ognyanova, Irina. "Religion and Church in the Ustasha Ideology (1941–1945)." *CCP* 64 (2009): 157–159.

Oldstone, Michael. *Viruses, Plagues, & History.* New York: Oxford University Press, 2010.

Olmsted, Frederick Law. "Letter to Regimental Commanders on the Strict Observance of Camp Police Rules, Washington, D.C., 1861." Library of Congress, Printed Ephemera Collection, Portfolio 204, Folder 26. Accessed June 20, 2017. https://www.loc.gov/item/rbpe.20402600.

Ormrod, W. Mark. *Edward III.* New Haven, CT: Yale University Press, 2011.

Ormrod, W. Mark. "The English Crown and the Customs, 1349–63." *EcHR*, New Series 40, no. 1 (February 1987): 27–40.

Ormrod, W. Mark. "The English Government and the Black Death of 1348–49." In *England in the Fourteenth Century: Proceedings of the 1985 Harlaxton Symposium*, edited by W. Mark Ormrod. Rochester, NY: Boydell Press, 1986.

Ormrod, W. Mark. "The Protecolla Rolls and English Government Finance, 1353–1364." *English Historical Review* 102, no. 404 (July 1987): 622–632.

Orosius. *Seven Books of History against the Pagans: The Apology of Paulus Orosius.* Translated by Irving Woodworth Raymond. New York: Columbia University Press, 1936.

Osborne, John B. "The Lancaster County Cholera Epidemic of 1854 and the Challenge to the Miasma Theory of Disease." *Pennsylvania Magazine of History and Biography* 133, no. 1 (January 2009): 5–28. Accessed May 14, 2017. http://www.jstor.org/stable/40543519.

Oxford, J. S., R. Lambkin, A. Sefton, R. Daniels, A. Elliot, R. Brown, and D. Gill. "A Hypothesis: The Conjunction of Soldiers, Gas, Pigs, Ducks, Geese and Horses in Northern France during the Great War Provided the Conditions for the Emergence of the 'Spanish' Influenza Pandemic of 1918–1919." *Vaccine* 23 (2005): 940–945.

Oxford, J. S., A. Sefton, R. Jackson, W. Innes, R. S. Daniels, and N. P. A. S. Johnson. "World War I May Have Allowed the Emergence of 'Spanish' Influenza." *The Lancet: Infectious Diseases* 2 (2002): 111–114.

Page, D. L. "Thucydides' Description of the Great Plague at Athens." *Classical Quarterly* 3 (1953): 109–110. Accessed August 31, 2017. http://www.jstor.org/stable/637025.

Palmer, Robert C. *English Law in the Age of the Black Death.* Chapel Hill: University of North Carolina Press, 2001.

Paltzer, Seth. "The Other Foe: The U.S. Army's Fight against Malaria in the Pacific Theater, 1942–45." *On Point* (April 30, 2016). Accessed September 7, 2017. https://armyhistory .org/on-point.

Papagrigorakis, Manolis J., C. Yapijakis, and P. Synodinos. "Ancient Typhoid Epidemic Reveals Possible Ancestral Strain of *Salmonella enterica* Serovar Typhi." *Infection, Genetics and Evolution* 7 (2007), 126–127.

Papagrigorakis, Manolis J., Christos Yapijakis, Philippos N. Synodinos, and Effie Baziotopoulou-Valavani. "E. DNA Examination of Ancient Dental Pulp Indicates Typhoid Fever as a Probable Cause of the Plague of Athens." *International Journal of Infectious Diseases* 10 (2006): 206–214.

Papagrigorakis, Manolis J., P. N. Synodino, A. Stathi, C. L. Skevaki, and L. Zachariadou. "The Plague of Athens: An Ancient Act of Bioterrorism?" *Biosecurity and Bioterrorism: Biodefense Strategy, Practice, and Science* 11, no. 3 (September 2013): 228–229.

Pappenheimer, A. M., Jr., and D. Michael Gill. "Diphtheria." *Science, New Series* 182, no. 4110 (October 26, 1973): 353–358. Accessed September 2, 2017. http://www.jstor .org/stable/1737276.

Parker, H. M. D. *A History of the Roman World from A.D. 138 to 337.* London: Methuen & Co. Ltd., 1958.

Parkman, Francis. *The Conspiracy of Pontiac and the Indian War after the Conquest of Canada.* 6th ed. Vol. 2. Boston: Little, Brown, 1886.

Parry, Adam. "The Language of Thucydides' Description of the Plague." *Bulletin of the Institute of Classical Studies* 16 (1969): 106–118. Accessed August 31, 2017. http://onlinelibrary .wiley.com/doi/10.1111/j.2041-5370.1969.tb00667.x/abstract.

Pašić, Lana. "Political and Social Consequences of Continuing Displacement in Bosnia and Herzegovina." *Forced Migration Review* 50 (September 2015): 7–8. Accessed August 13, 2017. http://www.fmreview.org/dayton20/pasic.html.

Patrick, Adam. "A Consideration of the Nature of the English Sweating Sickness." *Medical History* 9, no. 3 (July 1965): 272–279.

Pearcy, Lee T. "Diagnosis as Narrative in Ancient Literature." *American Journal of Philology* 113, no. 4 (Winter 1992): 595–616. Accessed August 31, 2017. http://www.jstor.org /stable/295542.

Perri, Timothy J. "The Evolution of Military Conscription in the United States." *Independent Review* 17, no. 3 (2013): 429–439.

Petri, William A. "Epidemic Typhus." *Merck Manual.* Accessed September 2, 2017. www.merck manuals.com/professional/infectious-diseases/rickettsiae-and-related-organisms /epidemic-typhus.

Pfister, Christian, Rudolf Brazdul, and Mariano Barriendos. "Reconstructing Past Climate and Natural Disasters in Europe Using Documentary Evidence." *PAGES Past Global Changes News* 10, no. 3 (December 2002): 6–8.

Phillips, Howard. "The Recent Wave of 'Spanish' Flu Historiography." *Social History of Medicine* 27, no. 4 (2014): 789–808.

Pierce, John R., and James V. Writer. *Yellow Jack: How Yellow Fever Ravaged America and Walter Reed Discovered Its Deadly Secrets.* Hoboken, NJ: John Wiley & Sons, Inc., 2005.

Pinault, Jody Ruben. "Hippocrates and the Plague." *Hippocratic Lives and Legends.* Leiden, the Netherlands: E. J. Brill, 1992.

Pinault, Jody Ruben. "How Hippocrates Cured the Plague." *Journal of History of Medicine and Allied Sciences* 41, no. 1 (1986): 52–75. doi:10.1093/jhmas/41.1.52.

Poole, J. C. F., and A. Holladay. "Thucydides and the Plague of Athens." *Classical Quarterly* 29 (1979): 282–300.

Porter, Katherine Anne. *Pale Horse, Pale Rider.* Orlando, FL: Harcourt Brace & Company, 1939.

Porter, William D. "Imported Malaria: 50 Years of U.S. Military Experience." *Military Medicine* 171 (October 2006): 925–928.

Power, Samantha. *A Problem from Hell: American and the Age of Genocide.* New York: Basic Books, 2002.

Powers, Ramon, and James N. Leiker. "Cholera among the Plains Indians: Perceptions, Causes, Consequences." *Western Historical Quarterly* 29, no. 3 (Autumn 1998): 317–340.

Preeta, Kutty, Jennifer Rota, William Bellini, Susan B. Redd, Albert Barskey, and Gregory Wallance. "Measles." *Manual for the Surveillance of Vaccine-Preventable Diseases.* Centers for Disease Control and Prevention. Accessed September 2, 2017. https://www.cdc.gov/vaccines/pubs/surv-manual/chpt07-measles.html.

Prentice, Michael B., and L. Rahalison. "Plague." *The Lancet* 369, no. 9568 (April 7, 2007): 1196–1207.

Prescott, William. *History of the Conquest of Mexico.* Reprint. New York: Bantam Books, 1964. First Published in 1843.

Price-Smith, Andrew T., and John L. Daly. "Downward Spiral: HIV/AIDS, State Capacity, and Political Conflict in Zimbabwe." *Peaceworks* No. 53 (Washington, D.C.: United States Institute of Peace, 2004). Accessed September 18, 2017. https://www.usip.org/publications/2004/07/downward-spiral-hivaids-state-capacity-and-political-conflict-zimbabwe.

Prinzing, Friedrich. *Epidemics Resulting from Wars.* Edited by Harald Westergaard. Oxford: Clarendon Press, 1916.

"The Progress of Science: William Crawford Gorgas." *Scientific Monthly* 11, no. 2 (August 1920): 187–190.

Prunier, Gerard. *Africa's World War: Congo, the Rwandan Genocide, and the Makings of a Continental Catastrophe.* New York: Oxford University Press, 2009.

Purcell, David W., Christopher H. Johnson, Amy Lansky, Joseph Prejean, Renee Stein, Paul Denning, Zaneta Gaul, Hillard Weinstock, John Su, and Nicole Crepaz. "Estimating the Population Size of Men Who Have Sex with Men in the United States to Obtain HIV and Syphilis Rates." *Open AIDS Journal* 6 (2012): 98–107.

Quammen, David. *Spillover: Animal Infections and the Next Human Pandemic.* New York: W. W. Norton & Company, 2012.

Radusin, Milorad. "The Spanish Flu—Part II: The Second and Third Wave." *History of Medicine* 69, no. 10 (2012): 917–927.

Ramsay, James H. *A History of the Revenues of the Kings of England 1066–1399.* Vol. 2. Oxford: Clarendon Press, 1925.

Reff, Daniel T. *Disease, Depopulation, and Culture Change in Northwestern New Spain, 1518–1764.* Salt Lake City: University of Utah Press, 1991.

Reid, Ann H., Jeffery K. Taubenberger, and Thomas G. Fanning, "The 1918 Spanish Influenza: Integrating History and Biology." *Microbes and Infection* 3 (2001): 81–87.

Reyntjens, Fiilip. *The Great African War: Congo and Regional Geopolitics, 1996–2006.* New York, Cambridge University Press, 2009.

Ricard, Robert. *Spiritual Conquest of Mexico.* Translated by Lesley Byrd Simpson. Berkeley: University of California Press, 1966.

Rice, Geoffrey W., and Edwina Palmer. "Pandemic Influenza in Japan, 1918–19: Mortality Patterns and Official Responses." *Journal of Japanese Studies* 19, no. 2 (Summer 1993): 389–420. Accessed September 2, 2017. http://www.jstor.org/stable/132645.

Ring, Natalie J. "Mapping Regional and Imperial Geographies: Tropical Disease in the U.S. South." In *Colonial Crucible: Empire in the Making of the Modern American State*, edited by Alfred W. McCoy and Francisco A. Scarano. Madison: University of Wisconsin Press, 2009: 297–308.

Robb, Amanda. "Yellow Fever Virus: Structure and Function." Study.com. Accessed September 2, 2017. http://study.com/academy/lesson/yellow-fever-virus-structure-and-function.html.

Roberts, Kenneth. *March to Quebec: Journals of the Members of Arnold's Expedition.* New York: Doubleday, 1938.

Robles, Theodore F., Ronald Glaser, and Janice K. Kiecolt-Glaser. "Out of Balance: A New Look at Chronic Stress, Depression, and Immunity." *Current Directions in Psychological Science* 14, no. 2 (April 2005): 111–115. Accessed September 6, 2017. http://www.jstor.org/stable/20182999.

Ross, Ronald. *The Prevention of Malaria.* New York: E. P. Dutton & Co., 1910.

Rowse, Alfred L. *Bosworth Field: From Medieval to Tudor England.* Garden City, NY: Doubleday & Company, 1966.

Rubin, Richard. *The Last of the Doughboys: The Forgotten Generation and Their Forgotten World War.* Boston: Houghton Mifflin Harcourt, 2013.

Ruffin, Edmund, ed. "On Malaria: Extracts from Three Lectures on the Origin and Properties of Malaria and Marsh Miasma." *The Farmer's Register* 2, no. 1 (June 1834): 20–23.

Rupp, Stephanie, Phillipe Ambara, Victor Narat, and Tamara Giles-Vernick. "Beyond the Cut Hunter: A Historical Epidemiology of HIV Beginnings in Central Africa." *EcoHealth* 13, no. 4 (2016): 661–671.

Russell, Ephraim. "The Societies of the Bardi and the Peruzzi and Their dealings with Edward III." In *Finance and Trade under Edward III*, edited by George Unwin. Manchester, UK: Manchester University Press, 1918: 93–135.

Russell, Francis. "Journal of the Plague: The 1918 Influenza." *Yale Review* 47 (1957): 223–224.

Sahagun, Bernardino de, comp. *Florentine Codex: General History of Things of New Spain.* Translated by Arthur J. O. Anderson and Charles E. Dibble. 2nd ed. Santa Fe, NM: School of American Research and University of Utah, 1975.

Sarasomboth, S., N. Banchuin, T. Sukosol, B. Rungpitarangsi, and S. Manasatit. "Systemic and Intestinal Immunities after Natural Typhoid Infection." *Journal of Clinical Microbiology* 25, no. 6 (1987): 1088–1093.

Šarić, Velma. "Demographics of Bosnian War Set Out." *Global Voices, TRI*, no. 739 (May 4, 2012). Accessed August 13, 2017. https://iwpr.net/global-voices/demographics-bosnian-war-set-out.

Sartin, Jeffrey S. "Infectious Diseases during the Civil War: The Triumph of the 'Third Army.'" *Clinical Infectious Diseases*16, no. 4 (April 1993): 580–584. Accessed September 7, 2017. http://www.jstor.org/stable/4457020.

Schmid, Boris V., Ulf Büntgen, W. Ryan Easterday, Christian Ginzler, Lars Walløe, Barbara Bramanti, and Nils Chr. Stenseth. "Climate-Driven Introduction of the Black Death and Successive Plague Reintroductions in Europe." *Proceedings of the National Academy of Sciences of the United States of America* 112, no. 10 (January 2015): 3020–3025.

Schnerb, Bertrand. "Vassals, Allies and Mercenaries: The French Army before and after 1346." In *The Battle of Crécy, 1346*, edited by Andrew Ayton and Philip Preston. Rochester, NY: Boydell & Brewer, Ltd., 2005: 265–272.

Schuck-Paim, Cynthia, G. Dennis Shanks, Francisco E. A. Almeida, and Wladimir J. Alonso. "Exceptionally High Mortality Rate of the 1918 Influenza Pandemic in the Brazilian Naval Fleet." *Influenza and Other Respiratory Viruses* 7, no. 1 (2013): 27–34.

Schuenemanna, Verena J., Kirsten Box, Sharon DeWitte, Sarah Schmedes, Joslyn Jamieson, and Alissa Mittnik, *Scriptores Historia Augustae*. Translated by David Magien. Cambridge, MA: Harvard University Press, 1991.

Schultz, M. G. "Imported Malaria." *Bull World Health Organ* 50 (1974): 329–336.

Seacole, Mary. *Wonderful Adventures of Mrs. Seacole in Many Lands.* Edited by W. J. S. with introduction by W. H. Russell. London: James Blackwood, Paternoster Row, 1857.

Sells, Michael. "Crosses of Blood: Sacred Space, Religion, and Violence in Bosnia-Hercegovina." *Sociology of Religion* 64, no. 3 (2003): 309–331. Accessed August 12, 2017. http://www.jstor.org/stable/3712487.

Sepsis Alliance. "Sepsis and Pneumonia." Accessed August 27, 2017. http://www.sepsis.org/sepsis-and/pneumonia.

Shah, Sonia. *Pandemic: Tracking Contagions, from Cholera to Ebola and Beyond.* New York: Sarah Crichton Books, Farrar, Straus and Giroux, 2016.

Shah, Sonia. *The Fever: How Malaria Has Ruled Humankind for 500,000 Years.* New York: Sarah Crichton Books, 2010.

Shanks, G. Dennis. "Measles Epidemics of Variable Lethality in the Early 20th Century." *American Journal of Epidemiology* 179, no. 4 (February 15, 2014): 413–422. Accessed September 2, 2017. https://academic.oup.com/aje/article/179/4/413/128401/Measles-Epidemics-of-Variable-Lethality-in-the.

Shapiro, Beth. "No Proof That Typhoid Caused the Plague of Athens (A Reply to Papagrigorakis et al.)." *International Journal of Infectious Diseases* 10 (2006): 334–340. Accessed August 31, 2017. http://ac.els-cdn.com/S1201971206000531/1-s2.0-S1201971206000531-main.pdf?_tid=481bc36e-8f24-11e7-82c9-00000aacb362&acdnat=1504277345_278565821f4a0200da459ae9aaf906c9.

Shilts, Randy. *And the Band Played On: Politics, People, and the AIDS Epidemic.* New York: St. Martin's Press, 1987.

Shryock, Richard H. "A Medical Perspective on the Civil War." *American Quarterly* 14, no. 2 (Summer 1962): 161–173.

Shulimson, Jack. "Marines in the Spanish-American War." In *Crucible of Empire*, 127–157. Annapolis, MD: Naval Institute Press, 1993.

Siler, Joseph F. *The Medical Department of the United States Army in the World War.* Vol. 9, *Communicable and Other Diseases.* Washington, D.C.: GPO, 1928: 5–170, 233–262, 311–386, 409–472, 511–528, 551–558.

Slack, J. Andrew, and Roy R Doyon. "Population Dynamics and Susceptibility for Ethnic Conflict: The Case of Bosnia and Herzegovina." *Journal of Peace Research* 38, no. 2 (March 2001): 139–161. Accessed August 12, 2017. ww.jstor.org/stable/425492.

Slater, Leo Barney. *War and Disease: Biomedical Research on Malaria in the Twentieth Century.* New Brunswick, NJ: Rutgers University Press, 2009.

Slavin, Philip. "The Great Bovine Pestilence and Its Economic and Environmental Consequences in England and Wales, 1318–50." *EcHR* 65, no. 4 (2012): 1239–1266.

Smallman-Raynor, Matthew, and Andrew D. Cliff. "Epidemic Diffusion Processes in a System of U.S. Military Camps: Transfer Diffusion and the Spread of Typhoid Fever in the Spanish-American War, 1898." *Annals of the Association of American Geographers* 91, no. 1 (March 2001): 71–91. Accessed July 30, 2017. http://www.jstor.org /stable/3651192.

Smallman-Raynor, Matthew, and Andrew Cliff. "The Spread of Human Immunodeficiency Virus Type 2 into Europe: A Geographical Analysis." *International Journal of Epidemiology* 20, no. 2 (1991): 480–489.

Smallman-Raynor, Matthew, and Andrew D. Cliff. "The Geographical Spread of Cholera in the Crimean War: Epidemic Transmission in the Camp Systems of the British Army." *Journal of Historical Geography* 30, no. 1 (Jan. 2004): 32–69.

Smiley, Anthony W. "The Homefront: World War One at Home." Air Command and Staff College thesis, Air University, 2000.

Smith, Dale C. "Military Medical History: The American Civil War." *OAH Magazine of History* 19, no. 5, Medicine and History (September 2005): 17–19. Accessed August 27, 2017. http://www.jstor.org/stable/25161973?seq=1&cid=pdf-reference#references _tab_contents.

Smith, Digby. *An Illustrated Encyclopedia of Uniforms of the Napoleonic Wars.* London: Lorenz Books, 2008.

Smith, Joseph. *The Spanish-American War: Conflict in the Caribbean and the Pacific, 1895–1902.* London: Longman, 1994.

Smocovitis, Vassiliki Betty. "Desperately Seeking Quinine: The Malaria Threat Drove the Allies' WWII Cinchona Mission." *Modern Drug Discovery* 6, no. 5 (May 2003): 57–58.

"Some Sketches from the Present War." *Advocate of Peace* 11, no. 12 (December 1854): 185–188. Accessed September 16, 2017. www.jstor.org/stable/27891349.

Soper, George A. "The Influenza Pneumonia Pandemic in the American Army Camps during September and October, 1918." *Science* 48, no. 1245 (November 1918): 451–456.

Soubbotitch, Voyislav. "A Pandemic of Typhus in Serbia in 1914 and 1915." *Proceedings of the Royal Society of Medicine* 11 (1918): 31–39.

Spence, Karen. "The Epidemic That Killed Pericles: Contextual and Paleopathological Analysis of the 5th Century BCE Plague of Athens via Primary Resources and Modern DNA Sequence-Based Identification Strategies of Dental Pulp from a Mass Grave at Kerameikos: A Novel Offering of Compelling Evidence of Avian Influenza as the Causative Agent of the Plague of Athens." Master's thesis, University of Leicester, 2013.

Spickelmier, Roger K. *Training of the American Soldier during World War I and World War II.* Fort Leavenworth, KS: U.S. Army Command and General Staff College, 1987.

Spiegel, Paul B. "HIV/AIDS among Conflict-Affected and Displaced Populations: Dispelling Myths and Taking Action." *Disasters* 28, no. 3 (2004): 322–339.

"Spokane, Washington." *Influenza Encyclopedia: The American Influenza Epidemic of 1918–1919, a Digital Encyclopedia.* University of Michigan Center for the History of Medicine and Michigan Publishing. Accessed September 2, 2017. http://www.influenzaarchive .org/cities/city-spokane.html#.

Stark, Richard B. "Immunization Saves Washington's Army." *Surgery, Gynecology and Obstetrics* 144 (1977): 425–431.

Starr, Isaac. "Influenza in 1918: Recollections of the Epidemic in Philadelphia." *Annals of Internal Medicine* 145, no. 2 (July 2006): 138–140.

Steiner, Paul E. *Disease in the Civil War: Natural Biological Warfare in 1861–1865.* Springfield, IL: Charles C Thomas.

Stokes, Joseph. "Mumps." *Preventive Medicine in World War II.* Vol. 4, *Communicable Diseases Transmitted Chiefly through Respiratory and Alimentary Tracts*, edited by Ebbe Curtis

Hoff and Phebe M. Hoff. Washington, D.C.: U.S. Army Medical Department, Office of Medical History, 1958. 135–140.

Sudhoff, Karl. "Pestschriften aus den ersten 150 Jahren nach der Epidemie des 'schwarzen Todes' 1348." *Archiv für Geschichte der Medizin (AGM)* 5 (1912).

Sumption, Jonathan. *The Hundred Years War I: Trial by Battle.* Philadelphia: University of Pennsylvania Press, 1990.

Sumption, Jonathan. *The Hundred Years War II: Trial by Fire.* Philadelphia: University of Pennsylvania Press, 1999.

Svoboda, Elizabeth. "Deep in the Rain Forest, Stalking the Next Pandemic." *The New York Times* (October 20, 2008). https://mobile.nytimes.com/2008/10/21/health/research/21prof.html.

Talty, Stephan. *The Illustrious Dead: The Terrifying Story of How Typhus Killed Napoleon's Greatest Army.* New York: Crown Publishers, 2009.

Tankard, Danae. "Protestantism, the Johnson Family and the 1551 Sweat in London." *London Journal* 29, no. 2 (2004): 1–16.

Taubenberger, Jeffery K., Johan V. Hultin, and David M. Morens. "Discovery and Characterization of the 1918 Pandemic Influenza Virus in Historical Context." *Antiviral Therapy* 12, no. 4, pt. B (2007): 581–591.

Taubenberger, Jeffery K., and David M. Morens. "1918 Influenza: The Mother of All Pandemics." *History* 12, no. 1 (January 2006). Accessed September 2, 2017. https://wwwnc.cdc.gov/eid/article/12/1/05-0979_article.

Taubenberger, Jeffery K., Ann H. Reid, Thomas A. Janczewski, and Thomas G. Fanning. "Integrating Historical, Clinical and Molecular Genetic Data in Order to Explain the Origin and Virulence of the 1918 Spanish Influenza Virus." *Philosophical Transactions: Biological Sciences* (2001): 1829–1839.

Taunbenber, Jeffery K., Ann H. Reid, Amy E. Krafft, Karen E. Bijwaard, and Thomas G. Fanning. "Initial Genetic Characterization of the 1918 'Spanish' Influenza Virus." *Science*, New Series 275, no. 5307 (March 21, 1997): 1793–1796. Accessed September 2, 2017. http://www.jstor.org/stable/2892709.

Temperley, Gladys. *Henry VII.* Reprint. Westport, CT: Greenwood Press, 1971. First published in 1914.

Thayer, Thomas C., ed. *A Systems Analysis View of the Vietnam War 1965–1972, Casualties and Losses.* Vol. 8. AD A051613. Department of Defense, OASD (SA) RP Southeast Asia Intelligence Division, February 18, 1975.

Thompson, Angela. "To Save the Children: Smallpox Inoculation, Vaccination, and Public Health in Guanajuato, Mexico, 1797–1840." *The Americas* 49, no 4 (April 1993): 431–455.

Thompson, Tommy. "'Dying like Rotten Sheepe': Camp Randall as a Prisoner of War Facility during the Civil War." *Wisconsin Magazine of History* 92, no. 1 (Autumn 2008): 2–15. Accessed September 7, 2017. http://www.jstor.org/stable/25482093.

Thorpe, Vanessa. "Black Death Skeletons Reveal Pitiful Life of 14th-century Londoners." *The Observer* (March 29, 2014). Accessed September 16, 2017. https://www.theguardian.com/science/2014/mar/29/black-death-not-spread-rat-fleas-london-plague.

Thucydides. *History of the Peloponnesian War to 411 BCE.* Translated by Rex Warner. Reprint. London: Penguin Books, 1972. First published in 1954.

Thucydides. "Plague of Athens." In *History of the Peloponnesian War*, edited by A. Peabody and translated by Benjamin Jowett. Boston: Lothrop & Co., 1883.

Thucydides. "The Plague." *Thucydides.* Translated by Benjamin Jowett. Oxford: Clarendon Press, 1900. Accessed September 16, 2017. http://www.perseus.tufts.edu/hopper/text?doc=Thuc.+2.47&fromdoc=Perseus%3Atext%3A1999.04.0105.

Thursfield, Hugh. "Smallpox in the American War of Independence." *Annals of Medical History.* Series 3, 2 (1940): 312–318.

Thwaites, Guy, Mark Taviner, and Vanya Gant. "The English Sweating Sickness, 1485 to 1551." *New England Journal of Medicine* 336, no. 8 (February 1997): 580–582.

Thwaites, Guy, Mark Taviner, and Vanya Gant. "The English Sweating Sickness, 1485–1551: A Viral Pulmonary Disease?" *Medical History* 42 (1998): 96–98.

Timberg, Craig, and Daniel Halperin. *Tinderbox: How the West Sparked the AIDS Epidemic and How the World Can Finally Overcome It.* New York: Penguin, 2012.

Tiwari, Tejpratap S. P., MD. "Diptheria." In *VDP Surveillance Manual.* 5th ed. (2011): 1–9. Accessed September 2, 2017. https://www.cdc.gov/vaccines/pubs/surv-manual/chpt01-dip.pdf.

Toderich, Kristina, Munimjon Abbdusamatov, and Tsuneo Tsukatani. "Water Resources Assessment, Irrigation and Agricultural Developments in Tajikistan." Kier Discussion Paper Series. Kyoto Institute of Economic Research, no. 585 (March 2004). Accessed September 2, 2017. https://repository.kulib.kyoto-u.ac.jp/dspace/bitstream/2433/129519/1/DP585.pdf.

Tonkin Gulf Resolution. Public Law 88-408, 78. Stat. 384. August 10, 1964.

Tout, T. F. *Chapters in Administrative History.* Vol. 4. Manchester, UK: Manchester University Press, 1928.

The Trans-Atlantic Slave Trade Database. Accessed September 2, 2017. www.slavevoyages.org/voyage/33528/variables.

"The Treatment of Pneumonia." *Scientific American* 55, no. 8 (August 21, 1886): 119. Accessed August 27, 2017. http://www.jstor.org/stable/26093152.

Trevelyan, George Otto. *George the Third and Charles Fox: The Concluding Part of the American Revolution.* New York: Longmans, Green& Co, 1912.

Tuchman, Barbara. *A Distant Mirror: The Calamitous 14th Century.* New York: Ballantine Press, 1978.

Underwood, E. Ashworth. "Milestones in Medicine: 11, The Sweating Sickness." *Health Education Journal* 8 (1950): 127–128.

United Nations. "HIV/AIDS, Malaria and Other Diseases," Accessed September 2, 2017. http://www.rw.one.un.org/mdg/mdg6.

U.S. Army, Surgeon-General's Office. *Report of the Surgeon-General of the Army to the Secretary of War for the Fiscal Year Ending June 30, 1899.* Washington, D.C.: U.S. Government Printing Office, 1899.

U.S. Army Medical Department. "Medical Mobilization and the War." *JAMA* 71, no. 1 (September 14, 1918): 909–915.

U.S. Army Medical Department. *Preventive Medicine in World War II.* Vol. 8, *Civil Affairs/Military Government Public Health Activities.* Part 3, *The Mediterranean.* Washington, D.C., 1976.

U.S. Army Medical Department, Office of Medical History. "Thomas Lawson." Accessed August 27, 2017. http://history.amedd.army.mil/surgeongenerals/T_Lawson.html.

U.S. Army Medical Department, Office of Medical History. "William A. Hammond." Accessed August 27, 2017. http://history.amedd.army.mil/surgeongenerals/W_Hammond.html.

van Hartesveldt, Fred R. "The Doctors and the 'Flu': The British Medical Profession's Response to the Influenza Pandemic of 1918–1919." *International Social Science Review* 85, no. 1-2 (2010): 28–39.

Vaughan, Victor C. "Communicable Diseases in the National Guard and National Army of the United States during the Six Months from September 29, 1917 to March 29, 1918." *Journal of Laboratory and Clinical Medicine* 3, no. 11 (August 1918): 635–718.

Vaughan, Victor C. *Epidemiology and Public Health: A Text and Reference Book for Physicians, Medical Students and Health Workers.* Vol. 1. St. Louis, MO: C. V. Mosby Company, 1922. Accessed September 2, 2017. https://books.google.com/books?id=J4saAAAAMAAJ.

Vaughan, Warren T., and Truman G. Schnabel. "Pneumonia and Empyema at Camp Sevier." *Archives of Internal Medicine* 22, no. 4 (1918): 440–465.

Vega, Garcilaso de la, El Inca. *Royal Commentaries of the Inca and General History of Peru.* Translated by H. V. Livermore. Austin: University of Texas Press, 1966.

Verano, John W., and Douglas H. Ubelaker. "Health and Disease in the Pre-Columbian World." In *Seeds of Change: A Quincentennial Commemoration*, edited by Herman J. Viola and Carolyn Margolis. Washington, D.C.: Smithsonian Institution Press, 1991: 209–223.

Vergil, Polydore. *Anglica Historia.* Edited and translated by Denys Hat. Reprint. London: Offices of the Royal Historical Society, 1950. First published in 1513, 1537.

Verwimp, Philip. "Machetes and Firearms: The Organization of Massacres in Rwanda." *Journal of Peace Research* 43, no. 1 (2006): 5–22. Accessed September 18, 2017. http://journals.sagepub.com/doi/pdf/10.1177/0022343306059576.

Villanueva, Jaime. "Viage Literario a las Iglesias de Espana XI Viage a Gerona." In *The Black Death*, edited and translated by Rosemary Horrox. Manchester, UK: Manchester University Press, 1984: 270–271.

Vitek, Charles R., Erika Y. Bogatyreva, and Melinda Wharton. "Diphtheria Surveillance and Control in the Former Soviet Union and the Newly Independent States." *Journal of Infectious Diseases* 181 (Supplement 1): S23–S26. Accessed September 16, 2017. https://academic.oup.com/jid/article/181/Supplement_1/S23/842014/Diphtheria-Surveillance-and-Control-in-the-Former.

Volo, Dorothy Denneen, and James M. Volo. *Daily Life in Civil War America.* Westport, CT: Greenwood Press, 1998.

Walker, H. K., W. D. Hall, and J. W. Hurst, eds. *Clinical Methods: The History, Physical, and Laboratory Examinations.* 3rd ed. Boston: Butterworths, 1990).

Wallace, Mark R., Braden R. Hale, Gregory C. Utz, Patrick E. Olson, Kenneth C. Earhart, Scott A. Thornton, and Kenneth C. Hyams. "Endemic Infectious Disease of Afghanistan." *Clinical Infectious Diseases* 34, Supplement 5, "Afghanistan: Health Challenges Facing Deployed Troops, Peacekeepers, and Refugees" (June 15, 2002): S171–S207. Accessed on September 2, 2017. http://www.jstor.org/stable/4461994.

Wang, Haidong and the GBD 2015 Collaborators. "Estimates of Global, Regional, and National Incidence, Prevalence, and Mortality of HIV, 1980–2015: The Global Burden of Disease Study 2015." *The Lancet HIV* 3, no. 8 (2016): 361.

Warner, Israel. "Letter to Henry Stephens, January 15, 1846." *Proceedings of the Vermont Historical Society* 11 (June 1943).

Washington, George. Papers. Founders Online, National Archives.

Washington, George. "George Washington to the New York Convention, February 10, 1777." *Founders Online, National Archives.* Accessed September 2, 2017. http://founders.archives.gov/documents/Washington/03-08-02-0320.

Washington, George. "To George Washington from Brigadier General Samuel Holden Parsons, 6 March 1777." Accessed September 2, 2017. http://founders.archives.gov /documents/Washington/03-08-02-0553.

Washington, George. "To George Washington from Major General Horatio Gates, 29 July 1776." Accessed September 2, 2017. http://founders.archives.gov/documents /Washington/03-05-02-0369.

Washington, George. "To George Washington from Major General Horatio Gates, 7 August 1776." Accessed September 2, 2017. http://founders.archives.gov/documents/Washing ton/03-05-02-0451.

Watson, Patricia A. *The Angelic Conjunction: Preacher-Physicians of Colonial New England.* Knoxville: University of Tennessee Press, 1991.

Wax, Emily. "Cycle of War Is Spreading AIDS and Fear in Africa." *Washington Post*, November 13, 2003. Accessed September 2, 2017. https://www.washingtonpost.com/archive /politics/2003/11/13/cycle-of-war-is-spreading-aids-and-fear-in-africa/6736e773 -5817-4cce-ab07-742a1c82f873/?utm_term=.852b9c6f6940.

Welford, Mark, and Brian J. Bossak. "Revisiting the Medieval Black Death of 1347–1351: Spatiotemporal Dynamics Suggestive of an Alternate Causation." *Geography Compass* 4, no. 6 (June 2010): 561–575.

Wheelis, Mark. "Biological Warfare at the 1346 Siege of Caffa." *Emerging Infectious Diseases* 8, no. 9 (September 2002): 971–975. Accessed September 2, 2017. https://wwwnc .cdc.gov/eid/article/8/9/pdfs/01-0536.pdf.

Whitmore, Thomas. *Disease and Death in Early Colonial Mexico: Simulating Amerindian Depopulation.* Boulder, CO: Westview Press, 1992.

Wiley, Bell Irvin. *The Life of Billy Yank: A Common Soldier of the Union.* Baton Rouge: Louisiana State University Press, 1987.

Wilkinson, Ray. "Heart of Darkness." *Refugees Magazine* 110 (December 1, 1997). Accessed September 2, 2017. http://www.unhcr.org/3b6925384.html.

Willard, James Field. *Parliamentary Taxes on Personal Property 1290 to 1334.* Cambridge, MA: Medieval Academy of America, 1934.

Williams, Ralph Chester, MD. *The United States Public Health Service, 1798–1950.* Washington, D.C.: Commissioned Officers Association of the United States Public Health Service, 1951.

Wolf, Eric. *Sons of the Shaking Earth: The People of Mexico and Guatemala—Their Land, History, and Culture.* Chicago: University of Chicago Press, 1959.

Wolfe, Nathan D., Peter Daszak, A. Marm Kilpatrick and Donald S. Burke. "Bushmeat Hunting, Deforestation, and Prediction of Zoonotic Disease." *Emerging Infectious Disease* 11, no. 12 (2005): 1822–1827.

Woodbury, F. T. "Model Barrack for Prevention of Respiratory Disease in the Army." *JAMA* 72, no. 17 (1919): 1212–1214.

Woodward, Joseph Janvier. *Outlines of the Chief Camp Diseases of the United States Armies: As Observed during the Present War.* Philadelphia: J. B. Lippincott & Co., 1863.

World Health Organization. *Expert Committee on Malaria.* Sixth Report. WHO/Mal/180, June 28, 1956.

World Health Organization. "Plague—Madagascar" (November 21, 2014). Accessed September 2, 2017. http://www.who.int/csr/don/21-november-2014-plague/en.

Wrench, Ed. M. "The Lessons of the Crimean War." *British Medical Journal* 2, no. 2012 (July 22, 1899): 205–208. Accessed June 26, 2017. http://www.jstor.org/stable/20261303.

Wright, Thomas, ed. *Political Poems and Songs.* Vol. 1. London: Longman, Green, Longman and Roberts,1859.

Wylie, John A. H., and Leslie H. Collier. "The English Sweating Sickness (Sudor Anglicus): A Reappraisal." *Journal of the History of Medicine and Allied Sciences* 36, no. 4 (1981): 425–445.

Yarrison, James L. "The U.S. Army in the Root Reform Era, 1899–1917." US Army Center of Military History. Accessed September 2, 2017. http://www.history.army.mil/documents /1901/Root-Ovr.htm.

"Yellow Fever: Cause for Concern?" *British Medical Journal (Clinical Research Edition)* 282, no. 6278 (May 1981): 1735–1816.

Yip, Ka-che. *Disease, Colonialism, and the State: Malaria in Modern East Asian History.* Hong Kong: Hong Kong University Press, 2009.

Young, Alvin Lee. *The History, Use, Disposition and Environmental Fate of Agent Orange.* New York: Springer, 2009.

Ziegler, Philip. *The Black Death.* Stroud, Gloucestershire: Sutton Publishing Ltd., 1969.

Zinsser, Hans. *Rats, Lice, and History.* Boston: Little, Brown and Company, 1963.

Zwierzchowski, Jan, and Ewa Tabeau, "The 1992–1995 War in Bosnia and Herzegovina: Census-Based Multiple System Estimation of Casualties' Undercount." Conference Paper for the International Research Workshop on "The Global Costs of Conflict." Households in Conflict Network and German Institute for Economic Research. February 1–2, 2010, Berlin.

About the Editor and Contributors

Editor

Rebecca M. Seaman is dean of social sciences and humanities at Olympic College, Bremerton, Washington. A professor of history, she specializes in colonial, Native American, trans-Atlantic, and military history. Previous works include *Conflict in Early America: An Encyclopedia of the Spanish Empire's Aztec, Inca and Mayan Conquests* (2013) and editor for the *Journal of the North Carolina Association of Historians* (2012–2016); "John Lawson, the Outbreak of the Tuscarora Wars and 'Middle Ground' Theory," in *JNCAH*; and "Enslavement of Native American's during The War of the Spanish Succession," in *From Captivity to Freedom: Themes in Ancient and Modern Slavery*.

Contributors

Jillion Becker graduated from Texas Woman's University with an MA in history and a minor in health studies. Additionally, she has a degree in biochemistry. Her article on "In Flew Enza: Public Memory of the Influenza Epidemic of 1918 in Pennsylvania" was published in *Ibid: A Student History Journal* and received an award from the Texas Regional Phi Alpha Theta Conference. Her master's thesis was titled "Licking Polio: An Investigation of the Use of Social Mobilization in the Years 1938–2000 in Global Polio Eradication."

Arthur (Art) Boylston graduated from Yale College and Harvard Medical School, and he is a fellow of the Royal College of Pathologists. A retired professor of pathology and an experiential immunologist, he is now a senior teaching fellow in the Nuffield Department of Clinical Laboratory Sciences at Oxford University. He is the author of a history of variolation titled *Defying Providence*.

Christopher Davis is a doctoral candidate in U.S. history at the University of North Carolina at Greensboro. He received his BA in international studies from Elon University and MA in history from the University of North Carolina at Greensboro. He specializes in American history during the World War I era, as well as Haitian history, and is currently conducting research into the history of American missionaries in Haiti during the U.S. occupation (1915–1934).

Sarah Douglas completed her PhD in 2015 at the Ohio State University. In addition to authoring several articles and serving as coeditor for a *Festschrift* volume in honor of Dr. Guilmartin, her dissertation, "The Price of Pestilence: England's Response to the Black Death in the Face of the Hundred Years War," will be ready for publication in 2018. Dr. Douglas is now lecturing for the OSU Department of History and Central State University's Department of Humanities, teaching courses on European history, world history, and military history.

Larry Grant studied history at the University of California, San Diego. He served 23 years as a U.S. Navy officer in a variety of positions at home and globally. Following his retirement, he volunteered with the South Carolina Historical Society and works as an adjunct professor of history at The Citadel, Charleston, South Carolina. There, he conducts interviews for the college's oral history program and archives. In 2010, he edited Maj. Gen. Johnson Hagood's post–World War I memoir of the U.S. occupation of the German Rhineland. He has written on the U.S. Army during World War I and other military subjects.

Hilary Green is an assistant professor of history in the Department of Gender and Race Studies at the University of Alabama. Dr. Green is the author of *Educational Reconstruction: African American Schools in the Urban South, 1865–1890* (2016). She has served as book review editor for the *Journal of the North Carolina Association of Historians* for the past five years.

Christopher Howell is an archaeologist and ancient historian. He has served as a professor of world history and anthropology at Red Rocks College in Denver, Colorado, for the past 15 years. His research centers on prehistory and comparative world history. Topics include war and society, seafaring, disease variables in world history, Colombian Exchange, mythology, and ancient India.

Wesley Renfro is an associate professor of political science and legal studies at St. John Fisher College in Rochester, New York. He teaches and writes on a range of topics, including empire, American foreign policy, presidential decision making and international conflict, and the politics of the Middle East. His work has appeared in numerous journals and edited volumes. He is the also the coauthor of a forthcoming book on the Middle East.

Joshua M. Seaman is an independent historian. He earned his BA in history from Gonzaga University and MA in American history from Norwich University. He briefly served in the U.S. Army infantry, which prompted his interest in military history. His areas of focus include colonial through early U.S. history, military history, and the Catholic Church in America.

Brenda Thacker received her BA in ancient studies from Webster University in 2010 and her MA in history from the University of Missouri–St. Louis in 2016, where she taught courses on world systems and Western civilization. She currently works for the St. Louis Public Library and Washington University in St. Louis, and she is working on starting her own consulting business. She also volunteers for the Missouri Historical Society as a researcher. Her areas of interest include the history of disease, late antiquity, public and digital history/humanities, archaeology, and material culture.

Angela Thompson is a historian of Latin America at East Carolina University. Dr. Thompson's principal area of research is the social history of Mexico in the 18th and 19th centuries. Most of her publications deal with the social history of the important silver mining region of Guanajuato, Mexico, but also the history of demography; family, children, and women; labor, and epidemics, public health, and education.

Sonia Valencia is a graduate student of history at Eastern Carolina University in the Maritime Studies graduate program. Studying under Dr. Angela Thompson and Dr. Lynn Harris, she presented research on the topic of how measles affected the transport ships and crews during World War I at the North Carolina Association of Historian's Annual Conference. She has also collaborated with Coast Guard historians and archaeologists of the North Carolina Maritime Museum in research for the location of the Revenue Service Cutters *Diligence III* and *Governor Williams*.

John Jennings White III hails from the Piedmont region of North Carolina. He graduated with a bachelor's degree and master's in history from the University of North Carolina at Greensboro, where he specialized in military history. Mr. White is currently the historian for a major U.S. corporation.

Edwin Wollert earned his PhD in history of science from Oregon State University in 2017, with a dissertation about Tudor England. He previously taught philosophy and history for the University of Alaska Anchorage. He owns a small publishing operation in Oregon and is at work on his next novel and academic articles. He is also proficient or fluent in several languages, including Latin, Spanish, German, and Welsh.

Index

Page numbers in *italics* indicate figures, and those in **bold** indicate tables.